TIME AND BODY

Time and Body promotes the application of phenomenological psychopathology and embodied research to a broad spectrum of mental disorders. In a new and practical way, it integrates the latest research on the temporal and intersubjective constitution of the body, self, and its mental disorders from phenomenological, embodied, and interdisciplinary research perspectives. The authors investigate how temporal processes apply to the contribution of embodiment and selfhood, as well as to their destabilization, such as in eating disorders and borderline personality disorders, schizophrenia, depression, social anxiety, or dementia. The chapters demonstrate the applicability of phenomenological psychopathology to a range of illnesses and its relevance to treatment and clinical practice.

CHRISTIAN TEWES is Adjunct Professor (Privatdozent) of Philosophy at the University of Jena, Germany, and he is currently working at the Section of Phenomenological Psychopathology and Psychotherapy, Department of General Psychiatry, University of Heidelberg. His research interests comprise embodiment theories, phenomenology, philosophy of mind, and anthropology.

GIOVANNI STANGHELLINI is a psychiatrist, Chair of the School of Phenomenological-Dynamic Psychotherapy, and Professor of Dynamic Psychology at G. d'Annunzio University of Chieti, Italy.

Endorsements for *Time and Body*

"This is a masterful and timely contribution to our understanding of mental disorders. With essays from leading experts, it shows how psychopathologies are embedded in the world and shaped by the complex intertwining of temporality, embodiment, and intersubjectivity. It will be an authoritative resource in phenomenological psychopathology for years to come."

Kevin Aho, Professor of Philosophy, Florida Gulf Coast University, USA, and author of *Contexts of Suffering*

"This book is a wide-ranging analysis of how some of the principles of phenomenological philosophy cast light on dementia, anorexia nervosa, social anxiety, and borderline personality disorder. It is a welcome addition to the growing interest in phenomenological psychopathology among psychiatrists, psychologists, and philosophers."

John Cutting, licensed psychiatrist and honorary Senior Lecturer, Kings College Hospital, UK

"In this volume, the editors bring together a remarkable group of researchers from philosophy, psychiatry, and psychology to advance our understanding of embodied and temporal experience in mental illness. This collection should be read by anyone working at the intersection of philosophy and mental health."

Anthony Vincent Fernandez, Postdoctoral Research Fellow of Philosophy, University of Oxford, UK, and Assistant Professor of Philosophy, Kent State University, USA

"A veritable tour de phenomenological force! This is a sparkling collection of the brightest and best in contemporary phenomenology, and a timely celebration of Thomas Fuchs' uniquely important contributions to the future of this rapidly expanding field."

Bill (KWM) Fulford, Fellow of St Catherine's College and Member of the Philosophy Faculty, Oxford University, UK

"This is an exciting collection of state-of-the-art phenomenological psychopathology essays. It contains excellent contributions from leading theorists who show how phenomenology and embodied, enactive theories offer new insights in psychopathology (and vice versa). The authors address depression, eating disorders, borderline personality disorder, and schizophrenia – honouring Thomas Fuchs' own influential contributions."

Sanneke de Haan, Researcher, Tilburg University, the Netherland and author of *Enactive Psychiatry*

(*cont. on page* 406)

TIME AND BODY

Phenomenological and Psychopathological Approaches

Christian Tewes
University of Heidelberg

Giovanni Stanghellini
G. d'Annunzio University of Chieti

CAMBRIDGE
UNIVERSITY PRESS

CAMBRIDGE
UNIVERSITY PRESS

University Printing House, Cambridge CB2 8BS, United Kingdom

One Liberty Plaza, 20th Floor, New York, NY 10006, USA

477 Williamstown Road, Port Melbourne, VIC 3207, Australia

314–321, 3rd Floor, Plot 3, Splendor Forum, Jasola District Centre, New Delhi – 110025, India

79 Anson Road, #06-04/06, Singapore 079906

Cambridge University Press is part of the University of Cambridge.

It furthers the University's mission by disseminating knowledge in the pursuit of education, learning, and research at the highest international levels of excellence.

www.cambridge.org
Information on this title: www.cambridge.org/9781108489355
DOI: 10.1017/9781108776660

First published 2021

A catalogue record for this publication is available from the British Library.

Library of Congress Cataloging-in-Publication Data

Names: Tewes, Christian, 1972- editor. | Stanghellini, Giovanni, editor.
Title: Time and body : phenomenological and psychopathological approaches / [edited by Christian Tewes, Giovanni Stanghellini].
Description: Cambridge ; New York, NY : Cambridge University Press, 2020. | Includes bibliographical references and index.
Identifiers: LCCN 2020024659 (print) | LCCN 2020024660 (ebook) | ISBN 9781108489355 (hardback) | ISBN 9781108702355 (paperback) | ISBN 9781108776660 (ebook)
Subjects: LCSH: Psychology, Pathological. | Phenomenological psychology. | Time–Psychological aspects. | Mind and body.
Classification: LCC RC454 .T483 2020 (print) | LCC RC454 (ebook) | DDC 616.89–dc23
LC record available at https://lccn.loc.gov/2020024659
LC ebook record available at https://lccn.loc.gov/2020024660

ISBN 978-1-108-48935-5 Hardback
ISBN 978-1-108-70235-5 Paperback

The book is dedicated to Thomas Fuchs' enduring work in phenomenological psychopathology and embodied research, and to his sixtieth anniversary. Its thematic fields cover his wide-ranging and decades-long research on time, body, and the intersubjective constitution of psychopathology. In dedicating the book to him we wish the jubilarian the best of health and many further years researching these and related fields!

Cover Picture: Caspar David Friedrich, “Der Mönch am Meer”.
bpk / Nationalgalerie, SMB / Andres Kilger

Contents

Part III Borderline Personality and Eating Disorders

Part IV Depression, Schizophrenia, and Dementia

Figures

Contributors

VALERIA BIZZARI Section of Phenomenological Psychopathology and Psychotherapy, Department of General Psychiatry, University of Heidelberg

ANNA BORTOLAN Department of Political and Cultural Studies, Swansea University

NATALIE DEPRAZ Department of Philosophy, University of Rouen Normandy

OTTO DOERR-ZEGERS Department of Psychiatry East, University of Chile and Center for Studies on Phenomenology and Psychiatry, Diego Portales University, Santiago de Chile

ERIK NORMAN DZWIZA-OHLSEN a.r.t.e.s. Graduate School for the Humanities Cologne, University of Cologne

TOM FROESE Embodied Cognitive Science Unit, Okinawa Institute of Science and Technology Graduate University

THOMAS FUCHS Section of Phenomenological Psychopathology and Psychotherapy, Department of General Psychiatry, University of Heidelberg

SHAUN GALLAGHER Department of Philosophy, University of Memphis
School of Liberal Arts, University of Wollongong, Australia

LORENZO GILARDI Independent Scholar, Como, Italy

ALLAN KØSTER Department of Communication and Psychology, University of Aalborg

STEFAN KRISTENSEN Visual Arts – Faculty of Arts, University of Strasbourg

JOEL KRUEGER Department of Sociology, Philosophy, and Anthropology, University of Exeter

DOROTHÉE LEGRAND Archives Husserl, CNRS, Ecole normale supérieure, Paris Sciences et Lettres Research University, Paris.

EDWARD A. LENZO Department of Philosophy, University of Memphis

MILENA MANCINI Department of Psychological, Health and Territorial Sciences, G. d'Annunzio University of Chieti

ADRIAN P. MUNDT Medical Faculties, Diego Portales University and University of Chile

LUCY OSLER Department of Sociology, Philosophy, and Anthropology, University of Exeter

HÉCTOR PELEGRINA-CETRAN Faculty of Philosophy and Letters, Autonomous University of Madrid

MATTHEW RATCLIFFE Department of Philosophy, University of York

LANEI M. RODEMEYER McAnulty College and Graduate School of Liberal Arts Philosophy, Duquesne University

PHILIPP SCHMIDT Department of Philosophy, Technical University of Darmstadt; Department of Philosophy, University of Würzburg

PASCAL SIENAERT Academic Center for ECT and Neuromodulation, Catholic University of Leuven

ADRIAN SPREMBERG Department of Psychiatry, University of Campinas

GIOVANNI STANGHELLINI Department of Psychological, Health and Territorial Sciences, G. d'Annunzio University of Chieti

SHOGO TANAKA Center for Liberal Arts, Tokai University

CHRISTIAN TEWES Section of Phenomenological Psychopathology and Psychotherapy, Department of General Psychiatry, University of Heidelberg

SAMUEL THOMA Department for Psychiatry and Psychotherapy, Immanuel Klinik Rüdersdorf, Berlin, Brandenburg Medical School

WOLFGANG TSCHACHER Department of Psychotherapy, University Hospital of Psychiatry, University of Bern

ZENO VAN DUPPEN Psychiatry Department, Catholic University of Leuven

DITTE WINTHER-LINDQVIST Danish School of Education, Aarhus University

I

Introduction – Time and Body
Phenomenological and Psychopathological Approaches

Christian Tewes and Giovanni Stanghellini

Research on the embodied mind has gained an ever increasing significance in recent decades. It is no longer an outsider position in the cognitive sciences but has made an impact on mainstream science, being applied not only in the biological and psychological realm but also in the cultural sphere (Durt, Fuchs, & Tewes, 2017; Etzelmüller & Tewes, 2016). One particular strand of embodiment research, "classical enactivism," aims at integrating the first-person perspective of experience into the exploration of the human mind – alongside explorations of autopoiesis and dynamical systems theory. In this regard, phenomenological methods and insights are not only a heuristic tool for studying the intertwinement of mind and world but a necessary ingredient for research on subjective experience (Thompson, 2007).

The fundamental distinction made in the phenomenological tradition between the *subject-body* and the *object-body* points to the need to incorporate different research methods and perspectives into an exploration of the embodied human mind. Thus, the "subject-body," considered in sensorimotor terms, refers to the smooth integration of action and perception into meaningful Gestalts by means of sense-making activities. In the undisturbed flow of interactions, the body functions as a medium by means of its intentional capacities and experiential perspective on the lifeworld (Merleau-Ponty, 1945/2005). The "object-body," by contrast, refers to the entangled double structure of the body, which is also disclosed at the experiential level of description (Plessner, 1928/1975). When we get exhausted or injured, the body can become an explicit obstacle for the constant flow of interaction with the environment and lifeworld. We can also *objectify* the living-body by means of our reflexive capacities and specify its organismic processes or its biochemical ingredients (the physical body).

Such capacities are not acquired in solitary ways by individuals separated from the social environment, but have a constitutional basis in the intersubjective cultural realm. Enactivism has defined this intersubjective foundation as a form of "participatory sense-making." Such processes are based on the regulated interaction of two or more autonomous agents. One can also describe them as processes of coordination and synchronizing, e.g., when two people take their cues from each other in conversation or adjust their steps when walking side by side. It is a somewhat fleeting (not perfectly symmetrical) synchronization, but it engages them in a mutual adjustment of intentional movements (Dumas, Kelso, & Nadel, 2014, pp. 1–2). When engaging in such coupled actions, the interactors are still involved in individual sense-making processes. But what is decisive is "the coordination of intentional activity in interaction, whereby individual sense-making processes are affected and new domains of social sense-making can be generated that were not available to each individual on her own" (De Jaegher & Di Paolo, 2007, p. 497). What emerges in these interactions is a form of mutually shared meaning or sense-making that leads to an enculturated form of understanding, one that is shaped by the "unfolding of the social engagement" (Di Paolo & De Jaegher, 2017, p. 90).

Famously, the way such processes shape the object-body at the level of social engagement was explored by Jean-Paul Sartre (1943/1956). Sartre differentiates between three ontological dimensions of body constitution. The first dimension comes close to what we have called the subject-body: In everyday interactions I can use things as objects and tools, but my body is not itself an object for me ("I exist my body" Sartre, 1943/1956, p. 351). In the second dimension, my body is also known and "used" by others. This interrelation of Self and Other is then specified in the third dimension: It is where the other is disclosed to me as a subject for whom I am the object. In Sartre's words: "I exist for myself as a body known by the Other. This is the third ontological dimension of my body" (Sartre, 1943/1956, p. 351).

A significant research field in phenomenological psychopathology is the attempt to explicate and analyze at different levels of constitution the experiential shift between the subject- and object-body in psychopathological disorders. Severe depression, for instance, has been explored at the first-person level of experience in terms of how it affects the double structure of the body. In this context, Thomas Fuchs has coined the term "corporification": In severe depressive episodes, the patient's body loses its spontaneous fluidity and becomes an obstacle (it is sometimes felt as heavy or inflexible); every movement requires a disproportionate effort. It can even feel as if the entire body is solidified, as in cases of the so-called depressive stupor (Fuchs, 2016, p. 432).

Another constitutional aspect of the object-body comes into play when one uses phenomenological psychopathology to analyze eating disorders.

It has been shown that eating disorders can depend on an internalized distorted *body image*, an idea that recalls Sartre's third dimension of the object-body constitution. Thus, anorexia in its various forms can have a foundation in a normatively laden body image resulting from social expectations (the "ideal body shape" one is pressured to conform to). It involves an internalized "objectifying gaze" of the other toward the individual's own body that can lead to life-threatening illness (Stanghellini, 2019; Svenaeus, 2013).

It has already been indicated in enactive and dynamic terms that time plays a major role in constituting the body at the subjective and intersubjective levels of description. In the tradition of phenomenological psychopathology too, temporality has been a major issue since the work of Binswanger (1960), Blankenburg (1992), Minkowski (1970), Straus (1960), Tellenbach (1980), and von Gebsattel (1954), who in turn drew upon the philosophical works of Bergson, Husserl, and Heidegger. These authors analyzed psychopathological disturbances in the patient's experience of time, specifically in severe depression, obsessive-compulsive disorder, and schizophrenia. Due to the complex interplay between the subject- and the object-body, the various types of psychopathological disorders affect quite different constitutional levels of temporality. Crucially, such concepts may also be applied to psychopathological disorders that display temporal dissociations or damage to embodied interpersonal synchrony. Mental disorders are not only accompanied by the interruption of the continuity of daily life, but frequently by a destabilization of the temporal constitution of the Self too. This becomes obvious in cases such as *dementia* where patients progressively lose their autobiographical or declarative memory (Hydén, 2014; Lindemann, 2014). But it is also detectable in *schizophrenia* where phenomenological analyses reveal a *temporal fragmentation* of self-experience (Stanghellini et al., 2016).

Let us explain these temporal dimensions in a bit more detail. In dementia, the *explicit* temporal integration of the narrative self is fragmented and ultimately lost. This means a gradual loss of the capacity to integrate biographical items from linear time (one's birthday, schooldays, date of marriage, etc.) with episodic memories. In persons affected by major depression, empirical findings confirm the relevance of distinctive features of abnormal time experiences, supporting the hypothesis of an intrinsic disordered temporal structure in depressive symptoms (Stanghellini et al., 2017). In schizophrenia, by contrast, the *implicit* micro-temporal order of inner time consciousness (including what Husserl [1969] termed the "passive synthesis" of "presentation," "retention," and "protention") is disturbed, creating the so-called micro-gaps of awareness and disconnected fragments which may be experienced as inserted thoughts or voices (Fuchs, 2013, p. 86). These fragmented experiences are often described by schizophrenic patients as extraneous to their sense of selfhood (ipseity) (Stanghellini, 2009). This exemplifies the constitutive function of temporality for the continuity of the embodied Self.

As already indicated, phenomenological and embodied dynamical approaches to time consciousness have the potential to help us analyze mental disorders in terms of their co-constituting intersubjective dimensions. Thus, any psychopathological destabilization of the human mind has repercussions for intersubjective temporal relations, as in the case of depression, where an individual's shared intersubjective time is *desynchronized*, leading to a loss of bodily resonance, and culminating in depressive delusions where the patient is unable to take the perspective of others (Fuchs, 2013, p. 99). Likewise, *traumatic experiences* that are deeply entrenched in body memory can also have effects on the (re)organization of autobiographical memories, resulting in the further destabilization of social interaction (Brown & Reavey, 2015). Both of these examples indicate the intertwinement of individual and interpersonal temporal factors in psychopathological disorders.

Moreover, research has shown that these concepts can be extended to psychotherapeutic encounters as well. Thus, interpersonal synchrony is itself highly significant for the successful outcome of psychotherapeutic treatment at different levels of study, such as synchronic movements or the regulation of emotions between patient and therapist (Fuchs, Messas, & Stanghellini, 2019; Koole & Tschacher, 2016, pp. 10–11). Today, researchers in the field have further differentiated and analyzed the properties of time consciousness and begun to apply them in a diagnostic and explanatory way to a broader range of mental disorders (Stanghellini & Aragona, 2016).

It is the aim of the present volume to sharpen and deepen an understanding of the intertwinement of time and bodily experience and to contribute to the further development of an embodiment-based phenomenological psychopathology. To this end, the volume elaborates and discusses key notions and findings from the research fields mentioned above. Each of the authors uses the methods and insights of *phenomenology* and *embodiment research* to explore the interrelation between psychopathology, temporality, and the embodied mind. They investigate how temporal processes contribute to the constitution of embodiment and selfhood, as well as to their destabilization in psychopathological disorders. Thus, it is the aim of the volume to present new insights from phenomenological psychopathology and enactive research while demonstrating these research fields' applicability to different illnesses and their relevance to treatment and clinical practice.

The volume begins with an introductory chapter on the interrelations between time, embodiment, and intersubjectivity in psychopathology by Thomas Fuchs, who is one of the leading researchers in phenomenological psychopathology and enactivism. Each of the following chapters in the book is supplemented with a commentary to discuss questions raised, controversies, or further prospects for research. The volume is divided into four parts.

Part I, *Body and Time: General Aspects*, explores the key concepts of the volume in more detail. In Chapter 3, Dorothée Legrand considers the intersubjective constitution of the "body" and its role in clinical practices, drawing upon the ideas of Maurice Merleau-Ponty and Jacques Lacan. Legrand explores the body not only as the lived-body but also as the body that incarnates otherness. Otherness is explained in a twofold way: On the one hand, the body as a living organism is a generality and its functioning hosts a "germ of depersonalization"; on the other hand, the body is that which keeps another subject away from me, separate from me, and irreducible to me. According to this approach, the body is both a concretion of alterity and of singularity. On this basis, Legrand outlines the possibility of developing a clinical practice informed by the ideas of both Merleau-Ponty and Lacan.

In Chapter 4, Giovanni Stanghellini offers a detailed phenomenological analysis of the various manifestations of corporeality in order to show how the body is apprehended in different psychopathological conditions. He argues for a distinction between the "body-object," the "lived-body," and the "living body." He defines the latter as the immediately felt, pathic, non-representational, experiential, and invisible manifestation of one's corporeality. A further manifestation of corporeality is the "body-for-others" that is the experience of feeling one's corporeality when looked at by another person. Stanghellini proceeds to relate these different profiles of corporeality to specific anomalous psychopathological conditions, for example, the body as restricted, inhibited, and rigid in melancholia or the body apprehended through the gaze of the other as in eating disorders.

In Chapter 5, Natalie Depraz examines different aspects of the peculiar temporality of "chronic time" considered in light of its pathological dimensions. She does so by applying different methods and resources and interweaving them: clinical literature on the topic, conceptual philosophical frameworks, and first-person micro-phenomenological interviews. The inquiry is based on a research program at the University of Rouen Normandy which investigates three chronic diseases in teenagers: diabetes, anorexia, and schizophrenia. The broad hypothesis of her contribution is that chronicity may be not only a property of these illnesses but also a more global pathology with social and civilizational consequences.

Wolfgang Tschacher develops a quantitative approach to the exploration of psychotherapy on the basis of dynamic systems theory. Tschacher notes how high-resolution time series allow the mapping of therapeutic processes at a timescale of seconds, the "here-and-now," the present moment. The demand for high-resolution data can be satisfied with the help of measurements such as body movement or physiological signals. As the embodiment approach has shown, mental processes are reciprocally connected to bodily variables, so that the mind can be analyzed via the body. Tschacher gives the example of the time series of respiratory activity measured in naturalistic psychotherapy sessions. From this data, he shows how the nonverbal synchrony of the present moment can be derived.

In Part II, the phenomena of *Grief and Anxiety* are investigated from existential and phenomenological perspectives. Allan Køster's contribution focuses on the experiences of persons who have been bereaved of an intimate other and left with profound feelings of emptiness. Feelings of emptiness are, however, difficult to specify in detail and are not exclusive to bereavements (they are reported across a range of psychopathological conditions, such as schizophrenia and borderline personality disorder). Køster provides an existential-phenomenological analysis of feelings of emptiness, arguing that in the context of bereavement such feelings should in no way be interpreted as merely metaphorical, but rather as (often profoundly embodied) feelings of actually being emptied. This is not meant as an experience of abstract nothingness but a profound vacancy in the absence of a concrete presence.

In Chapter 8, Shogo Tanaka focuses on the relationship between social anxiety, bodily experiences, and interpersonal contact with others. He starts by revisiting the phenomenology of bodily experiences and clarifies the difference between the body-as-subject and the body-as-object. Tanaka distinguishes the experience of one's body-as-object for others from those of one's body-as-object for oneself. As already pointed out, among phenomenologists, Sartre emphasized the former aspect of bodily experiences, calling it the "third ontological dimension of the body." On the basis of this notion, Tanaka develops a phenomenology of social anxiety and its disorders.

Part III concentrates on the psychopathological conditions of borderline personality disorder (BPD) and eating disorders. Matthew Ratcliffe and Anna Bortolan start with a contribution on BPD by examining the phenomenology of emotion dysregulation. They emphasize how emotions ordinarily arise within the context of a structured experiential world, how they play a role in maintaining, repairing, and reshaping that world, and how both the world's stability and the workings of emotion processes depend on our being able to relate to other people in certain ways. Ratcliffe and Bortolan go on to show how emotion dysregulation (of the kind associated with BPD) is *implied* by way of experiencing and relating to the social world as a whole. Given that other people play essential roles in sustaining a structured, practically meaningful world and regulating the emotions that arise within it, emotion regulation and dysregulation turn out to be interpersonal, rather than wholly intrapersonal, in structure.

In Chapter 10, Philipp Schmidt addresses how three kinds of instability associated with BPD, namely, instability in identity, affect, and interpersonal relationships, display aspects of disturbed self-experience in relation to the body. He emphasizes the ways in which these aspects of disturbed self-experience are experientially interconnected and interwoven. He also discusses how the experience of the body features in these aspects of disturbed self-experience and suggests that BPD involves a fourth kind of instability: a significant instability in embodiment. Finally, he shows how an analysis of the experiential interconnections between BPD-related phenomena and the bodily dimension of disturbed self-experience not only helps us describe and understand BPD experience but also allows significant insights into how the clinical picture of BPD emerges and persists over time. This can lend support to a holistic understanding of BPD: a Gestalt-like complex of intertwined experiential structures.

In Chapter 11, Lanei M. Rodemeyer argues that there are several levels to the constitution of experience presented in Husserl's phenomenology and that they are much more systematically treated in his work than it might first appear. After providing an overview of each of these levels, Rodemeyer argues that a Husserlian view of phenomenological constitution can help us understand the experience of gender and, more specifically, the gendered character of eating disorders. In doing so, Rodemeyer demonstrates that these different levels of experiential constitution can be applied to areas beyond phenomenology, providing frameworks and terminology that can, for instance, have therapeutic application.

Otto Doerr-Zegers and Héctor Pelegrina-Cetran offer an analysis of the intertwinement of the anorexic patient with their body and the world. According to their approach, three fundamental anthropological dimensions are severely disturbed in anorexia nervosa: corporeality, spatiality, and temporality. The authors explore how these dimensions constitute an existential form of anorexia that presents the self-image of a disembodied subject in a purely physical world of rationalistic thoughts.

In Part IV, the authors focus on illnesses such as depression, schizophrenia, and *dementia*. Edward A. Lenzo and Shaun Gallagher offer a phenomenologically inspired enactivist interpretation of how disordered temporal experience relates to the structure of intrinsic temporality, which much of phenomenological psychopathology takes as its starting point. They point to a long-standing view in phenomenological psychopathology, reinforced by empirical studies, which understands depression in terms of a disruption to the intrinsic human experience of time. A growing consensus in the field now links psychopathologies to disorders of affect, affordances, and the narrative aspects of experience. Lenzo and Gallagher interpret these links in terms of enactive approaches to cognition and dynamical systems theory.

In Chapter 14, Tom Froese and Joel Krueger address the peculiarity that people with schizophrenia not only report feelings of dissociality but also the opposite: an unusual fluidity of the self-other boundary as expressed in experiences of ambiguous body boundaries, intrusions, and even merging with others. Here the person has not lost access to the socially extended mind but has instead become lost in it, possibly due to a weakened sense of self. Froese and Krueger argue that this neglected aspect of schizophrenic social dysfunction can be usefully approached via the concept of "genuine intersubjectivity": One normally participates in a shared experience with another person by implicitly co-regulating how the interaction unfolds. This co-regulation integrates the dynamical bases of each person's experience into one interpersonal process and gives the interaction an ambiguous second-person character. The upshot is that reports of abnormal self-Other fluidity are not indicative of hallucinations without any basis in reality, but of a heightened sensitivity and vulnerability to processes of interpersonal alignment and mutual incorporation that form the normal basis of social life. Froese and Krueger conclude by discussing implications of this view both for the science of consciousness and for intervention and therapy.

In Chapter 15, Zeno Van Duppen and Pascal Sienaert deal with the psychopathological phenomenon of catatonia: a severe psychiatric syndrome characterized by specific motor abnormalities such as immobility, mutism, staring, rigidity, or psychomotor agitation. Until recently, catatonia was often thought of as a subtype of schizophrenia. Today it is recognized that it can be a symptom of different medical and psychiatric illnesses, as well as occurring independently of them. Despite the fact that catatonia is encountered remarkably often by clinicians, and has been a subject of study for decades, it remains poorly understood. Until now, phenomenological psychopathology has also devoted little attention to the phenomenon. To redress this imbalance, Van Duppen and Sienaert investigate the phenomenology of catatonia, i.e., its subjective and intersubjective presentation. The authors present a clinical vignette and clarify its phenomenology with emphasis on fear, embodiment, and temporality. Indirectly, their investigation sheds new light on how trauma can affect subjectivity, in both its embodied and temporal dimension.

In Chapter 16, Christian Tewes explores the intertwinement of embodied selfhood and personal identity over time in dementia. According to the cognitivist picture of personal identity prevalent in the scientific literature and public debate, severe cases of dementia, where there is a loss of declarative memory, linguistic capacities, and social orientation, effectively turn the patient from a person into a non-person. After critically analyzing the arguments and assumptions behind this view, Tewes introduces the concept of "embodied selfhood" as a counterview. He argues that even in severe cases of dementia – such as late-stage Alzheimer's disease – the manifold expressive forms of embodied selfhood justify the continued ascription of embodied personal selfhood in its qualitative and temporal dimensions.

Acknowledgment

We are grateful to the Marsilius-Kolleg of the University of Heidelberg and the Protestant Institute for Interdisciplinary Research (FEST) in Heidelberg for supporting the work on this anthology. We thank Mailin Hebell-Dowthwaite, Lukas Iwer, Damian Peikert, Daniel Vespermann, Dr. Adrian Wilding, and the publisher Cambridge University Press for their invaluable help and cooperation in preparing the manuscript for publication.

References

Binswanger, L. (1960). *Melancholie und Manie: Phänomenologische Studien* [Melancholy and mania: Phenomenological studies]. Pfullingen, Germany: Neske.

Blankenburg, W. (1992). Zeitigung des Daseins in psychiatrischer Sicht [Temporalization of being in psychiatric view]. In E. Angehrn, H. Fink-Eitel, C. Iber, & G. Lohmann (Eds.), *Dialektischer Negativismus* [Dialectical negativism] (pp. 130–155). Frankfurt am Main, Germany: Suhrkamp.

Brown, S. D., & Reavey, P. (2015). Turning around on experience: The 'expanded view' of memory within psychology. *Memory Studies*, 8(2), 131–150. doi: 10.1177/1750698014558660

De Jaegher, H., & Di Paolo, E. A. (2007). Participatory sense-making: An enactive approach to social cognition. *Phenomenology and the Cognitive Sciences*, 6(4), 485–507. doi: 10.1007/s11097-007-9076-9

Di Paolo, E., & De Jaegher, H. (2017). Neither individualistic nor interactionist. In C. Durt, T. Fuchs, & C. Tewes (Eds.), *Embodiment, enaction, and culture: Investigating the constitution of the shared world* (pp. 87–105). Cambridge, MA: Massachusetts Institute of Technology Press.

Dumas, G., Kelso, J. A. S., & Nadel, J. (2014). Tackling the social cognition paradox through multi-scale approaches. *Frontiers in Psychology*, 5, 1–4. doi: 10.3389/fpsyg.2014.00882

Durt, C., Fuchs, T., & Tewes, C. (Eds.). (2017). *Embodiment, enaction, and culture. Investigating the constitution of the shared world*. Cambridge, MA: MIT Press.

Etzelmüller, G., & Tewes, C. (Eds.). (2016). *Embodiment in evolution and culture.* Heidelberg, Germany: Mohr Siebeck.

Fuchs, T. (2013). Temporality and psychopathology. *Phenomenology and the Cognitive Sciences*, 12(1), 75–104. doi: 10.1007/s11097-010-9189-4

Fuchs, T. (2016). Anthropologische und phänomenologische Aspekte psychischer Erkrankungen [Anthropological and phenomenological aspects of psychiatric disorders]. In H.-J. Möller, G. Laux, & H. P. Kampfhammer (Eds.), *Psychiatrie, Psychosomatik, Psychotherapie* [Psychiatry, psychosomatics, psychotherapy] (pp. 417–431). Berlin, Germany: Springer. doi: 10.1007/978-3-642-45028-0_16-1

Fuchs, T., Messas, G. P., & Stanghellini, G. (2019). More than just description: Phenomenology and psychotherapy. *Psychopathology*, 52(2), 63–66. doi: 10.1159/000502266

Husserl, E. (1969). *Zur Phänomenologie des inneren Zeitbewusstseins (1893–1917)* [On the phenomenology of the consciousness of internal time] (R. Boehm, Ed.). The Hague, Netherlands: Martinus Nijhoff.

Hydén, L.-C. (2014). How to do things with others: Joint activities involving persons with Alzheimer's disease. In L.-C. Hydén, H. Lindemann, & J. Brockmeier (Eds.), *Beyond loss. Dementia, identity, personhood* (pp. 137–154). Oxford, UK: Oxford University Press.

Koole, S. L., & Tschacher, W. (2016). Synchrony in psychotherapy: A review and an integrative framework for the therapeutic alliance. *Frontiers in Psychology*, 7, 1–17. doi: 10.3389/fpsyg.2016.00862

Lindemann, H. (2014). Second nature and the tragedy of Alzheimer's. In L.-C. Hydén, H. Lindemann, & J. Brockmeier (Eds.), *Beyond loss. Dementia, identity, personhood* (pp. 11–23). Oxford, UK: Oxford University Press.

Merleau-Ponty, M. (2005). *The phenomenology of perception* (C. Smith, Trans.). Abingdon-on-Thames, UK: Taylor and Francis e-Library. (Original work published 1945)

Minkowski, E. (1970). *Lived time: Phenomenological and psychopathological studies.* Evanston, IL: Northwestern University Press.

Plessner, H. (1975). *Die Stufen des Organischen und der Mensch* [Levels of organic life and the human]. Berlin, Germany: De Gruyter. (Original work published 1928)

Sartre, J.-P. (1956). *Being and nothingness* (H. E. Barnes, Trans.). New York, NY: Philosophical Library. (Original work published 1943)

Stanghellini, G. (2009). Embodiment and schizophrenia. *World Psychiatry*, 8(1), 56–59. doi: 10.1002/j.2051-5545.2009.tb00212.x

Stanghellini, G. (2019). The optical-coenaesthetic disproportion in feeding and eating disorders. *European Psychiatry*, 58, 70–71. doi: 10.1016/j.eurpsy.2019.02.005
Stanghellini, G., & Aragona, M. (Eds.). (2016). *An experiential approach to psychopathology. What is it like to suffer from mental disorders?* Berlin, Germany: Springer.
Stanghellini, G., Ballerini, M., Presenza, S., Mancini, M., Northoff, G., & Cutting, J. (2017). Abnormal time experiences in major depression: An empirical qualitative study. *Psychopathology*, 50(2), 125–140. doi: 10.1159/000452892
Stanghellini, G., Ballerini, M., Presenza, S., Mancini, M., Raballo, A., Blasi, S., & Cutting, J. (2016). Psychopathology of lived time: Abnormal time experience in persons with schizophrenia. *Schizophrenia Bulletin*, 42(1), 45–55. doi: 10.1093/schbul/sbv052
Straus, E. (1960). Das Zeiterleben in der Depression und in der psychopathischen Verstimmung [Temporal experience in depression and psychopathic upset]. In E. Straus (Ed.), *Psychologie der menschlichen Welt* [Psychology of the human world] (pp. 126–140). Berlin, Germany: Springer.
Svenaeus, F. (2013). Anorexia nervosa and the body uncanny: A phenomenological approach. *Philosophy, Psychiatry, & Psychology*, 20(1), 81–91. Retrieved from https://muse.jhu.edu/article/511263
Tellenbach, H. (1980). *Melancholy. History of the problem, endogeneity, typology, pathogenesis, clinical considerations* (E. Eng, Trans.). Pittsburgh, PA: Duquesne University Press.
Thompson, E. (2007). *Mind in life. Biology, phenomenology, and the sciences of mind*. Cambridge, MA: Harvard University Press.
von Gebsattel, E. (1954). Zeitbezogenes Zwangsdenken in der Melancholie [Time-related compulsive thinking in melancholia]. In E. von Gebsattel (Ed.), *Prolegomena einer medizinischen Anthropologie* [Prolegomena of a medical anthropology] (pp. 1–18). Berlin, Germany: Springer.

2

Time, the Body, and the Other in Phenomenology and Psychopathology

Thomas Fuchs

Introduction

The phenomenology of temporality has usually taken as its basis the analysis of consciousness (Husserl, 1991) or of human existence (Heidegger, 1962). Only first steps have been made by Maurice Merleau-Ponty (1945/1962), Michel Henry (1975/2012), or Dan Zahavi (1999) toward concepts of bodily subjectivity and intersubjectivity that include their temporal dimension as well. A fundamental investigation into the interconnection of temporality, embodiment, and their interpersonal embeddedness is still missing (see Fuchs, 2013b, 2017, 2018b for steps in this direction). In what follows, I intend to give an overview of such connections and their significance for mental disorders, not least with the goal to stimulate and structure further research on these issues. I will start with the interrelation of embodiment and temporality, then in Part II extend the view to their connection with intersubjectivity. Part III is dedicated to the analysis of major mental disorders such as autism, schizophrenia, depression, and posttraumatic stress disorder from the perspective of temporality and embodiment.

Embodiment and Temporality

The relations between corporeality and temporality reach from the microstructure of conscious experience to the enactment of human existence. First, the prereflective internal time consciousness is marked by the *rhythmicity* of vital processes (heartbeat, respiratory rhythm, daily periods, etc.) as well as by cyclically recurrent drives, urges, and needs, which may be subsumed under the term *conation*.[1] Furthermore, the body

[1] From the Latin *conatus* = endeavor, effort, drive, urge. The concept dates back to Stoic philosophy and was later used by Hobbes and Spinoza in particular to denote the living being's striving for self-preservation (*conatus sese conservandi*), in close connection with affective–volitional life.

forms an extract of sensorimotor and affective experiences that sediment in *implicit or body memory*, thus shaping an individual's capacities and dispositions. Finally, *biographical* and *existential temporality* are essentially characterized by the vital processes of birth, growth, aging, and dying; on this level, embodiment also underlies the explicit, linear time perspective that arises with the reflective awareness of one's life and its course. In what follows, I will take a closer look at these interrelations of body and time.

Body Time

As is well known, Husserl regarded time as the core structure of pure consciousness, conceiving it as an intertwinement of protentions, primary impressions, and retentions. On the other hand, the embodiment of the subject remained for him but an additional correlate of consciousness, not being constitutive of time experience; he considered the body mainly from a spatial point of view, as the zero point of orientation (Husserl, 1952). However, if subjectivity is conceived as essentially bodily in Merleau-Ponty's sense, then the living, sensing, and moving body should also be regarded as the basis of the stream of consciousness. On this condition, the pure transcendental form of time turns into a bodily stream and sense of time, though only as a "lived time" which does not yet become explicit or conscious as such. As an implicit or prereflective "body time," temporality becomes a manifestation of the process of life itself, which underlies the continuity of the embodied subject (Fuchs, 2017, 2018b).

Evidence for such a basis of temporality may be seen, on the one hand, in the microtemporality of experience, for which periodical bodily processes play a formative, if not a constitutive, role. Thus, respiratory movement and heartbeat produce a constant underlying rhythmization of the stream of consciousness, even if this is for the most part not consciously recognized. On a neurobiological level, recent research suggests that the continuous central integration of such rhythmic bodily signals forms the basis of our sense of the duration of time (Craig, 2009; Wittmann, 2013, 2015). Thus, the interoceptive experience of one's own body not only provides a prereflective self-awareness but also seems to underlie the diachronic continuity of the embodied self (Fuchs, 2017).

The rhythmic nature of prereflective temporality also becomes manifest in the units of experienced *presence*: They do not form a linear continuum, but intervals, in which events are rhythmically combined into meaningful groups (Kiverstein, 2010). Various findings point to an interval duration of the experienced present of approximately three seconds (see Pöppel, 1997, 2000, pp. 59–73). This is noticeable, for instance, in the spontaneous segmentation that occurs when one listens to the regular ticking of a metronome. Through accentuation, beats of twos or threes emerge in our minds (1-2, 1-2, or 1-2-3, 1-2-3, etc.). However, this grouping only works up to an interval of two to three seconds between the beats; beyond that only single beats can be heard, and grouping is no longer possible (Szelag, von Steinbüchel, Reiser, Gilles de Langen, & Pöppel, 1996). Similarly, the perspectival perception of ambiguous or bistable figures, such as the Necker cube, or the gestalt perception of Rubin's vase (is it a vase or two faces?), switches around every three seconds spontaneously (Kornmeier, Ehm, Bigalke, & Bach, 2007). Last, spontaneous speech is also rhythmically structured, so that the average duration of a verse line is about three seconds (Pöppel, 2000, pp. 85–86). Thus, one could say that meaningful units of conscious experience are grouped in intervals that approximate the rhythm of breathing.

Finally, the subjective experience of the duration of time varies depending on the motivation, arousal, or relaxation of the body, which manifests itself in heart and breathing rates, muscle tension, or blood pressure (Wittmann, 2015). Sympathicotonic arousal (as in anxiety) and parasympathicotonic relaxation (as in resting or lethargy) occur with different experiences of time. Above all, the increase of vital drive in manic states as well as the inhibition of drive in depression lead to changes in time experience, namely, to a felt acceleration in one case and to a stretching of time in the other (Bschor et al., 2004; Fuchs, 2013b). Subjective time is thus closely related to the overall arousal level and drive of the body. This will become even more obvious in the following section.

Conation and the Future

A further connection of temporality and embodiment consists in the fact that the bodily drives, urges, and needs, which may be subsumed under the term *conation*, crucially determine the future-directed temporality of primary experience (Fuchs, 2013b). The periodical states of lack and shortage undergone by the organism require instinctual impulses such as thirst, hunger, the motor, or the sex drive, which aim at compensating the occurrent lack. With this instinctual direction, the felt "not yet" of possible fulfillment awakens as well (Jonas, 1963, pp. 99–107). In striving and anticipated satisfaction lies a central root of the experience of time: Deficiency and need open up a time differential or "time span," which is primarily experienced as an appetitive tension toward what-is-to-come or to-be-achieved and its final fulfillment.

Moreover, the intentional arcs directed toward specific objects are supported by the embodied *emotions*, which bridge the delay of satisfaction in experience and accompany the movement toward the desired object. Thus, hunting is motivated by desire and aggression; flight, conversely, by avoidance and fear (Jonas, 1963, p. 101). Emotions, through their bodily resonance (interoceptive sensations and movement tendencies), also lend vital meanings to objects in the environment, making them appear enticing, comforting, repellent, threatening, and so forth (Fuchs & Koch, 2014). In this way, they impart an affective character to the protentions (i.e., prereflective anticipations of the future), which again testifies to the conative and affective roots of time experience: Every striving and seeking, but also every attention and interest manifest the appetitive directedness of the body toward the immediate future.

The recurrent dynamic of lack, urge, expectation, desire, and fulfillment is both the subjective side and the motivating force of the processes of self-preservation that constitute animal life, driving it forward into the future. Though embodiment and conation constitute the basis of temporal experience, this basis has a *rhythmic and cyclical*, not a linear character.[2] It is characterized by periodically recalled processes, cycles of lack and fulfillment, expenditure and regeneration, waking and sleeping, as well as by rhythmic processes such as heartbeat, breathing, walking, or chewing. On a wider scale, we find the rhythms of hormone secretion, body temperature, sleep–wake cycles, and energy balance to be synchronized to the day period. Hence, as living beings, we share the sense and rhythm of temporal becoming with the ambient world, as Minkowski stated:

> It is not only that we feel a general progression, in us as well as outside us, but rather a unique rhythm common to us and to ambient becoming that makes me feel that I am advancing in my life simultaneously with time. (Minkowski, 1970, pp. 69–70)

Understanding consciousness as embodied, thus, leads to the following thesis: The primary and implicit form of time experience reveals the rhythmic-dynamic structure of the lived body and of the processes of life that underlie this very experience. Of course, life also means a continuous movement from birth to death. Nevertheless, the prereflective experience of time has a cyclical structure, and it is only when this primary experience is overlaid by an explicit reference to the anticipated future or the remembered

[2] Although the recurrent achievement of drive goals includes (usually short) linear sequences of time, these do not coalesce into a continuous linear time perspective.

past that an overarching linear time perspective is opened up for the subject. This linear perspective then spans recurrent temporal episodes by the awareness of one's biography as a whole, of one's finitude, and of the course of the world even beyond one's own life (Fuchs, 2018b).

Body Memory

The bodily basis of temporality is not restricted to recurrent episodes or cycles, however, but in itself also shows a continuous and long-term structure. It consists in the history and habituality of the lived body, that means, its capacity to form a lasting memory of repeated experiences, which I call *implicit or body memory* (Casey, 1984; Fuchs, 2012, 2019a). This memory is radically different from explicit, autobiographical memory, or remembering: While the latter directs itself back to the past where the experiences line up sequentially, body memory, by contrast, consists in the repetition or "reenactment" of what has been experienced, learnt, or habitualized, without the past being still remembered as such. It comprises all the individual's capacities, habits, and dispositions, which are actualized automatically, without explicit intent – it is our *lived past.*

Repetition and practice are the primary ways in which habits of movement, perception, and behavior anchor themselves in body memory, starting with walking upright, through learning to read and write, to the use of instruments such as playing the violin or typing with a keyboard. Bodily learning consists mainly in the gradual *forgetting* of what has been trained explicitly in the beginning, namely, to the extent that learned action becomes a part of one's tacit knowing how – becomes part of our "flesh and blood." Repetition results in *automatization*, a process that integrates single movements within a uniform temporal gestalt, which is incorporated in the form of unreflective bodily enactments (Fuchs, 2012). One then no longer knows how one does what one self-evidently does – such as driving a car or dancing a waltz. The knowing how lies in the limbs and senses of the body, on which we come to rely. This melting of repeated experiences into body memory is particularly favored by rhythmic repetition, be it in melodies, meter, or rhyming, or be it in the rhythmic forms of movement such as walking, dancing, or skiing. It is no coincidence that rhythmic and repetitive interactions (singing, rhyming, playing, rituals) are an essential feature of children's early socialization. Thus, in body memory, we find again the rhythmic-periodical structure of immediate bodily enactment. Yet this structure is now integrated within an overarching, reenacting, and malleable structure, namely, in the habituality of the body. It conveys our fundamental experience of familiarity with the world, and our experience of sameness and recurrence in the change of situations. Primarily formed in early childhood, bodily habituality modifies and alters itself in the course of life – body memory displays a lifelong, if waning, plasticity. Nevertheless, the temporality of existence remains always bound to a basic cyclical structure – it is also repetition in every moment, the recurrence of the familiar and the similar. The surprising and the new can only emerge against this given background.

Temporality of Existence

Finally, embodiment plays a major role for *existential temporality*, opened up through one's relation to life as a whole, which is essentially characterized by the vital processes of birth, growth, aging, and dying. Existence means to be given to oneself through birth, as captured both by Hannah Arendt's "natality" and Heidegger's "thrownness" (Arendt, 1958; Heidegger, 1962): to emerge from a primordial ground which is neither retrievable nor at one's disposal, and which nevertheless remains the basis of all activities and projects throughout one's life. Being such a bodily being, with this size, this sex, these endowments, or these disabilities, sets the inescapable framework of one's existence, a framework one has to deal or to cope with, whether one likes it or not.

Subjective temporality in early life is characterized by the cyclical structure of body time. With the development of autobiographical memory beginning in the second year of life, the perspective of time broadens; memories of the past become possible as well as anticipations of the more distant future (Markowitsch & Welzer, 2009). Gradually, one's own lifespan enters consciousness as a continuum. Biographical time arises along with the reflective awareness of oneself as both being a body (body-as-subject) and having a body (body-as-object); a body one is bound to, a body that one is dependent upon, which will finally succumb to illness and death. Using a crucial term of Plessner (1928), it is the self-reflective or "excentric position" of humans, placing them in a virtual position outside of their bodily center, which creates this ambiguity of the body.

The dialectic of being and having a body unfolds in the course of life. It requires taking a stance toward one's bodily existence, its needs, and its changes. On the one hand, existence means constant growth, carried by the body's life process, which, as we have seen, incorporates all experiences in body memory and turns them into acquired skills and dispositions. In this way, growth continues in the form of cumulative experience even beyond adolescence, throughout one's life. On the other hand, bodily changes also mean transition, aging, and decline, gradually restricting the scope of remaining possibilities, which is caused by physical or mental impairment as well as by the mere contraction of residual lifetime. Numerous existential challenges – and corresponding neurotic disorders – result from our awareness of existing as mortal living beings, whose days are counted. Finally, it is our body that renders us inherently vulnerable and exposed to illness, both physical and mental, for mental disorders are always disorders of one's embodied existence as well. Vulnerability to illness and death is part of our predicament as living, bodily beings.

In sum, embodiment may be considered as constitutive for prereflective or lived time as well as for autobiographical time. This becomes manifest (1) in the microtemporality of conscious experience, which is based on the interoception of rhythmic processes; (2) in the bodily dynamics of drive and conation, creating an appetitive tension toward the future that is present even in the slightest attention and protention; (3) in the habitual structure of body memory, which forms an extract of past experiences as the basis of bodily capacities and dispositions; and (4) in the diachronic continuity of the embodied self, which undergoes the changes of the life process – birth, growth, maturation, aging, and dying – and thus underlies the biographical time of existence. Hence, as living, embodied beings, we are essentially temporal beings: The embodiment and the temporality of the subject are equally manifestations of the life process. As self-conscious and stance-taking subjects, persons then face the task of dealing with the basic, autonomous processes of their bodily life and its changes in growth and aging – not least of dealing with its fundamental vulnerability, disposition to illness, and mortality.

Embodiment, Temporality, and Intersubjectivity

Body, time, and intersubjectivity are equally interconnected. Starting in the child's early development, interbodily resonance and interaffectivity establish the primary experience of the shared present. Thus, a basic *co-temporality* emerges, which later continues in explicit *synchronization* and timing arrangements as the basis of social life. However, this temporal alignment and harmonization is also subject to *desynchronizations*, for example, in backlogs of tasks, in guilt, remorse, or grief – situations and feelings that fix the subject on the past and require processes of psychosocial *resynchronization*. Thus, intersubjective time constitutes itself on the level of implicit co-temporality as well as on the level of explicit social organization. This will be explained in more detail below.

Interbodily Resonance and Basal Co-temporality

The rhythmic and recurrent character of lived time lends itself quite naturally to various phenomena of bodily *resonance*. This may be defined as the tendency of the body to synchronize with external processes such as musical rhythms or, on a larger timescale, with the circadian rhythm.[3] A particular form of resonance also emerges in interpersonal encounters, namely, *interbodily resonance*. It may be described, on the one hand, in enactivist terms, namely, as a dynamical coupling and coordination of embodied agents (1), on the other hand, in phenomenological terms, as mutual incorporation or intercorporeality (2). This prereflective synchronization creates the experience of a shared presence; it is the basis of the fundamental sense of being-with-others in a common time.

(1) Numerous analyses of social interactions and conversations have shown that participants unconsciously coordinate their movements and utterances, most often in a rhythmic way (Condon, 1986; Gill, 2012; Issartel, Marin, & Cadopi, 2007; Laroche, Berardi, & Brangier, 2014). For instance, listeners synchronize their movements, however tiny, with the changes in speed, direction, and intonation of the speaker's utterances (Davis, 1982). Speech rates tend to converge (Street, 1984), and a close temporal coupling is even observed in breathing during turn-taking (McFarland, 2001). Studies on the way musicians work together while playing show similar coordinations (Maduell & Wing, 2007). These findings suggest that in general, interactors are coupled with each other by perception–action loops, thus being entrained toward a shared timing. Enactivist accounts of intersubjectivity describe the autonomy of this process, which gains a certain independence from the partners' prior dispositions and intentions, as "participatory sense-making" (De Jaegher & Di Paolo, 2007; Fuchs & De Jaegher, 2009).

(2) In phenomenological terms, interacting partners experience each other empathically through the mutual affection of their lived bodies. Mediated through eye contact, facial expressions, voice, touch, gesture, and other movements, they enter into a dyadic bodily state. Their body schemas expand and in a sense incorporate the perceived body of the other. This creates a dynamical interplay, which forms a phenomenal basis of social understanding and may be described as "mutual incorporation" (Fuchs &

[3] The endogenous sleep–wake cycle is a bit longer than twenty-four hours, but it is synchronized to the environment by external timekeepers, mainly by light; the same happens of course in the case of intercontinental travels (Czeisler et al., 1999).

De Jaegher, 2009; Leder, 1990, p. 94). Looked at more closely, the emotions felt by one partner are visible and sensible in his own bodily resonance and expression; this turns into a bodily impression or affection experienced by the other. Now both sense the changes they induce in the other's experience with their own body: The lived body's impression or reaction on the one side becomes a living body's expression for the other, and vice versa (Froese & Fuchs, 2012). The mutual affection experienced by each other's gaze creates an especially strong sense of interpersonal presence.

Infant research has shown how interbodily resonance shapes the child's primary experience: The communication between infant and mother is characterized by rhythmic–melodic interactions, mutual resonance of facial expression and gesture, creating an affective attunement (Stern, 1985). Already in the first months of life, dyads show regular turn-taking in vocalization or other expressive gestures at a pace of two to three seconds and thereby experience a shared present (Malloch, 1999; Malloch & Trevarthen, 2009). These reciprocal interactions are confined to response latencies or contingencies within the range of 200–800 milliseconds – otherwise desynchronization will occur (Nadel, Carchon, Kervella, Marcelli, & Réserbat-Plantey, 1999). The rhythmic or musical nature of early intercorporeality is also highlighted by Stern's concept of "vitality affects," meaning the intensity contours of mutual bodily expressions such as surging, bursting, accelerating, slowing down, and fading away, which are mostly bound to a time frame of one to three seconds as well (Stern, 2010).

Thus, from the very beginning the microdynamics of interaction entail a synchronization that is usually not conscious – it rather conveys the tacit feeling of being temporally connected with others, of living with them in a *basic co-temporality*. The intersubjective "now" is constituted through the presence of the other, in particular through our simultaneous referral to the world, as in pointing or looking at, shared attention or joint action. It may of course be made explicit by the use of indexical words such as "here," "this," and "now"; however, all use of indexicals is based on the participants' primary intercorporeality.

Social Synchronization

Intersubjective synchronization becomes also explicit in the various forms of social coordination or "timing": in shared daily and weekly routines, time scheduling, appointments, punctuality – in a broader sense, in all mutual commitments and arrangements. In this way, an individual's own time is more or less coupled with the social or world time. Synchronization also marks the changes and developments that occur in various phases of life. Important biographical transitions (entering school, starting work, marriage, steps of career, retirement, etc.) are more or less standardized and bind together the individuals of a cohort. Finally, there is the contemporaneity of people belonging to the same culture with their specific history, values, styles, forms of behavior, etc.

Social synchronization does not remain constant but repeatedly passes through phases of *desynchronization*, in which the individual lags behind the common time of the others, such as in backlogs of tasks, in grief, guilt, or remorse (Fuchs, 2001, 2013b). Thus, grief reflects a break in one's synchronicity with others – the mourner cannot detach him- or herself from the shared past, whereas the general or world time keeps going on. Guilt, the failure to meet expectations or obligations, also has a retarding structure inasmuch as it fixes the individual to past omissions. Finally, mental illness usually means a deceleration, a loss of ability to act, and thus a partial exclusion from the life of others as well. Not only individuals, however, but also social groups may lose their synchronization with the general development of society and experience themselves as decoupled or disadvantaged, often resulting in collective anger and resentment.

To summarize: Intersubjective time is neither a mere co-presence in physical space, nor a mere simultaneity of activities that can be observed from an external point of view. Rather, being together in time is primarily based on the interbodily resonance and coordination of individuals in face-to-face encounters. Together, they enact a dynamical landscape of intertwined bodily expressions and impressions that enable the experience of a shared present as well as a basic empathic understanding of each other. On a more explicit level, intersubjective time can be considered a relation of individual and social processes characterized by synchronizations and desynchronizations. While lived or implicit time is basically associated with synchrony – when we are fully immersed in an activity or interaction, time usually does not come to awareness as such – the experience of explicit time arises particularly in desynchronized states, as a "too early" or "too late" in the relation of individual and world time (Fuchs, 2013b).

Embodiment, Temporality, and Psychopathology

The interconnections between embodiment, temporality, and intersubjectivity may undergo various kinds of disturbances which crucially impact on the emergence and course of mental disorders. I will demonstrate this by the paradigmatic examples of

(1) the loss of interbodily resonance and affective attunement, as in autism and schizophrenia;
(2) the biological and social desynchronization that is a crucial characteristic of major depression;
(3) the disturbances of body memory in posttraumatic stress disorder; and
(4) the existential relation to one's changing body in anorexia nervosa.

As I will try to show by these examples, mental illnesses may to a large extent be described as *disturbances of embodied and intersubjective temporality*: What psychiatric patients essentially lack is fully sharing the present with others, interacting with them in an implicit, empathic way, and experiencing their own agency through the resonance it creates in others.

Autism

According to current cognitive theories of autism, the disorder is due to a difficulty to "read other people's minds," to imagine what they are thinking or feeling, or in other words, to a lack of theory of mind (ToM). However, many autistic symptoms such as lack of emotional contact, lack of interest in others, agitation, and anxiety are already present in the first years of life, that means, long before the supposed age to acquire a ToM which is around four years. From a phenomenological viewpoint, autism should therefore rather be conceived as a *disorder of embodied intersubjectivity* (De Jaegher, 2013; Gallagher, 2004). This includes basic disturbances of embodiment found in children with autism, namely, a lack of sensorimotor integration and holistic perception as well as disturbances of motor coordination (Gepner & Mestre, 2002). These conditions are bound to impair especially the perception, interactive understanding, and imitation of others' expressions and bodily behavior. As a result, children with autism lack interbodily resonance and interaffectivity with others, which leads to a variety of social, communicative, and cognitive deficits, among them a disturbed development of higher-order capacities such as perspective taking and language acquisition.

Moreover, autistic children show problems in establishing *perceptual and situational coherence*: They focus on single parts or elements rather than perceiving the gestalt of objects, and they tend to treat things and events decontextualized, thus missing their particular meaning provided by the situation as a whole (Frith, 1989; Happé, 1995). The expression of a face, for example, is a holistic phenomenon: It is only perceived when we do not focus on a single feature or detail. However, eye tracking studies have shown that children with autism focus on peripheral features of faces, and on irrelevant details of interactive situations while missing the relevant social cues (Klin, Jones, Schultz, & Volkmar, 2003). This failure of holistic cognition significantly interferes with the development of social understanding. Generally, autistic children therefore prefer to attend to inanimate objects over living beings or humans (Klin, Lin, Gorrindo, Ramsay, & Jones, 2009). They neglect or avoid in particular the other's gaze (Jones, Carr, & Klin, 2008), thus missing the meeting of gazes and the awareness of being the object of another's attention; however, both are crucial bridges for establishing a shared intersubjective present.

Regarding interactive coordination, a lack of synchronicity during interactions has been retrospectively observed already in eleven-month-old autistic infants (Trevarthen & Daniel, 2005). Research also suggests that children with autism have problems in establishing shared rhythms, for example, tapping in synchrony with an auditory stimulus (Sheridan & McAuley, 1997). The general lack of interbodily resonance and rhythmicity leads to a failure of affect attunement and to a missing readiness to imitate others as well as to identify with them (Hobson & Lee, 1999; Smith & Bryson, 1994). Hence, for autistic children, the others remain rather enigmatic or foreign beings, which their body cannot resonate with. The patterns of everyday interactions such as greeting or farewell are usually impoverished (Hobson & Lee, 1998). On the other hand, people with autism often report a need to adhere to strict routines or rituals in order to avoid the unpredictability of social encounters. They are not able to get involved in the spontaneity of interaction that creates the "intersubjective now," or a shared temporality. What autistic children lack is thus not a theoretical concept of other minds but a primary sense of bodily being-with-others.

Schizophrenia

Minkowski was the first to describe schizophrenia in terms of a disturbed temporality, implying a fundamental desynchronization from the shared world: The patients lose their vital contact with reality, the resonance with others, and, thus, their participation in collective or ambient becoming (Minkowski, 1958). This view may be connected to the concept of schizophrenia as a *disembodiment*, or a basic disturbance of the embodied self, which has been developed in recent phenomenological psychopathology. This includes a weakening of the basic sense of self, a disruption of implicit bodily functioning, and a disconnection from the intercorporeality with others (Fuchs, 2005; Sass & Parnas, 2003; Stanghellini, 2004). These alterations are also bound to compromise the temporal attunement to the shared world.

As we saw, it is the lived body that conveys the practical knowledge of how to interact with others, how to understand their expressions and actions on the background of the shared situation. If this embodied involvement in the world is disturbed, it will result in a fundamental alienation of intersubjectivity: The basic sense of being-with-others is replaced by a sense of detachment that may pass over into a threatening alienation. Accordingly, it has been shown that schizophrenic patients lack primary or bodily empathy, that means, they have problems with perceiving facial and gestural expressions of others (Amminger et al., 2012; Edwards, Jackson, & Pattison, 2002; Kington, Jones, Watt, Hopkin, & Williams, 2000). Further, patients often show a lack of implicit social understanding, manifesting itself in a subtle "loss of natural self-evidence" (Blankenburg, 1971). The sense of proportion for what is appropriate, likely, and relevant in the social context is missing:

> I don't really grasp what others are up to … I constantly observe myself while I am together with people, trying to find out what I should say or do. It's easier when I am alone or watching TV. (Quotation from a patient with schizophrenia, Psychiatric Clinic, Heidelberg)

In the intercorporeal encounter, the patient's emotional expressions and verbal utterances do not seem to correspond to each other or to the context (parathymia). Bodily movements and expressions are not integrated to form a harmonious whole through which the person could manifest himself. As a result, others will tend to experience the patient more as an object-body than as an expressive body. This impression – equivalent to the well-known "praecox-feeling" (Rümke, 1941/1990) – corresponds to the experiential disembodiment of the schizophrenic person.

In addition to disembodiment and the resulting disturbances of intersubjectivity, schizophrenia is also characterized by a *fragmentation of lived time*: The intentional arc of directed attention, thought, or action may become discontinuous, interrupted by sudden breaks or gaps, and renders goal-directed performance difficult or impossible. Particularly the protentional function or immediate anticipation of the "next-to-come" seems to be weakened, leading to a failure of the connecting of experiences that is constitutive for the intentional arc (Fuchs, 2007, 2013b; Gallagher, 2005). As a result, overarching meaningful units of thought or action are no longer available as a matter of course, as becomes manifest in formal thought disorder (including thought blockages or thought withdrawal), disturbances of listening or speaking, and last but not least in a loss of implicit, automatic bodily functioning:

> I found recently that I was thinking of myself doing things before I would do them. If I am going to sit down, for example, I have got to think of myself and almost see myself sitting down before I do it. It's the same with other things like washing, eating, and even dressing—things that I have done at one time without even bothering. (McGhie & Chapman, 1961, p. 107)

The patients may attempt to compensate for these disturbances on the explicit level, namely, by trying to put the sentences or actions together deliberately from single words or movements – described as "morbid rationalism" by Minkowski (1970). Rather than *living* time, the patient may thus attempt to *construct* his own temporality in an explicit and intellectual manner. However, this results in an even greater loss of spontaneity or fluidity of actions and thoughts, and in hyperreflexivity of various kinds (Fuchs, 2011; Sass, 1992). It affects in particular the temporal synchronization with others, rendering fluent social interactions difficult or impossible. The patient loses the security of being in a common time, in atmospheric presence or syntony with others.

As a result, many patients withdraw into isolation. The complexity and subtlety of common sense, that is, the implicit rules of social conduct, are too difficult for them to manage. This may lead them to construct "algorithms" – logical or even mathematical rules of adequate behavior that they derive from observing others. Autistic withdrawal can be understood as an attempt to reduce the burden of these complex social interactions. Another possibility is the minimization of change: When the flow of time consciousness is fragmented, repetitiveness and even monotony of the surrounding world may help the patient to create a substitute for the lacking inner continuity (Fuchs, 2013b).

The fragmentation of implicit time is also what Stanghellini et al. (2016) have found in their recent qualitative research on altered time experience in schizophrenia. The main temporal alteration in their investigation is, more specifically, the emergence of subsequent "split moments," for example, the world as a series of fragmented snapshots. In such a discontinuous succession of moments, the identity of the subject over time becomes dubious and uncertain, and the patient may even wonder whether he still is the same person as he was before:

> I constantly have to ask myself "who am I really?" It is hard to explain … most of the time I have this very strange thing: I watch myself closely, like how am I doing now and where are the "parts".… I think about that so much that I get to nothing else. It is not easy when you change from day to day. As if you were a totally different person all of a sudden. (Quotation from a patient diagnosed with schizophrenia, De Haan & Fuchs, 2010, p. 329)

As can be seen, the fragmentation of lived time in schizophrenia may also affect the sense of continuity of the self.

Affective Disorders

In contrast to the fragmentation of temporality in schizophrenia, affective disorders show a *retardation* or *acceleration* of lived time, subjectively experienced as time "slowing down" in depression or "speeding up" in mania (Bschor et al., 2004). This may be considered as a result of a lack of bodily conation, on the one hand, and its excess on the other. Moreover, both depression and mania are characterized by the fact that the organism's cyclical processes are derailed and the rhythmization of everyday life no longer functions (Fuchs, 2013b).

In manic states, the movement of life accelerates and constantly overruns the cyclical time of the body and its diurnal rhythms, favoring instead linearly accelerated time. Manic patients ignore the needs of their body, do not grant themselves any sleep, and ignore the signs of developing exhaustion. The body is exploited mercilessly, turned into a mere vehicle and instrument of the inflated drive. The loss of the present time of the body is also manifest in the fact that manic patients only fleetingly enter into contact with the world and others, and in their restlessness cannot tarry in the present. For them, the present is indeed determined by what is missing or what could be possible. Manic patients, therefore, live beyond their means and exhaust their biological and social resources. The rhythmic, and therefore also retarding, moment of existence is no longer perceived, but rather repressed or overrun.

The counterpart of mania, *depression*, is characterized by a loss of rhythmical temporality as well, obviously not through acceleration, but by deceleration. Depressive patients typically complain about how slowly time passes for them, how agonizingly the day stretches out, and in experimental studies, they tend to estimate the duration of a given time interval as longer than it really is (Bech, 1975; Bschor et al., 2004; Kitamura & Kumar, 1982). In addition to this, there is a disturbance of the hormonal diurnal rhythm, of the sleep–wake cycle, of drive, appetite, and interest, resulting in a loss of the cyclical-bodily structure of time up to the point of complete lethargy, inaction, and aboulia (i.e., the absence of volition).[4]

These alterations amount to a fundamental *desynchronization* of the depressed person from the environment or from the world time. This applies both to the organismic and the psychological level, where depression is experienced as a lagging behind or "remanence," as Tellenbach (1980) has described it. Vain attempts to keep up with events and obligations reinforce the patient's feeling of remanence. To this is added the loss of interbodily resonance and emotional attunement with others. The continuous synchronization of bodily gestures and gazes, that normally accompanies interaction, breaks down. The patients feel unable to emotionally communicate their experience; moreover, their own empathic perception and resonance with the other's body is lacking (Bourke, Douglas, & Porter, 2010). The inability to empathize with other people, to be addressed or affected by them, is often described by the patients themselves as a "feeling of not-feeling"; it can also be seen as an *affective depersonalization* (Fuchs, 2000). Thus, the failure of conative-affective dynamics is accompanied not only by a loss of basic co-temporality with others but also by a profound alienation from oneself.

Posttraumatic Stress Disorder

Emotional trauma confronts us with another kind of embodied temporality, one which is crucially mediated by body memory. The traumatic event is an experience that may not be appropriated and integrated into a meaningful context; it often does not partake in explicit, autobiographical memory. As Merleau-Ponty writes, the trauma

> does not leave us but remains constantly hidden behind our gaze instead being displayed before it. The traumatic experience does not survive as a representation in the mode of objective consciousness and as a "dated" moment; it is of its essence to survive only as a manner of being and with a certain degree of generality. (Merleau-Ponty, 1945/1962, p. 83)

4 Recent research even points to disturbances of the rhythmic gene activity in the brain of patients with major depressive disorder (MDD): Li et al. found that in terms of this activity, "the circadian rhythms of MDD cases were not synchronized ('entrained') normally to the solar day" (Li et al., 2013, p. 9953).

The trauma thus withdraws from conscious recollection, but remains all the more virulent in the memory of the lived body that carries it into the environment. Traumatized persons become hypersensitive to threatening, shaming situations similar to the trauma in some manner, even if this similarity is not consciously known, and try to circumvent them. All the same, at every step, they may encounter something that reawakens the trauma. Victims of accidents may panic when the present traffic situation somehow resembles the former traumatic circumstances (Hackmann, Ehlers, Speckens, & Clark, 2004). The former pains of a torture victim may reappear in a present conflict and correspond exactly to the body parts that were exposed to the torture. The body recollects the trauma as if it were happening anew (Van der Kolk, 2014).

Thus, the victim reexperiences feelings of pain, anxiety, and terror again and again, combined with fragments of intense images. Moreover, the injury has penetrated the body of the subject and has left behind a constant responsiveness, a readiness to defend oneself. Often it happens that a permanent predisposition develops to react with fear and nervousness, to become alarmed every time the doorbell rings, a feeling of being followed or observed by unknown people. Most of all, the intercorporeal memory of the traumatized person has changed deeply: They retain a sense of being defenseless, always exposed to a possible assault. The felt memory of an alien intrusion into the body has irreversibly shaken the primary trust into the world; every unknown person is turned into a potential threat. Jean Améry, himself a victim, writes that the survivor of the torture will no more be able to feel at home, secure, and familiar anywhere in the world (Améry, 1977, p. 58).

The after effects of trauma may also serve as a paradigm for reconceiving the *unconscious* in terms of embodiment (Fuchs, 2019a). As we have seen earlier, what is mediated and enabled by body memory is mostly forgotten in terms of explicit memory; through automatization, it has become "unconscious." This also applies to former interpersonal experiences that shape the person's lived body and lived space in a certain way, be it as dispositions of openness and approximation or of fear and avoidance. The latter is obviously the case in posttraumatic stress disorder, where the victim is both attracted by trauma-related cues and tries to avoid them. One may recall here that Freud for the first time described the neurotic "repetition compulsion" in relation to traumatic neurosis (Freud, 1975, pp. 288ff.). What is meant here is the unconscious tendency to relive or even reenact unmastered experiences of the past, be it in thought, dreams, actions, games, or relationships. The individual is entrapped time and again in the same dysfunctional patterns of behavior and relationships, even though they may try to avoid this by all means on the conscious level.

If, for example, the early childhood of a person is marked by abuse and violent experiences, then this motif can determine their later relationships in such a way that they unconsciously keep creating abusive situations. This means that it is not just pleasant relations that are sought or looked for, but particularly harmful and painful situations are also recreated. The explanation for this lies in the unconscious fixations of body memory, which contains unfavorable patterns of perception and behavior as kinds of stage directions, tending toward their actualization even if they are no longer appropriate to current circumstances. The cyclical time structure of the unconscious overlays later, similar situations and repeats an old pattern, similar to an old vinyl record on which the needle was stuck.

Hence, unconscious fixations resemble distortions or restrictions in a person's lived space, caused by a past that continues to be implicitly present in the memory and dispositions of the body (Fuchs, 2019a). Its traces can be noticed in the "blind spots," gaps, or recesses of a patient's lived space: in the actions or objects that they avoid, or in the interactive patterns into which they fall even against their conscious intentions. The patient's conduct of life itself manifests a reverse side, an alterity hidden to themselves. From a phenomenological point of view, the unconscious is thus not a hidden intrapsychic entity, located in some depth "below consciousness," or in a vertical dimension. It rather manifests itself in the *horizontal* dimension of the phenomenal field, as Merleau-Ponty remarked:

> This unconscious is to be sought not at the bottom of ourselves, behind the back of our "consciousness," but in front of us, as articulations in our field. It is "unconscious" by not being object but by being that through which objects are possible, it is the constellation from which our future may be read. (Merleau-Ponty, 1964/1968, p. 180)

Anorexia Nervosa

Anorexia may finally serve as an example of a disorder that is related to embodiment and existential temporality: The process of bodily and social maturation does not proceed naturally, but is disturbed by a reflective, controlling, and rejecting attitude. Triggered by the awareness of the other's look on one's own maturing and possibly sexual body, this body becomes an alienated and finally repulsive object. "With the Other's look the 'situation' escapes me. I am no longer master of the situation" (Sartre, 1969, p. 265). The anorexic patient desperately tries to regain control by subjugating her body.[5] Thus, the conflict between *being* a body-subject and *having* one's body as an object becomes the core of the disorder (see also Legrand, 2010).

The anorectic patient refuses the dependence on the prereflective, natural body with its uncontrollable change and obscure becoming, its threatening impulses, and cravings – in particular hunger and sexual desire – which may only be quenched by external supply. This self-willed, appetent body now becomes an alienated, repulsive object that may even arouse disgust. The patients thus not only reject their hungry, growing body but also deny the maturation of their female, swelling, and sexual body. Gaining independence from it, and turning it into an object of control and mastery, becomes a source of grandiose triumph (Waller, Sines, Meyer, Foster, & Skelton, 2007). Thus, the implicit sense of bodily ownership is replaced by an explicit appropriation of the body aimed at perfect control and maximal suppression of desire.

Although the cultural ideal of the slender figure and corresponding distortions of body image can play a role as a trigger, such external aspects do not constitute the actual source of the disorder. Instead, the patients attempt to compensate for their profound lack of self-esteem and identity by successfully controlling and modeling their body (Gaete & Fuchs, 2016). The anorexic adopts the societal ideal of *body image*, yet at the same time inverts it, for she is no longer concerned with the body-for-others; quite the contrary, through the body's submission, she tries to become independent from everyone else. "I don't feel hungry, I have no desire" – for her this means: I am self-sufficient and no longer need anything from outside (Dignon, Beardsmore, Spain, & Kuan, 2006). In fact, she rejects precisely the sexualization of the body and associated feminine identity options, and thus ultimately the separation from childhood, which is supposedly "sexless." Her ideal is the nonbodily, asexual, angelic body; her actual role model is not the model on the catwalk, but the saint.

In the desperate striving for perfection, the anorexic alienates herself from her earthly, bodily being. The tension of being a body and having a body becomes a radical dualism that is reminiscent of the Platonic and Christian ideas of the body as the prison of the soul:

> It was as if I had to punish my body. I hate and detest it. If I let it be normal for a few days, then I would have to deprive it again. I feel caught in my body—as long as I keep it under rigid control, it can't betray me. (Kaplan, 1984, p. 278)

[5] The description is restricted to female anorexia, which constitutes the vast majority of cases.

In sum, anorectic patients try to escape the cyclic, autonomous processes of need, drive, and satisfaction that rule their bodies; on a deeper level, this means the attempt to arrest the course of biological life, which leads to maturation and sexuality. Thus, the example of anorexia shows that the bodily processes of growth, maturation, aging, and dying are always also existential tasks to be taken up and coped with.

Conclusion

The aim of this introductory chapter was to point out the complex interrelations of temporality, embodiment, and intersubjectivity, and to show, using the examples of several major illnesses, how they may contribute to a deeper understanding of psychopathology. If humans are essentially bodily, temporal, and social beings, then psychic illness must equally manifest itself in all three existential dimensions. However, their disturbances are always more than only psychopathological symptoms. They rather represent more or less fundamental disruptions in the most basic human functions, and since all three dimensions also structure the experience of the self, mental illness always means a self-disturbance, even though in various degrees and on different levels.

I have pointed out how the microstructure of *embodied temporality* may become dissolved in schizophrenia, leading to disruptions of the continuity of self-experience, as well as to a fragmentation of the intentional arc of perceiving, thinking, and acting. Further, the microstructure of *bodily resonance* characteristic of social interactions may also be disturbed, as is the case in autism and schizophrenia, entailing a lack of empathic understanding and "sensus communis" or social sense (Thoma & Fuchs, 2018). The *loss of conation* in depression has a similar impact on the affectability of the body, resulting in emotional numbness and a loss of interaffectivity. On a larger time scale, the desynchronization in depression encompasses experiences of backlog and remanence in relation to social or world time.

We have further seen how the *memory of the body* may harbor residuals of emotional trauma that resist the course of biographical time and fixate the person on a past that does not pass. Indeed, the realm of the unconscious as a whole may be regarded as a deeper level of temporality which accompanies conscious life, namely, in the form of embodied dispositions to strive for, or to avoid, situations once experienced in the past. On the other hand, the unconscious also contains hints for future development, which may be used in psychotherapy as a bodily "felt sense" of what the person is to discover about his or her further potentialities (Gendlin, 2012).

Finally, the temporality of the body in its lifelong change of growth, maturation, aging, and decline underlies the *existential challenges* that the person has to cope with. It frequently leads into "limit situations" in the sense of Jaspers (1919), in which the necessary changes required by the course of life may overburden the individual's capacities of adaptation. I have given the example of anorexia nervosa as a disorder of existential temporality, which is related to both the development of the body and to the social changes connected with it. In similar ways, the existential tasks and crises arising from the interrelations of embodiment, temporality, and intersubjectivity may be regarded as a crucial basis for understanding disturbances that were traditionally ascribed to the neurotic domain or to personality disorders (Fuchs, 2013a).

Understanding psychiatric disturbances as alterations of embodiment, temporality, and intersubjectivity will substantially change the current mainstream approach to psychopathology as well as to treatment. If psychic life extends into the world, then psychiatric disorders should not be localized "within" the individual, be it in the psyche or the brain. They should rather be regarded as disturbances of being-in-the-world, and of interacting with others in accordance to one's needs for resonance and response. In other words, psychopathology changes from an individualistic to a relational, from an internalist to an (inter-)enactive framework (De Haan, 2020; Fuchs & Schlimme, 2009; Nielsen & Ward, 2018). So-called mental disorders are actually disturbances of bodily and interbodily existence, to which social dynamics contribute in significant ways. Hence, the biomedical view of psychiatric illness has to be extended and integrated into overarching ecological concepts (see, e.g., Fuchs, 2018a).

This will also have an impact on treatment approaches that are suitable to address the complex interrelations of the three existential dimensions. A conceptual and practical integration of body-oriented, interactive, social, and existential approaches would be a desideratum for the further development of phenomenological and enactive psychiatry. Thus, body-oriented and dance movement therapies have been successfully applied for the treatment of schizophrenia (Martin, Koch, Hirjak, & Fuchs, 2016; Röhricht & Priebe, 2006) as well as autism (Hildebrandt, Koch, & Fuchs, 2016; Koch, Mehl, Sobanski, Sieber, & Fuchs, 2015). Similarly, "assertive community treatment" and "open dialogue" approaches focusing on the patients' social interactions outside of institutional confines (Seikkula, Alakare, & Aaltonen, 2011) have proven successful in preventing relapse of schizophrenia. For the treatment of depression, the perspectives of embodiment and temporality suggest principles for a "resynchronization therapy" (Fuchs, 2019b), which can integrate various methods into an overarching framework. These are but a few examples of how the concepts presented in this chapter and in this volume may usefully inform psychiatric treatment to the benefit of the patients.

A final look shall be given to the therapeutic encounter as the core of treatment: It is the place where all three existential dimensions converge. As we have seen, the reciprocity of embodied interaction, for which synchronization and resonance are essential, often breaks down in psychic illness. Establishing a shared present through focusing on the here and now of the encounter, through attention on the interbodily resonance, last but not least through mindful listening, which does not seek for quick diagnostic classification and intervention, but first of all "lets the other be" (De Jaegher, 2019) – all this contributes significantly to overcoming the patient's alienation and isolation. *Being together in time*, or the present moment (Stern, 2004), is an essential remedy for the desynchronization occurring in psychic illness. Hence, we should further investigate the therapeutic effects of restoring intersubjective presence and rhythmic patterns of interaction (Ramseyer & Tschacher, 2011), not only in psychotherapeutic settings but in every clinical context, even during the first diagnostic process. Every clinical encounter entails this opportunity, and any kind of intervention should above all bring forth a truly lived experience with the patient – a shared co-temporality.

References

Améry, J. (1977). *Jenseits von Schuld und Sühne. Bewältigungsversuche eines Überwältigten* [Beyond guilt and expiation. Attempts to overcome of someone overcome]. Munich, Germany: dtv.

Amminger, G., Schäfer, M. R., Papageorgiou, K., Klier, C. M., Schlögelhofer, M., Mossaheb, N., … McGorry, P. D. (2012). Emotion recognition in individuals at clinical high-risk for schizophrenia. *Schizophrenia Bulletin*, 38(5), 1030–1039. doi:10.1093/schbul/sbr015

Arendt, H. (1958). *The human condition*. Chicago, IL: University of Chicago Press.

Bech, P. (1975). Depression: Influence on time estimation and time experience. *Acta Psychiatrica Scandinavia*, 51(1), 42–50. doi:10.1111/j.1600-0447.1975.tb00211.x

Blankenburg, W. (1971). *Der Verlust der natürlichen Selbstverständlichkeit* [The loss of natural self-evidence]. Berlin, Germany: Springer.

Bourke, C., Douglas, K., & Porter, R. (2010). Processing of facial emotion expression in major depression: A review. *Australian and New Zealand Journal of Psychiatry*, 44(8), 681–696. doi:10.3109/00048674.2010.496359

Bschor, T., Ising, M., Bauer, M., Lewitzka, U., Skerstupeit, M., Müller-Oerlinghausen, B., & Baethge, C. (2004). Time experience and time judgment in major depression, mania and healthy subjects. A controlled study of 93 subjects. *Acta Psychiatrica Scandinavica*, 109(3), 222–229.

Casey, E. S. (1984). Habitual body and memory in Merleau-Ponty. In J. N. Mohanty (Ed.), *Phenomenology and the human sciences* (pp. 39–57). Dordrecht, Netherlands: Springer.

Condon, W. S. (1986). Communication: Rhythm and structure. In J. R. Evans & M. Clynes (Eds.), *Rhythm in psychological, linguistic and musical processes* (pp. 55–77). Springfield, IL: Charles C. Thomas.

Craig, A. D. (2009). Emotional moments across time: A possible neural basis for time perception in the anterior insula. *Philosophical Transactions of the Royal Society of London: Biological Sciences, B*, 364(1525), 1933–1942. doi:10.1098/rstb.2009.0008

Czeisler, C. A., Duffy, J. F., Shanahan, T. L., Brown, E. N., Mitchell, J. F., Rimmer, D. W., … Kronauer, R. E. (1999). Stability, precision, and near-24-hour period of the human circadian pacemaker. *Science*, 284(5423), 2177–2181. doi:10.1126/science.284.5423.2177

Davis, M. (Ed.). (1982). *Interaction rhythms. Periodicity in communicative behavior.* New York, NY: Human Sciences Press.

De Haan, S. (2020). *Enactive psychiatry.* Cambridge, UK: Cambridge University Press.

De Haan, S., & Fuchs, T. (2010). The ghost in the machine: Disembodiment in schizophrenia. Two case studies. *Psychopathology*, 43(5), 327–333. doi:10.1159/000319402

De Jaegher, H. (2013). Embodiment and sense-making in autism. *Frontiers in Integrative Neuroscience*, 7, 1–19. doi:10.3389/fnint.2013.00015

De Jaegher, H. (2019). Loving and knowing: Reflections for an engaged epistemology. *Phenomenology and the Cognitive Sciences*. Advance online publication. doi:10.1007/s11097-019-09634-5

De Jaegher, H., & Di Paolo, E. (2007). Participatory sense-making: An enactive approach to social cognition. *Phenomenology and the Cognitive Sciences*, 6(4), 485–507. doi:10.1007/s11097-007-9076-9

Dignon, A., Beardsmore, A., Spain, S., & Kuan, A. (2006). 'Why I won't eat': Patient testimony from 15 anorexics concerning the causes of their disorder. *Journal of Health Psychology*, 11(6), 942–956. doi:10.1177/1359105306069097

Edwards, J., Jackson, H. J., & Pattison, P. E. (2002). Emotion recognition via facial expression and affective prosody in schizophrenia: A methodological review. *Clinical Psychology Review*, 22(6), 789–832. doi:10.1016/S0272-7358(02)00130-7

Freud, S. (1975). Jenseits des Lustprinzips [Beyond the pleasure principle]. In A. Mitscherlich, A. Richards, & J. Strachey (Eds.), *Studienausgabe (Vol. 3). Psychologie des Unbewußten* [Psychology of the unconscious] (pp. 213–272). Frankfurt am Main, Germany: S. Fischer.

Frith, U. (1989). *Autism: Explaining the enigma*. Oxford, UK: Basil Blackwell.

Froese, T., & Fuchs, T. (2012). The extended body: A case study in the neurophenomenology of social interaction. *Phenomenology and the Cognitive Sciences*, 11(2), 205–236. doi:10.1007/s11097-012-9254-2

Fuchs, T. (2000). *Psychopathologie von Leib und Raum. Phänomenologisch-empirische Untersuchungen zu depressiven und paranoiden Erkrankungen* [Psychopathology of body and space. Phenomenological-empirical investigations in depressive and paranoid disorders]. Darmstadt, Germany: Steinkopff.

Fuchs, T. (2001). Melancholia as a desynchronization. Towards a psychopathology of interpersonal time. *Psychopathology*, 34(4), 179–186. doi:10.1159/000049304

Fuchs, T. (2005). Corporealized and disembodied minds. A phenomenological view of the body in melancholia and schizophrenia. *Philosophy, Psychiatry & Psychology*, 12(2), 95–107. Retrieved from https://muse.jhu.edu/article/190379

Fuchs, T. (2007). The temporal structure of intentionality and its disturbance in schizophrenia. *Psychopathology*, 40(4), 229–235. doi:10.1159/000101365

Fuchs, T. (2011). The psychopathology of hyperreflexivity. *Journal of Speculative Philosophy*, 24(3), 239–255. doi:10.1353/jsp.2010.0010

Fuchs, T. (2012). The phenomenology of body memory. In S. Koch, T. Fuchs, M. Summa, & C. Müller (Eds.), *Body memory, metaphor and movement* (pp. 9–22). Amsterdam, Netherlands: John Benjamins.

Fuchs, T. (2013a). Existential vulnerability. Toward a psychopathology of limit situations. *Psychopathology*, 46(5), 301–308. doi:10.1159/000351838

Fuchs, T. (2013b). Temporality and psychopathology. *Phenomenology and the Cognitive Sciences*, 12(1), 75–104. doi:10.1007/s11097-010-9189-4

Fuchs, T. (2017). Self across time: The diachronic unity of bodily existence. *Phenomenology and the Cognitive Sciences*, 16(2), 291–315. doi:10.1007/s11097-015-9449-4

Fuchs, T. (2018a). *Ecology of the brain. The phenomenology and biology of the embodied mind*. Oxford, UK: Oxford University Press.

Fuchs, T. (2018b). The cyclical time of the body and its relation to linear time. *Journal of Consciousness Studies*, 25(7–8), 47–65. Retrieved from www.ingentaconnect.com/content/imp/jcs/2018/00000025/f0020007/art00003

Fuchs, T. (2019a). Body memory and the unconscious. In R. Gipps & M. Lacewing (Eds.), *The Oxford handbook of philosophy and psychoanalysis* (pp. 457–470). Oxford, UK: Oxford University Press.

Fuchs, T. (2019b). The life-world of persons with mood disorders. In G. Stanghellini, M. Broome, A. Raballo, A. V. Fernandez, P. Fusar-Poli, & R. Rosfort (Eds.), *The Oxford handbook of phenomenological psychopathology* (pp. 617–633). Oxford, UK: Oxford University Press.

Fuchs, T., & De Jaegher, H. (2009). Enactive intersubjectivity: Participatory sense-making and mutual incorporation. *Phenomenology and the Cognitive Sciences*, 8(4), 465–486. doi:10.1007/s11097-009-9136-4

Fuchs, T., & Koch, S. (2014). Embodied affectivity: On moving and being moved. *Frontiers in Psychology*, 5, 1–12. doi:10.3389/fpsyg.2014.00508

Fuchs, T., & Schlimme, J. (2009). Embodiment and psychopathology: A phenomenological perspective. *Current Opinion in Psychiatry*, 22(6), 570–575. doi:10.1097/YCO.0b013e3283318e5c

Gaete, I. M., & Fuchs, T. (2016). From body image to emotional bodily experience in eating disorders. *Journal of Phenomenological Psychology*, 47(1), 17–40. doi:10.1163/15691624-12341303

Gallagher, S. (2004). Understanding interpersonal problems in autism: Interaction theory as an alternative to Theory of Mind. *Philosophy, Psychiatry & Psychology*, 11(3), 199–217. doi:10.1353/ppp.2004.0063

Gallagher, S. (2005). *How the body shapes the mind*. New York, NY: Oxford University Press.

Gendlin, E. T. (2012). *Focusing-oriented psychotherapy: A manual of the experiential method*. New York, NY: Guilford Press.

Gepner, B., & Mestre, D. (2002). Rapid visual-motion integration deficit in autism. *Trends in Cognitive Sciences*, 6(11), 455. doi:10.1016/S1364-6613(02)02004-1

Gill, S. P. (2012). Rhythmic synchrony and mediated interaction: Towards a framework of rhythm in embodied interaction. *AI & Society*, 27(1), 111–127. doi:10.1007/s00146-011-0362-2

Hackmann, A., Ehlers, A., Speckens, A., & Clark, D. M. (2004). Characteristics and content of intrusive memories in PTSD and their changes with treatment. *Journal of Traumatic Stress*, 17(3), 231–240. doi:10.1023/B:JOTS.0000029266.88369.fd

Happé, F. (1995). *Autism: An introduction to psychological theory*. Cambridge, MA: Harvard University Press.

Heidegger, M. (1962). *Being and time* (J. Macquarrie & E. Robinson, Trans.). New York, NY: Harper and Row.

Henry, M. (2012). *Philosophy and phenomenology of the body* (G. Etzkorn, Trans.). Berlin, Germany: Springer. (Original work published 1975)

Hildebrandt, M. K., Koch, S. C., & Fuchs, T. (2016). "We dance and find each other": Effects of dance/movement therapy on negative symptoms in autism spectrum disorder. *Behavioral Sciences*, 6(4), 1–17. doi:10.3390/bs6040024

Hobson, R. P., & Lee, A. (1998). Hello and goodbye: A study of social engagement in autism. *Journal of Autism and Developmental Disorders*, 28(2), 117–127. doi:10.1023/A:1026088531558

Hobson, R. P., & Lee, A. (1999). Imitation and identification in autism. *The Journal of Child Psychology and Psychiatry and Allied Disciplines*, 40(4), 649–659. doi:10.1111/1469-7610.00481

Husserl, E. (1952). *Ideen zu einer reinen Phänomenologie und phänomenologischen Philosophie. II. Phänomenologische Untersuchungen zur Konstitution*. [Ideas pertaining to a pure phenomenology and to a phenomenological philosophy. II. Studies in the phenomenology of constitution]. The Hague, Netherlands: Martinus Nijhoff.

Husserl, E. (1991). *On the phenomenology of the consciousness of internal time* (J. Brough, Trans.). Dordrecht, Netherlands: Kluwer Academic.

Issartel, J., Marin, L., & Cadopi, M. (2007). Unintended interpersonal coordination: "Can we march to the beat of our own drum?" *Neuroscience Letters*, 411(3), 174–179. doi:10.1016/j.neulet.2006.09.086

Jaspers, K. (1919). *Psychologie der Weltanschauungen* [Psychology of worldviews]. Berlin, Germany: Springer.

Jonas, H. (1963). *The phenomenon of life. Toward a philosophical biology*. New York, NY: Harper & Row.

Jones, W., Carr, K., & Klin, A. (2008). Absence of preferential looking to the eyes of approaching adults predicts level of social disability in 2-year-old toddlers with autism spectrum disorder. *Archives of General Psychiatry*, 65(8), 946–954. doi:10.1001/archpsyc.65.8.946

Kaplan, L. J. (1984). *Adolescence: The farewell to childhood*. New York, NY: Simon & Schuster.

Kington, J. M., Jones, L. A., Watt, A. A., Hopkin, E. J., & Williams, J. (2000). Impaired eye expression recognition in schizophrenia. *Journal of Psychiatric Research*, 34(4–5), 341–347. doi:10.1016/S0022-3956(00)00029-7

Kitamura, T., & Kumar, R. (1982). Time passes slowly for patients with depressive state. *Acta Psychiatrica Scandinavica*, 65(6), 415–420. doi:10.1111/j.1600-0447.1982.tb00865.x

Kiverstein, J. (2010). Making sense of phenomenal unity: An intentionalist account of temporal experience. *Royal Institute of Philosophy Supplements*, 67, 155–181. doi:10.1017/S1358246110000081

Klin, A., Jones, W., Schultz, R., & Volkmar, F. (2003). The enactive mind, or from actions to cognition: Lessons from autism. *Philosophical Transactions of the Royal Society of London. Series B: Biological Sciences*, 358(1430), 345–360. doi:10.1098/rstb.2002.1202

Klin, A., Lin, D. J., Gorrindo, P., Ramsay, G., & Jones, W. (2009). Two-year-olds with autism orient to non-social contingencies rather than biological motion. *Nature*, 459(7244), 257–261. doi:10.1038/nature07868

Koch, S. C., Mehl, L., Sobanski, E., Sieber, M., & Fuchs, T. (2015). Fixing the mirrors: A feasibility study of the effects of dance movement therapy on young adults with autism spectrum disorder. *Autism*, 19(3), 338–350. doi:10.1177/1362361314522353

Kornmeier, J., Ehm, W., Bigalke, H., & Bach, M. (2007). Discontinuous presentation of ambiguous figures: How interstimulus-interval durations affect reversal dynamics and ERPs. *Psychophysiology*, 44(4), 552–560. doi:10.1111/j.1469-8986.2007.00525.x

Laroche, J., Berardi, A. M., & Brangier, E. (2014). Embodiment of intersubjective time: Relational dynamics as attractors in the temporal coordination of interpersonal behaviors and experiences. *Frontiers in Psychology*, 5, 1–17. doi:10.3389/fpsyg.2014.01180

Leder, D. (1990). *The absent body*. Chicago, IL: University of Chicago Press.

Legrand, D. (2010). Subjective and physical dimensions of bodily self-consciousness, and their dis-integration in anorexia nervosa. *Neuropsychologia*, 48(3), 726–737. doi:10.1016/j.neuropsychologia.2009.08.026

Li, J. Z., Bunney, B. G., Meng, F., Hagenauer, M. H., Walsh, D. M., Vawter, M. P., … Bunney, W. E. (2013). Circadian patterns of gene expression in the human brain and disruption in major depressive disorder. *Proceedings of the National Academy of Sciences*, 110(24), 9950–9955. doi:10.1073/pnas.1305814110

Maduell, M., & Wing, A. M. (2007). The dynamics of ensemble: The case for flamenco. *Psychology of Music*, 35(4), 591–627. doi:10.1177/0305735607076446

Malloch, S. N. (1999). Mothers and infants and communicative musicality. *Musicae Scientiae*, 3(1, Suppl.), 29–57. doi:10.1177/10298649000030S104

Malloch, S. N., & Trevarthen, C. (Eds.). (2009). *Communicative musicality: Narratives of expressive gesture and being human*. Oxford, UK: Oxford University Press.

Markowitsch, H., & Welzer, H. (2009). *The development of autobiographical memory*. London, UK: Psychology Press.

Martin, L. M., Koch, S. C., Hirjak, D., & Fuchs, T. (2016). Overcoming disembodiment: The effect of movement therapy on negative symptoms in schizophrenia – A multicenter randomized controlled trial. *Frontiers in Psychology*, 7, 1–14. doi:10.3389/fpsyg.2016.00483.

McFarland, D. H. (2001). Respiratory markers of conversational interaction. *Journal of Speech, Language, and Hearing Research*, 44(1), 128–143. doi:10.1044/1092-4388(2001/012)

McGhie, A., & Chapman, J. (1961). Disorders of attention and perception in early schizophrenia. *British Journal of Medical Psychology*, 34(2), 103–116. doi:10.1111/j.2044-8341.1961.tb00936.x

Merleau-Ponty, M. (1962). *Phenomenology of perception* (C. Smith, Trans.). London, UK: Routledge and Kegan Paul. (Original work published 1945)

Merleau-Ponty, M. (1968). *The visible and the invisible* (A. Lingis, Trans.). Evanston, IL: Northwestern University Press. (Original work published 1964)

Minkowski, E. (1958). Findings in a case of schizophrenic depression. In R. May, E. Angel, & H. Ellenberger (Eds.), *Existence. A new dimension in psychiatry and psychology* (pp. 127–139). New York, NY: Basic Books.

Minkowski, E. (1970). *Lived time: Phenomenological and psychopathological studies* (N. Metzel, Trans.). Evanston, IL: Northwestern University Press.

Nadel, J., Carchon, I., Kervella, C., Marcelli, D., & Réserbat-Plantey, D. (1999). Expectancies for social contingency in 2-month-olds. *Developmental Science*, 2(2), 164–173. doi:10.1111/1467-7687.00065

Nielsen, K., & Ward, T. (2018). Towards a new conceptual framework for psychopathology: Embodiment, enactivism, and embedment. *Theory & Psychology*, 28(6), 800–822. doi:10.1177/0959354318808394

Plessner, H. (1928). *Die Stufen des Organischen und der Mensch* [Levels of organic life and the human]. Berlin, Germany: De Gruyter.

Pöppel, E. (1997). A hierarchical model of temporal perception. *Trends in Cognitive Sciences*, 1(2), 56–61. doi:10.1016/S1364-6613(97)01008-5

Pöppel, E. (2000). *Grenzen des Bewusstseins. Wie kommen wir zur Zeit, und wie entsteht Wirklichkeit?* [Limits of consciousness. How do we get to time and how does reality emerge?] Frankfurt am Main, Germany: Insel.

Ramseyer, F., & Tschacher, W. (2011). Nonverbal synchrony in psychotherapy: Coordinated body movement reflects relationship quality and outcome. *Journal of Consulting and Clinical Psychology*, 79(3), 284–295. doi:10.1037/a0023419

Röhricht, F., & Priebe, S. (2006). Effect of body-oriented psychological therapy on negative symptoms in schizophrenia: A randomized controlled trial. *Psychological Medicine*, 36(5), 669–678. doi:10.1017/S0033291706007161

Rümke, H. C. (1990). The nuclear symptom of schizophrenia and the praecox feeling (J. Neelman, *Trans.). History of Psychiatry*, 1(3), 331–341. (Original work published 1941) doi:10.1177/0957154X9000100304

Sartre, J.-P. (1969). *Being and nothingness: An essay on phenomenological ontology* (H. E. Barnes, Trans.). New York, NY: Routledge.

Sass, L. A. (1992). *Madness and modernism. Insanity in the light of modern art, literature, and thought.* New York, NY: Basic Books.

Sass, L. A., & Parnas, J. (2003). Schizophrenia, consciousness, and the self. *Schizophrenia Bulletin*, 29(3), 427–444. doi:10.1093/oxfordjournals.schbul.a007017

Seikkula, J., Alakare, B., & Aaltonen, J. (2011). The comprehensive open-dialogue approach in Western Lapland: II. Long-term stability of acute psychosis outcomes in advanced community care. *Psychosis*, 3(3), 192–204. doi:10.1080/17522439.2011.595819

Sheridan, J., & McAuley, J. D. (1997). *Rhythm as a cognitive skill: Temporal processing deficits in autism.* Paper presented at the Fourth Australiasian Cognitive Science Conference, Newcastle, NSW. Retrieved from http://citeseerx.ist.psu.edu/viewdoc/download;jsessionid=A0658E4D38992A0792D3F274AB602585?doi=10.1.1.54.4592&rep=rep1&type=pdf

Smith, I. M., & Bryson, S. E. (1994). Imitation and action in autism: A critical review. *Psychological Bulletin*, 116(2), 259–273. doi:10.1037/0033-2909.116.2.259

Stanghellini, G. (2004). *Disembodied spirits and deanimated bodies: The psychopathology of common sense.* Oxford, UK: Oxford University Press.

Stanghellini, G., Ballerini, M., Presenza, S., Mancini, M., Raballo, A., Blasi, S., & Cutting, J. (2016). Psychopathology of lived time: Abnormal time experience in persons with schizophrenia. *Schizophrenia Bulletin*, 42(1), 45–55. doi:10.1093/schbul/sbv052

Stern, D. N. (1985). *The interpersonal world of the infant: A view from psychoanalysis and developmental psychology.* New York, NY: Basic Books.

Stern, D. N. (2004). *The present moment in psychotherapy and everyday life.* New York, NY: W. W. Norton & Company.

Stern, D. N. (2010). *Forms of vitality: Exploring dynamic experience in psychology, the arts, psychotherapy, and development.* Oxford, UK: Oxford University Press.

Street, R. L. Jr. (1984). Speech convergence and speech evaluation in fact-finding interviews. *Human Communication Research*, 11(2), 139–169. doi:10.1111/j.1468-2958.1984.tb00043.x

Szelag, E., von Steinbüchel, N., Reiser, M., Gilles de Langen, E., & Pöppel, E. (1996). Temporal constraints in processing of nonverbal rhythmic patterns. *Acta Neurobiologiae Experimentalis*, 56(1), 215–225.

Tellenbach, H. (1980). *Melancholy. History of the problem, endogeneity, typology, pathogenesis, clinical considerations* (E. Eng, Trans.). Pittsburgh, PA: Duquesne University Press.

Thoma, S., & Fuchs, T. (2018). A phenomenology of sensus communis. Outline of a phenomenological approach to social psychiatry. In M. Englander (Ed.), *Phenomenology and the social context of psychiatry: Social relations, psychopathology, and Husserl's philosophy* (pp. 137–159). London, UK: Bloomsbury.

Trevarthen, C., & Daniel, S. (2005). Disorganized rhythm and synchrony: Early signs of autism and Rett syndrome. *Brain and Development*, 27(Suppl. 1), S25–S34. doi:10.1016/j.braindev.2005.03.016

Van der Kolk, B. (2014). *The body keeps the score: Mind, brain and body in the transformation of trauma*. London, UK: Penguin.

Waller, G., Sines, J., Meyer, C., Foster, E., & Skelton, A. (2007). Narcissism and narcissistic defenses in the eating disorders. *International Journal of Eating Disorders*, 40(2), 143–148. doi:10.1002/eat.20345

Wittmann, M. (2013). The inner sense of time: How the brain creates a representation of duration. *Nature Reviews Neuroscience*, 14(3), 217–223. doi:10.1038/nrn3452

Wittmann, M. (2015). Modulations of the experience of self and time. *Consciousness and Cognition*, 38, 172–181. doi:10.1016/j.concog.2015.06.008

Zahavi, D. (1999). *Self-awareness and alterity. A phenomenological investigation*. Evanston, IL: Northwestern University Press.

PART I

Body and Time: General Aspects

3

The Body – Another

Phenomenological and Psychoanalytic Perspectives

Dorothée Legrand

In this contribution, I consider what we call "body" and its role in clinical practices. My chapter draws upon the ideas of Maurice Merleau-Ponty and Jacques Lacan. This allows me to consider not only the body as a materiality structured by its finitude, not only the body as a locus of our lived experiences, not only the body as anchoring our actions but also the body as it incarnates otherness. Otherness is here understood as twofold: On the one hand, the body as a living organism is a generality and its functioning hosts a germ of depersonalization; on the other hand, and at the same time, the body is that which keeps any other subject away from me, separated from me, irreducible to me. It thus appears that the body is at once both a concretion of alterity and of singularity. On the basis of such a conceptualization of the body, I consider the possibility of designing a clinical practice informed by both Merleau-Ponty and Lacan.

Let us start with a long quote – which is modified here to read "body" where the original says "ego":

> Normally, there is nothing of which we are more certain than the feeling of our self, of our own [body]. This [body] appears to us as something autonomous and unitary, marked off distinctly from everything else.... The [body] seems to maintain clear and sharp lines of demarcation. There is only one state—admittedly an unusual state, but not one that can be stigmatized as pathological—in which it does not do this. At the height of being in love the boundary between [one body and another] threatens to melt away. Against all the evidence of his senses, a man who is in love declares that "I" and "you" are one, and is prepared to behave as if it were a fact. What can be temporarily done away with by a physiological function must also, of course, be liable to be disturbed by pathological processes. Pathology has made us acquainted with a great number of states in which the boundary lines between the [body] and the external world become

> uncertain or in which they are actually drawn incorrectly. There are cases in which parts of a person's own body, even portions of his own mental life—his perceptions, thoughts and feelings—, appear alien to him and as not belonging to his [body]; there are other cases in which he ascribes to the external world things that clearly originate in his own [body] and that ought to be acknowledged by it. Thus even the feeling of our own [body] is subject to disturbances and the boundaries of the [body] are not constant. Further reflection tells us that the adult's [body]-feeling cannot have been the same from the beginning … originally the [body] includes everything, later it separates off an external world from itself. Our present [body]-feeling is, therefore, only a shrunken residue of a much more inclusive—indeed, an all-embracing—feeling which corresponded to a more intimate bond between the [body] and the world about it. If we may assume that there are many people in whose mental life this primary [body]-feeling has persisted to a greater or less degree, it would exist in them side by side with the narrower and more sharply demarcated [body]-feeling of maturity, like a kind of counterpart to it.… But have we a right to assume the survival of something that was originally there, alongside of what was later derived from it? (Freud, 1930/1964, pp. 65–68)

The author's reply is instant and unequivocal: "Undoubtedly" (Freud, 1930/1964, p. 68). These words were written by Sigmund Freud after more than thirty years of practice and research in psychoanalysis. Freud's voice here seems to find some echo in Maurice Merleau-Ponty's conception of time. As Merleau-Ponty argues, notably in his lectures on passivity, human development "does not absolutely liquefy what preceded it" (Merleau-Ponty, 2010, p. 25). Rather, what we surpass is preserved. This preservation does not imply that our life develops along predetermined tracks. Instead, Merleau-Ponty says, it involves "the reaction of a history upon itself, and the originary implulsion of pre-maturation, institution does not absolutely liquefy what preceded it" (2010, p. 25). In particular, according to Merleau-Ponty, the "child's own body" is first perceived "by means of that of the parents, in a relation of identification with their bodies" (2010, p. 21). "Disappointment, frustration" are needed in order to "rupture" this "unity." Castration, says Merleau-Ponty, is what allows the "reduction of one's own body to one's own body" (2010, p. 21). Thus, what we name "our body" is not a given; rather, the "reduction" to one's own body is a late achievement, and in fact, it is never fully and definitely achieved, since the primary identification of one body with another here described by Merleau-Ponty, or the originary all-embracing state described by Freud, even if forgotten, is not eradicated but "instituted."

By "institution" Merleau-Ponty means continuation, temporal integration, and for him, "bodies are instituted life" (2010, p. 30). In particular, the impersonal functioning of the living body is continued, temporally integrated and instituted into the personal body, which is then lived consciously as one's own proper body. The impersonal and the personal dimensions of the body form an *indivisible intermeshing*. As a living organism the body is *common*, it is an all-embracing flesh that never fully singularizes itself, it is a general body that supports the conscious experience of *my own* body with "a margin of *almost* impersonal existence … to which I entrust the care of keeping me alive" (Merleau-Ponty, 2012, p. 86). "I have 'sense organs,' a 'body,' and 'psychic functions' comparable to those of others" (2012, p. 86). And in this sense "the subject of perception is never an absolute subjectivity.… Perception is always in the impersonal mode of the 'One'" (2012, p. 249). The all-embracing body, living impersonally, is most of the time nonconscious, and it is precisely here that Merleau-Ponty describes an "organic suppression [*refoulement organique*]" (2012, pp. 80, 86). Here, the term suppression is not to be understood in opposition to consciousness. On the contrary, for Merleau-Ponty, "organic repression" as the "advent of the impersonal" is *tied* to the personal (2012, p. 86). According to Merleau-Ponty, personal bodies are instituted impersonally and what ties together the subjectively lived body and the a-subjective living body is the unconscious: There is, he says, an "osmosis between the body's anonymous life and the person's official life" and to account for that it is "necessary to introduce something *between* the organism and our selves considered as a sequence of deliberate acts and explicit understandings. This [is] Freud's *unconscious*" (Merleau-Ponty, 2007, p. 194). Here, the unconscious is the link between, on the one hand, the possibility to be a singular subject and, on the other, the "anonymous *adversity*" (2007, p. 203) of life wherein "our initiatives get bogged down in the paste of the body, of language, or of that world beyond measure" (2007, p. 203). This unconscious is a glue allowing the "osmosis" between different dimensions of one's being, preventing the subject from being divided and pulled apart by antagonistic forces.

Relative to such an integrative unconsciousness, consciousness is a deficit: Unconsciously, what reigns is an osmotic "indivision of feeling" (Merleau-Ponty, 1988, p. 179, translation modified), and against this background, the *particularity* of what we perceive, Merleau-Ponty says, "is only what is lacking in order to the world to be everything" (Merleau-Ponty, 2010, p. 165, translation modified). In this sense, perceptual consciousness is always and endlessly lacunar. As any delimited object presents itself in consciousness, this presence cuts into the plenitude of the world as a whole.

Yet the plenitude of the world is always there, ready to be cut into bits and pieces, ready to be taken into the conscious realm. We could thus say that an object delimited in consciousness is an institution of the unlimited, unconscious, impersonal, all-embracing world – just as, to use Merleau-Ponty's metaphor, seaweed can be viewed as a concretion of the sea. Just as the ocean is inexhaustible, consciousness is always exceeded by what is *not yet* conscious, and this implies that there is *always more* to be conscious of. That is to say, consciousness is never-endingly carried away toward an unfulfillable totality.

To this extent, Merleau-Ponty's philosophy is a constant challenge to totality. In his phenomenology, and perhaps in phenomenology in general, there is one, and maybe only one *im*possibility: Actual totality is impossible. That is to say, the totalization of possibilities is impossible. The actuality of consciousness is always constitutively exceeded by further possibilities, and in such a way, consciousness is structured by its impossible totalization. However, and precisely because Merleau-Ponty is confronted by the impossibility of a total integration, the gesture that he executes untiringly is a "movement towards integration": "[A]ll that is partial is to be reintegrated," he says (1968, p. 64). And if his philosophy is indeed a resistance to any presupposition of totality, it is simultaneously a gesture toward totalization. That consciousness is never totally conscious here means consciousness is always open to more. Insofar as it is open, consciousness is exceeded: Perception of any intentional object "leads toward the whole" (Merleau-Ponty, 2010, p. 165).

We see here how Merleau-Ponty's philosophy is organized around an oxymoron: the notion of *a total part* (1968, p. 218). In his view, "the whole is primary" and "total parts" are "cuts" in an "encompassing" space:

> Consider the *two*, the *pair*, this is not *two acts, two syntheses*, it is a fragmentation of being, it is a possibility for separation (two eyes, two ears: the possibility for *discrimination*, for the use of the diacritical), it is the advent of difference. (Merleau-Ponty, 1968, p. 217)

Each part is *total* insofar as the "advent of difference" is grounded in a totality that is always already there and never perishes. Together with the parts, and *within* each of the parts, the whole remains, is preserved as a whole, as each part promises its possible integration into the whole.

To this extent, Merleau-Ponty's philosophy aims at the impossible, aims at totalization. In his own words, it is animated by an "appeal for totality" (Merleau-Ponty, 1968, p. 104). Consciousness is never total but always *promises* its totalization. And in particular, "the transcendence of the thing compels us to say that it is plenitude only by being inexhaustible, that is, by not being all actual under the look – but it promises this total actuality, since it is there" (1968, p. 191).

However, despite this call to totality, Merleau-Ponty is well aware of the danger inherent in osmotic totalization. From his earliest work onwards, he is explicit about this danger: As a total part, as it inherently promises its integration into the whole, "every sensation includes a seed of dream or depersonalization, as we experience through this sort of stupor into which it puts us when we truly live at the level of sensation" (Merleau-Ponty, 2012, p. 223). We must hear this *stupor*: the stupor of depersonalization, the stupor of drowning in the inhuman ocean. We must understand that this is what Merleau-Ponty's phenomenological ontology *may* lead to, as it aims at rupturing singularity in favor of generality. Indeed, according to Merleau-Ponty, it is necessary that both the "individuality" of the body and the "absolute universality of the subject" are "broken" and give way to a "dialectical movement"; it is necessary that, alongside the absolutely individual flux of subjectivity, "generalities can be precisely inscribed or encrusted" (2010, p. 121). This generality is what Merleau-Ponty has called inter-corporeity, and this, he says, is one of the most important lessons to be learned from psychoanalysis.

However, I believe psychoanalysis is precisely that which can *resist* generalization, *resist* depersonalization. Specifically, psychoanalysis is designed to singularize the subject. And this term – singularization – is, I believe, what captures the irreducible difference between phenomenology and psychoanalysis – a difference which does not prevent working with both phenomenology and psychoanalysis.

In particular, if Merleau-Ponty is animated by an "appeal for totality," Jacques Lacan replies with a call for *de*totalization and, following his lead, psychoanalysis can be defined as the clinical theory that works specifically with that which resists the subject's integration into totality (1998). Understood in this framework, the unconscious names a specific manner in which the subject composes a wholly unified totality neither with his own history, nor with his own body; nor does the subject compose a wholly unified totality with anyone or anything else. Both Lacan and Merleau-Ponty would argue that totality is irretrievable, but while Merleau-Ponty orients his philosophy toward ever greater totalization, Lacan assumes that totality has always been lost and that this loss is not a deficit but precisely what constitutes the subject as a singularity, against its integration into a depersonalizing totality.[1] This consideration touches the very core of psychoanalysis insofar as this clinical theory is inseparable from the singularity of the subject. As such, it cannot be coherently fitted into any theoretical framework that reduces or aims at reducing the singularity of the subject. The subject to whom the psychoanalyst opens his door and his ears is irreducibly singular.

Following Giorgio Agamben, we can consider that this singular subject, whoever he is, is one who matters,[2] and we must acknowledge that a violence is involved here, since no subject is exceptional: No exceptional quality justifies that this subject matters. To give unconditional hospitality to the subject involves transcending any of the subject's phenomenal qualities and acknowledging that, whoever one is, one matters *structurally* (Derrida, 2000). This subject is not exceptionally particular, this singular subject is each time unique (Derrida, 2001). If anyone has given a philosophical relevance to *this* subject it is Emmanual Levinas by defining the psyche as "a resistance to the totality" (1969, p. 54) and by underlining that

> here the unicity of the ego first acquires a meaning—where it is no longer a question of the ego, but of me. The subject which is not an ego, but which I am, cannot be generalized, is not a subject in general; we have moved from the ego to me who am me and no one else. (Levinas, 1991, pp. 13–14)

As for Levinas, so for the psychoanalyst – the subject is "me" without substitute, without equivalent, irreducibly singular, unique. The subject is infinitely excessive, it is an irreducible excess that is impossible to merge into totality. By contrast, Merleau-Ponty says that the other is the alter ego with whom I share the *same* world, the *same* flesh, this other is "the other in general … it is generality, not individuality.… Here the other is grafted onto the same" (1973, p. 140). For Merleau-Ponty, the encounter of one with another is thus a "sympathy of totalities" (1973, p. 140).

This sympathy of totalities notably occurs through the body, the intercorporeal body, the general body, the impersonal body, the all-encompassing body, the flesh that characterizes *whichever subject* can be substituted by any

[1] The all-embracing state Freud describes as in-division *leaves a trace*, a trace which remains *irremediable* (Freud, 1964). One may even conjecture that totality never existed originally – perhaps what we are tempted to take as a trace of totality has been constructed as such, as a trace, while no original totality ever existed. Perhaps totality is irremediably lost precisely because it never originally existed.

[2] Giorgio Agamben uses the expression "whatever being" to mean "it does not matter which" and to mean "being such that it always matters" (2007, p. 1).

other. The sympathy of totalities also happens with speech. Here, speech is not added to the body as butter to bread, Merleau-Ponty says – speech is not a layer of "psychic reality" that would be spread over materiality. Rather, speech is a total part of the body, the body is a total part of speech, or, better, speech and the body are total parts of the all-encompassing flesh, so that

> if we were to make completely explicit the architectonics of the human body, its ontological framework, … we would see that the structure of its mute world is such that all the possibilities of language are already given in it.… [T]he whole [body] is overrun with words as with an invasion, it is henceforth but a variant of speech. (Merleau-Ponty, 1968, p. 155)

"The common language which we speak is something like the anonymous corporeality which we share with other organisms" (Merleau-Ponty, 1973, p. 140). It follows from this intertwinement of speech and body that, just like inter-corporeity, "the simple use of this language … yields another only in general, diffused through my field, … a notion rather than a presence" (1973, p. 140). This is so because language is "the voice of no one, since it is the very voice of the things, the waves, and the forests" (Merleau-Ponty, 1968, p. 155). Indeed, insofar as language is intertwined with the body, it articulates a "mute language" into speech. Such language, Merleau-Ponty says, is "absolutely universal." "Language is everything." Perception itself is "structured as a language" (1968, p. 126) and Merleau-Ponty is here quoting explicitly some of Lacan's most famous words. However, Lacan says exactly the opposite. When he says that the unconscious is structured as a language (1981), he thereby specifically and systematically insists on the idea that language imposes *dis*continuities. Contrary to Merleau-Ponty, and contrary to the idea that a psychoanalyst would reduce everything to language, it must be underlined that Lacanian psychoanalysis developed by taking as seriously as possible the fact that language is *not* everything (1974–1975). Specifically, in psychoanalysis, language is a knife that cuts our bodies out of the impersonal flesh. Merleau-Ponty himself recognizes such a language but derides it when he writes of a manner of speaking that "cuts the continuous tissue that joins us vitally to the things and to the past and is installed between ourselves and that tissue like a screen" (1973, p. 140). As a "cut," language is not "everything" but is a "regional problem." Yet Merleau-Ponty favors a practice of language where "speaking and hearing are indiscernible" (1973, p. 140). For Lacan, by contrast, to speak is to impose a difference, a distance, a space between the speaker and the listener; to speak is to assume that one is not fully transparent and accessible for the other, that one must get out of oneself to reach the other. If we first consider speech in its concreteness, it appears right away that to speak is to break any immediate body-to-body bonding with another. To be a speaking body is thus to work *against* any immediate integration with another. To speak is to singularize one's body; whether we like it or not, it imposes upon the body the attempt to get out of the all-embracing ocean. In other words, and despite Merleau-Ponty, speaking is a process of singularization insofar as it ruptures totality.

This can be said not only with Lacan but with Levinas too: Speaking is necessarily speaking to another, and thus, according to Levinas, whenever I speak I necessarily

> interrupt the ultimate discourse in which all the discourses are stated, in saying it to the one that listens to it, and who is situated outside the said that the discourse says, outside all it includes. That is true of the discussion I am elaborating at this very moment. This reference to an interlocutor permanently breaks through the text that the discourse claims to weave in thematizing and enveloping all things. In totalizing being, discourse qua discourse thus belies the very claim to totalize. (1991, p. 170)

The very fact of speaking, Levinas says, necessitates and "maintains the distance between me and the Other," it opens and maintains "the radical separation asserted in transcendence which prevents the reconstitution of totality" (1969, p. 40). To speak is thus to be singular, it is to be separated from the other, it is to be different and non-in-different to the other. That is to say: To be singular is to be plural – plural, insofar as singularity involves a process of singularization and therefore the distinction between multiple singularities.

In this sense, strictly speaking, "the" body, "one" body does not exist. There are only bodies. As Jean-Luc Nancy puts it, "bodies are differences" (2008, p. 152). This is not merely to say that bodies are all *different* from each other. Rather, specifically, bodies are themselves *differences* in the sense that bodies "take place at the limit, *qua limit* – external border, the fracture and intersection of anything foreign in a continuum of sense, a continuum of matter. An opening, discreteness" (2008, p. 17). This is not to say that my body starts on this side of a limit and your body starts on the other side; rather, and more radically, our bodies start simultaneously at the limit, qua limit. What Jean-Luc Nancy proposes is not merely that bodies are *limited* but that bodies exist *as* limit. Of course, a limit cannot be thought without thinking at once both sides of the limit, one cannot detach one side of a limit from its other side without effacing the limit altogether; likewise, one body cannot be detached from the other bodies that limit it. One body alone does not exist as such, there exist only bodies at the limit, qua limit.

Jean-Luc Nancy also indicates that this limit is not a given. Bodies are accomplished in a continuous process of singularizing, differentiating, spacing, distancing, and estrangement between one and another. As Nancy incisively puts it, "Le corps *donne lieu* à l'existence" (2008, p. 14), which is translated (by Richard Rand) as "the body *makes room* for existence," but which could be translated more literally as "the body *gives space* to existence." The body exists insofar as it gives space to what singularizes oneself and another: an empty space between oneself and another. In this sense, "*the body is the plastic material of spacing*.... [Bodies are] where existences *take place*" (Nancy, 2008, p. 63). This sentence contains all the keywords needed to define what we name *body*: The body is *material*, it is not a delimited space but a material *process* of spacing, and as such it is *plastic*: The border between one body and another is not fixed once and for all.

Now some may find it reassuring to think that the body Nancy writes about here may be given empirical confirmation. It is well known that an infant is capable of distinguishing between a touch that comes from his own hand and a touch that comes from another person's hand; he distinguish a double touch from a single touch (Rochat, 2004). And yet, in and of itself, this result does not prove that the infant experiences the limit between his body and another in any fixed, clear, and distinct manner, nor that he experiences one body as independent from another. Indeed, it has been shown that, as an adult, if I experience my own body in synchrony with my experience of another's body, I will soon experience the other body as my own, I will integrate the two synchronous experiences into one, into mine. This has been demonstrated, for instance, with the experimental manipulation of the so-called rubber hand illusion (Botvinick & Cohen, 1998). Without going into the details of these experiments here, it can be underlined that these results cohere with the idea that our experience of our bodily boundaries fluctuates, our bodily limits are designed and redesigned over and again – they may be lost, and regained. There are only artificial, porous, and tenuous boundaries between bodies. If we follow Jean-Luc Nancy here, we can see that even though the boundaries between one body and another are not given but are constantly created and recreated, it does not undermine the idea that the body is constituted by its boundary, is constituted *as* a boundary, as a difference from another body. On such a reading, the boundary is *constitutive* of the body: Not only is the body enveloped by a skin, but specifically the body *is* a skin: "a skin, variously folded, refolded, unfolded, multiplied, invaginated, exogastrulated, orificed, evasive, invaded, stretched, relaxed, excited, distressed, tied, untied" (Nancy, 2008, p. 15). Bodily limits are moveable, malleable, and yet they are not dispensable.

Moreover, Nancy argues, since bodies are limits, there is "no connective tissue, no cement, no bridge [between bodies].... From one singular [body] to another, there is contiguity but not continuity" (2000, p. 5). Here, of course, one may disagree and argue for the opposite view: There would be not only *contiguity* but rather *continuity* between bodies. Likewise, you may agree that the boundary between one body and another is not a given, but is constantly created and recreated, yet you may infer from this that one and another body are originally, persistently, and authentically one and the same matter, the same flesh. One could ground such an interpretation in a reading of Merleau-Ponty and argue that if the boundary between oneself and another is a construct, it means that it ought to be *de*constructed in order to reach an original state of osmotic integration into the all-encompassing flesh of the world.

By contrast, following Lacan one could argue that if the boundary between oneself and another is not given but a construct then it is *artificial*, it is vulnerable and porous and thus it must constantly be *re*constructed anew, as we cannot be subjects without being singularized, we cannot be singular without being plural, we always need to rebuild boundaries, we always suffer their rupture and we always need to build them again, we always need to renew our bodies as limits between one and another.

Merleau-Ponty may object that such a limited body is not a natural body, is not the body of Nature (with a capital "N"). Lacan would agree and would reply that he specifically works with speaking bodies, bodies that are the prey of language, human bodies that are constitutively cut off from the impersonal flesh. This cut, according to the psychoanalyst, is painful for all of us, and for some of us it is unbearable. Yet, if osmosis is impossible for a speaking body, if osmosis is impossible precisely because the body is speaking, then this impossibility is not destined to entail sufferance. On the contrary, if one does not take osmosis or totalization or unification or integration as a normative ideal, as an aim to be reached, as a task to be undertaken, if one realizes that one *is* and that one needs to be separated, different, unintegrated, disunified, then one may accept being and remaining singularly plural – talkatively.

References

Agamben, G. (2007). *The coming community* (M. Hardt, Trans.). Minneapolis, MN: University of Minnesota Press.

Botvinick, M., & Cohen, J. (1998). Rubber hands 'feel' touch that eyes see. *Nature*, 391(6669), 756. doi:10.1038/35784

Derrida, J. (2000). *Of hospitality: Anne Dufourmantelle invites Jacques Derrida to respond* (R. Bowlby, Trans.). Palo Alto, CA: Stanford University Press.

Derrida, J. (2001). In P.-A. Brault & M. Naas, (Eds.), *The work of mourning* Chicago, IL: The University of Chicago Press.

Freud, S. (1964). Civilization and its discontents. In J. Strachey (Ed.), *The standard edition of the complete psychological works of Sigmund Freud* (Vol. XXI, 1927–1931, pp. 59–145). London, UK: Hogarth Press and the Institute of Psycho-analysis. (Original work published 1930).

Lacan, J. (1974–1975). *Séminaire XXII: R.S.I.* Unpublished.

Lacan, J. (1981). *The Four Fundamental Concepts of Psychoanalysis. The Seminar, Book XI, 1964* (A. Sheridan, Trans.). New York, London: W. W. Norton & Company.

Lacan, J. (1998). *Encore. On Feminine Sexuality, the Limits of Love and Knowledge, The Seminar, Book XX, 1972-1973* (B. Fink, Trans.). New York, London: W. W. Norton & Company.

Lacan, J. (2002a). "The Function and Field of Speech and Language in Psychoanalysis (1953)", in *Ecrits*, (B. Fink, Trans.), (pp. 197–268). New York, London: W. W. Norton & Company.

Lacan, J. (2002b). "The Direction of the Treatment and the Principles of Its Power (1958)", in *Ecrits*, (B. Fink, Trans.), (pp. 489–542). New York, London: W. W. Norton & Company.

Levinas, E. (1969). *Totality and infinity* (A. Lingis, Trans.). Pittsburgh, PA: Duquesne University Press.

Levinas, E. (1991). *Otherwise than being or beyond the essence* (A. Lingis, Trans.). Dordrecht, Netherlands: Kluwer Academic.

Merleau-Ponty, P. (1968). *The visible and the invisible. Followed by working notes* (A. Lingis, Trans.). Evanston, IL: Northwestern University Press.

Merleau-Ponty, P. (1973). *The prose of the world* (J. O'Neill, Trans.). Evanston, IL: Northwestern University Press.

Merleau-Ponty, M. (1988). Themes from the lectures at the Collège de France, 1952–1960 (J. O'Neill, Trans.). In J. Wild & J. Edi (Eds.), *In praise of philosophy and other essays* (pp. 69–199). Evanston, IL: Northwestern University Press.

Merleau-Ponty, M. (2007). Man and adversity. In T. Toadvine & L. Lawlor (Eds.), *The Merleau-Ponty reader* (pp. 189–240). Evanston, IL: Northwestern University Press.

Merleau-Ponty, M. (2010). *Institution and passivity: Course notes from the Collège de France (1954–1955)* (L. Lawlord & H. Massey, Trans.). Evanston, IL: Northwestern University Press.

Merleau-Ponty, M. (2012). *Phenomenology of perception* (D. A. Landes, Trans.). Abingdon, UK: Routledge.

Nancy, J.-L. (2000). *Being singular plural* (R. Richardson & A. O'Byrne, Trans.). Palo Alto, CA: Stanford University Press.

Nancy, J.-L. (2008). *Corpus* (R. Rand, Trans.). New York, NY: Fordham University Press.

Rochat, P. (2004). *The infant's world.* Cambridge, MA: Harvard University Press.

3.1

Commentary on "The Body – Another: Phenomenological and Psychoanalytic Perspectives"

Phenomenology and Psychoanalysis: Disruptive Speech in the Realm of the Flesh

Stefan Kristensen

The question of the most rigorous and best-grounded philosophical basis for psychoanalytical experience is a serious question, not simply because psychoanalysis became the most influential current in psychotherapy during the last century but also because it is the only current trying to offer an interpretation of what happens in the deeper layers of our affective life. This is why philosophers in the phenomenological tradition have had difficulties in their approach to psychodynamics: The psychoanalytic attention to depth entails a more or less speculative approach to interpretation, because of what it sees as the hidden aspects of the psyche. On the other hand, phenomenology and psychoanalysis are essentially bound together by their refusal to reduce the subject to any kind of objective being. Among the few philosophers to have attempted an articulation between the two traditions, the boldest was Merleau-Ponty: He unambiguously affirmed that the psychoanalytic idea of the unconscious comes close to his phenomenological idea of intercorporeity, inasmuch as both notions refer to a common substance from which human subjectivity originates and of which we always keep a subterranean memory.

Legrand mentions a claim by Merleau-Ponty from his 1955 lectures on institution and passivity to support the opposite view: "Psychoanalysis," she writes, "is precisely that which can *resist* generalization, *resist* depersonalization" (Legrand, 2021, p. 41). She claims that the purpose and function of psychoanalytical practice is to create the conditions for the subject to become a singular subject through the use of speech. The "irreducible difference between phenomenology and psychoanalysis" lies in the concept of singularization (Legrand, 2021, p. 47): Whereas phenomenology focuses on the dimension of belonging (of the subject to the world, to the flesh, to the community), psychoanalysis places the emphasis on separation, singularization. But she does not infer from this that the two approaches are incompatible; "the difference," she writes, "does not prevent working with both phenomenology and psychoanalysis. Merleau-Ponty's phenomenological ontology *may* lead to … rupturing singularity in favor of generality." She emphasizes the "may" (Legrand 2021, p. 47).

So, where is the point of rupture? Is there indeed such a point at all? Is it a question of one's point of view, of perspective? The argument hinges on the question of speech, of spoken language, and its relation to the realm of the flesh, understood as the undifferentiated realm where subject and world, ego and other, and body and mind are inchoate and contained in virtual form. In Merleau-Ponty's ontology, the body is precisely the chosen phenomenon where this commonality is best perceptible: The body is both subject in virtue of its perspectivity and belongs to the world in virtue of its materiality. In this connection, Merleau-Ponty explicates a claim of Freud, with which Legrand starts her chapter, where the founder of psychoanalysis reflects on certain states of consciousness and pathology where the boundaries between the self and the world are blurred, leading him to the hypothesis that our present "Ego-feeling" (*Ichgefühl*) is a residue of a more fundamental feeling of belonging of the ego to the world, "an all-embracing feeling that corresponded to a more intimate bond between the I and the environment" (Freud, 1930/1964, pp. 65–68 uses the term *Umwelt*). This idea is indeed central to Merleau-Ponty's ontology: He uses the presupposition of an originary totality that is never completely lost. The individual conscious experience, according to Merleau-Ponty, is always part of the totality of the world too; as Legrand puts it, the presence of the perceived object "cuts into the plenitude of the world as a whole" (Legrand 2021, p. 45). Consciousness is "carried away toward an unfulfillable totality," (p. 45) as she also writes, but this totality is at the same time unattainable. The ego/body is always in movement toward an impossible totality, that is, striving toward fusion with things and the world.

Phenomenology, according to Legrand, lacks the means to resist depersonalization because it considers language to be in continuity with perception. Perception is an experience of being next to the perceived thing, it is a process where the subject tends to forget themselves, and language is nothing other than an expressive relation to the world, which reproduces the proximity of perception, but from a certain distance. Therein lies the fundamental difference between phenomenology and psychoanalysis, or more precisely between Merleau-Ponty's conception of language and Lacan's conception of language. The difference lies in the function of language in the relation to the self, and therefore in the effect of linguistic activity: differentiating oneself from others. Lacan considers that language, as speech addressed to another, is essentially a "cut" between oneself and others, a "process of singularization" as Legrand formulates it (Legrand, 2021, p. 49–50).

Legrand's opposition between psychoanalysis and phenomenology hinges on the status and role of speech. On her reading, speech exists for Merleau-Ponty in continuity with perception, whereas for Lacan it is essentially a cut in being. For Lacan so it is for two fellow philosophers, Emmanuel Levinas and Jean-Luc Nancy, who, in a nutshell, consider that the effect of speech is to create the distance between the ego and the other necessary to let the ego be itself. But here one can introduce a distinction that helps us to see the various views in a different way: namely, a distinction between the *genesis* of speech and its *function*. One can admit that speech *originates* from perceptual activity and yet at the same time accepts that the *role* of speech, specifically in the case of humans, is to institute *both* a *separation* and a *bond* between subjects. The continuity has to do with the relation to the world and the descriptive dimension of expression, whereas the "cutting" function is tied to the performative and relational dimension of expression, specifically the addressed speech.

It seems to me that Merleau-Ponty's account of speech is also able to account for this "cutting" function, although it is certainly true that he often emphasizes the continuity between perception and language. Thus, he frequently uses the concept of sublimation[1] to convey that linguistic meaning is indeed structured in a way other than perceptual sense, such that going from the one to the other does not simply involve jumping a gap. At the same time, he also accounts for the performative function of speech, although he does claim that language is structured as a system of diacritical signs, analogous to the perceptual field. The diacritical theory of language accounts for the expressive power of each sign that signifies via its relations to all the other signs (to summarize his reception of Saussure's linguistics), but this does not preclude that speech might play the role of a "cutting" in the relation between human subjects. In Merleau-Ponty's reading of Saussure, the concept of speech (*parole*) is equally important, as an attempt to answer the question of how the body of language changes and new meanings and new words are instituted in its body. And Merleau-Ponty describes the process of creative expression in many texts, for example in the Preface to Signs: "The words have power to arouse thoughts and implant henceforth inalienable dimensions of thought; and that they put responses on our lips we did not know we were capable of, teaching us [...] our own thoughts" (Merleau-Ponty, 2007, p. 332). The power of words is the other side of the experiential fact that my speech is ahead of my thoughts,

[1] As I have shown in my book *Parole et subjectivité* (Kristensen, 2010).

and this means that the words participate in creating the meaning in the very process of being addressed to another. If this is true, it implies that a gesture of speech intended to express the content of someone's affective life will participate in shaping the very meaning of this content. It will, in other words, play a key role in singularizing the speaking subject.

And yet Merleau-Ponty does not emphasize this singularizing power of speech; rather, his point of departure is the opposite: that it is the other who is the mystery, that the difficult task is to account for the connection with the common flesh from which we all originate. This is exactly the opposite of his friend, Jacques Lacan, whose concern was to account for the process of escaping the flesh and its terrifying anonymity. In *The Phenomenology of Perception*, for example, Merleau-Ponty writes that "solitude and communication do not have to be the two terms of an alternative, but rather two moments of one single phenomenon, since, in fact, the other does exist for me" (Merleau-Ponty, 1945, p. 417; my translation). The other does exist for me, this is the fact that he starts out from. The philosophical task is to account for our common belonging to the world.

The issue around language and speech is, in my view, merely a question of perspective; but the question of the body is more than that. When Legrand quotes Jean-Luc Nancy's ideas concerning the body, she seems to adopt his claim of a reduction of the body to a surface of (possible) inscriptions. While Merleau-Ponty thinks about language as a diacritical field, analogous to the perceptual field, Nancy thinks about the sensing body as a surface for scripture. To think about the body as a surface and as a boundary means to reject the distinction between the inside and the outside, to reject the dimension of depth. "To be a speaking body is thus to work *against* any immediate integration with another," she writes (Legrand 2021, p. 50, emphasis in original), whereas simple touch is always at risk of cultivating the confusion with the other. The body always already speaks, which means that it is the body itself, as speaking, that carries the task of differentiating myself from the other. But to define the body as a speaking surface[2] precludes the possibility of confusion with the other. There still has to be a depth in the body, a depth that the subject can experience and in which they can lose themselves, and where speaking to another can make a difference. It should not be an alternative: It should be possible to think about the body as a being both with depths and unspeakable meanings and also with a connection to spoken speech in its most disruptive power.

2 "The body always is structured as a return to sense," Nancy (2008, p. 69) writes in *Corpus*.

But, of course, this relies on a description of the psychotherapeutic setting where the issue at stake is the process of becoming a subject.

References

Freud, S. (1964). Civilization and its discontents. In J. Strachey (Ed.), *The standard edition of the complete psychological works of Sigmund Freud* (Vol. XXI. 1927–1931, pp. 59–145). London, England: Hogarth Press and the Institute of Psychoanalysis. (Original work published 1930.)

Kristensen, S. (2010). *Parole et subjectivité. Merleau-Ponty et la phénoménologie de l'expression* [Speech and subjectivity. Merleau-Ponty and the phenomenology of expression]. Hildesheim, Germany: G. Olms.

Legrand, D. (2021). The body – another. Phenomenological and psychoanalytic perspectives. In C. Tewes and G. Stanghellini (Eds.), *Body and time* (pp. 43–54). Cambridge, England: Cambridge University Press.

Merleau-Ponty, M. (1945). *Phénoménologie de la perception* [Phenomenology of perception]. Paris, France: Gallimard.

Merleau-Ponty, M. (2007). In T. Toadvine and L. Lawlor (Eds.), *Merleau-Ponty reader* (p. 332). Evanston, IL: Northwestern University Press..

Nancy, J.-L. (2008). *Corpus* (R. Rand, Trans.). New York, NY: Fordham University Press.

4

The Heart of Darkness of the Living Body

Giovanni Stanghellini

Introduction

A detailed phenomenological analysis of the various manifestations of corporeality can help to grasp and make sense of how the body is apprehended in different psychopathological conditions. I will argue that once the body-object (the representational, explicit and ultimately visible manifestation of one's corporeality) is distinguished from the lived body (the proto-reflexive semiexperiential/semirepresentational manifestation of one's corporeality), the latter should be distinguished from what I will call the "living body." The living body is the immediately felt, pathic, purely impressive, prereflective, nonrepresentational, experiential, and invisible manifestation of one's corporeality. I will argue that the living body possesses two distinct profiles: self-affection or the primordial bodily chiasm enforcing one's feeling of belonging to oneself and to the world, and the sheer flesh or chaotic plurality of invisible bodily forces immediately felt without the intercession of a representation. A further manifestation of corporeality is the body-for-others, that is the experience of feeling one's corporeality when it is looked at by another person. In the final part of this chapter, I will match these different profiles of corporeality to specific anomalous psychopathological conditions, namely, the appearance of the sheer, chaotic flesh to the borderline person's form of existence; the body as a corporealized, restricted, inhibited, and rigid body to melancholia; the mechanic, robotic functioning object "out there" to schizophrenia; and finally the body apprehended through the gaze of the other to the existence of persons with eating disorders (EDs).

The Flesh

We do not have a single body. We have at least three, maybe even four bodies.

If we imagine a continuum of ways of experiencing one's body, at one pole, there is the coenaesthetic experience of my body; at the opposite pole, there is the body experienced from the outside, my body as it appears to me in a mirror, or as if it were another person's body. At the first pole of this continuum, there is *this* body *here*; at the other extreme, there is *that* body *there*. I *feel* this body here *from within*, I *see* that body there *from without*. But let's proceed in order, because there are numerous intermediate stations. Each of these epiphanies of the corporeality needs careful analysis, especially if we want to enlighten with them certain forms of psychopathological conditions as I will try to do in this chapter.

The first way of experiencing one's body is called the "body-I-am": the primitive and immediate experience of myself, direct and not mediated by the other senses, especially not mediated by sight. We can use the word "flesh" to talk about this epiphany of the body. As Merleau-Ponty (1968) puts it, the flesh is the chiasm between myself and the world as it "touches itself seeing and touching the things" (p. 146). The flesh is the original possibility to feel myself. The flesh is what I feel in the act of perceiving something through one of the five senses. "Flesh" is feeling myself while experiencing something, so feeling myself while seeing, hearing, touching, tasting, and smelling. When we see something, *sentimus nos videre* (we feel ourselves seeing) explains Descartes in his letter to Plempius from October 3, 1637 (as cited in Henry, 2000). The flesh performs one of the functions that Aristotle (1957) attributes to the sixth sense, that is, the *koiné aisthesis*, to the sense that synthesizes all the senses and joins them to the one who feels: The *koiné aisthesis* is the faculty to feel myself at the very moment when I experience an object in the outside world.

Yet the flesh is something less, and at the same time more than the Aristotelian coenaesthesia. It is original bodily, principle of experience, pure impressionability; and at the same time immanence to myself, the most intimate possibility of feeling myself, in which the one who feels and what is felt are one and the same thing. In flesh, writes Michel Henry, the Self

> feels itself in the certainty and irreducibility of this self-feeling that unites it with itself and makes itself the Self that it is. While feeling itself, it is in possession of itself, takes place in it, rests on itself as on a ground on which it can take hold. (Henry, 2000, p. 261; my translation)

In the flesh lies the possibility of feeling that *this* experience I'm undergoing is *my* experience. The experience I have of the world confirms my presence, my existence. The shaping of my nuclear sense of presence to myself is based on my feeling myself as I'm perceiving something: to perceive that I am perceiving is to perceive that I exist.

Thus, the flesh is what connects me to myself and to the world while connecting my Self to the world.

My sense of my own Self, even my sense of *being* a Self, is rooted in my experience of my flesh (Merleau-Ponty, 1962). The deepest layer of experience that I make of myself, sometimes called *ipseity* (from Latin *ipse* meaning "Self"), is sensory, belongs to the animal principle of the faculty of feeling. Being a Self is feeling embodied, rooted in one's own flesh. This primordial level of self-consciousness is *pathic* (from Greek *pathos* meaning "affection," i.e., a kind of sensitivity based on feeling rather than on reasoning) and prereflexive; and is to be kept well distinguished from another form of self-consciousness which is fundamentally cognitive and reflexive. Whereas in this cognitive-reflexive self-experience, I *perceive* and represent my *Self* as an object, that is, as something separate from me; in the pathic and prereflexive self-experience I *feel myself*, that is, the one who feels and the one who is felt are but one same thing.

From the point of view of the flesh, the Self responds to the logic of *intimacy*: I am intimate and in contact with my incarnate Self. In fact, talking about my experience of my flesh is extremely difficult. The flesh is quasi-ineffable. The reason is that this experience gives itself in a prelinguistic, tacit, implicit, and prereflective dimension of existence. This helps us to understand what is meant by coenaesthesia. Coenaesthesia is the experience (a prereflexive experience) in which Self and body are given as indiscernible, that is, the act in which I feel in touch with myself as this flesh-that-I-am. *I exist my body*: This is the first dimension of being a body, and at the same time the foundation of my Self.

The flesh, therefore, is the original rooting in one's Self: feeling fit or not, heavy or light, agile or slow, strong or weak, in a temporal continuity that embraces both one's past, what is happening at the moment, and what is on the point of happening. That is what I feel implicitly a moment before I can say "*I am my body.*" The flesh is the sentient body before it is the object of explicit perception, discourse, or categorization.

The Living Body as Distinct from the Lived Body

The flesh, so to say, has two experiential sides: the first is pure event, the feeling that something is happening to me. To use (or perhaps abuse) the language of phenomenology, the flesh we are talking about is *a living* body, to be distinguished from the *lived* body of which speaks phenomenology itself. The lived body, unlike the living body, is not the immediate feeling of my bodily self, but a *post hoc representation* of it (Stanghellini, 2018).

We would do well, therefore, to distinguish the *living body* (the first of the four dimensions of body experience) from the *lived body* (the second dimension of body experience). The flesh as a living body is *present participle*, impression and feeling here-and-now; where instead the lived body is *past participle* (this is also the case in French: *vecu*, and in Italian: *vissuto*), therefore body known, represented, signified (an in-depth discussion of the translations of the German word *Leib* can be found in the commentary to this chapter). The body called "lived," after all, is the object of a retrospective look that I cast on the feeling I had in my flesh. The flesh as living body is *here*, while the lived body *there* – not so far away from the present moment in which I experience the flesh, but still a little far away from me. As Erwin Straus (1963) would put it, the living body stands on the side of the nonrational dimension of *sensation*, whereas the lived body stands on that of *perception*, that is, of the rational organization of primary sense experience.

The flesh as the "original corporeality" is not "an *object* [emphasis added] of experience, rather the principle of experience" (Henry, 2000, p. 172; my translation). The weakening of this primordial bond of intimacy with myself as flesh – of this embryo of the unity of Self, body, and world – is the beginning of the drift in which my body detaches itself from my Self.

I become explicitly conscious of my body as a lived body. While experiencing my body as a lived body, I start becoming reflexively conscious of my body. The flesh, so to say, detaches itself from the implicit dimension – the world of shadow – and makes its way to the world of light, the realm of the visible body, at the threshold of the body-object. The lived body is the beginning of the drift in which I experience my corporeality as detached from my Self. It is only a separation that happens in the domain of *time*, not in space: I perceive my body *retrospectively*, as when I look back at a moment that has just passed. My body is not yet fully exteriorized in space as an *ob-jectum* external to my Self – rather, it is like an image of myself, a snapshot, or better a movie frame, the photogram of a scene that has just elapsed. Yet in looking back at this photogram, I remain – my Self remains – without a mooring in the flesh, and therefore must go in search of other landings, other anchors. Being a Self is no longer a given, it has become a task.

As we will see in detail in the next paragraph, the flesh is not only what secures my Self in my body; feeling my flesh as living body can be an *almost unbearable experience* (Deleuze, 2003). That's probably why we look for a shelter in the lived body. The flesh as living body is on the side of the un-form, of a chaos of forces and as such it exists before the subject can appropriate it, give it a form, a structure, a purpose, and a meaning. The flesh as living body lies on the side of *dépanse* (Bataille, 1988) – excess, expenditure, consumption, and dissipation – whereas the lived body on the side of *economy*; one is pure tension, whereas the other is action aimed to accomplish a given purpose with a given meaning. The living body, for this reason, always seems *poised between the fullness of life and the abyss of death.*

The Heart of Darkness of the Flesh

In the previous paragraph I tried to distinguish the living from the lived body, characterizing the first one as pure impressionability or *sensation* and the second as the beginning of a proto-reflexive *self-representation*. Now I shall attempt to make a further distinction between the two profiles of the flesh as living body. The flesh is not only the tacit background of my existence – the tacit dimension that grants my feeling rooted in myself and genuinely immersed in the world. Phenomenology emphasizes (perhaps overemphasizes) this side of the flesh called *self-affection* (Henry, 1965, 2000) at the expense of downplaying the other side of the flesh – sheer flesh, the dark side of the flesh.

If, on the one hand, the living body is matter that responds to the appeal of the unity of life rooting myself in my body; on the other is disorganized matter, fragment, dismemberment, and convulsion. Pure sensation and pure vibration. A "body without organs" (as Deleuze [2003, p. 39] would say), that is *dys-organic*: head without a face, spasm without movement, drive without action, a scream that exceeds the *vultus* – the flesh on the point of becoming *meat*. From this angle, the organism – that is, the organization of the organs – is not life, but what *imprisons* life. This side of the living body, overlooking the abyss of death, is the violence of a sensation, pure intensity of feeling not mitigated by reason, meaning, purpose, direction: "presence, interminable presence" (Deleuze, 2003, p. 44), and extreme, unusable, irrepressible presence. The motto of the living body as sheer flesh could therefore be: "Everything that kills me makes me feel alive!" (Tedder, 2013) And also: *Go out of yourself to be in yourself!*

When I am my sheer flesh, I may feel on the threshold of mystical ecstasy, excess, hit by the impersonal impact of the world, immersed in pure instantaneousness. This profile of the flesh is what is seen from the point of view of death: la *part maudite* – the accursed share (as Bataille [1988] would say) – of the flesh, its deepest and almost unlivable power. "I suffer from a burning, painful aspiration that persists in me as an unfulfilled desire" explains Bataille (1973, "Preface," sect. 1; my translation):

> My tension in a way resembles a mad desire to laugh and differs little from the passions of which Sade's heroes burn. And yet it is close to that of martyrs and saints....
>
> I cannot doubt this delusion manifests in me the human character. But, it must be said, it leads to imbalance and painfully deprives me of rest. I burn and disorient myself and finally remain empty. I can propose great and necessary actions but none enough to my fever....
>
> The states of glory, the sacred moments that reveal the immeasurable, go beyond the results to which it tended. Common morality places these results on the same level as the ends of sacrifice. A sacrifice explores the depths of being and the destruction that guarantees it reveals its tearing. But he is exalted for a trivial purpose. Morality always tends to the good of beings. (Bataille, 1973, "Preface," sect. 1; my translation)

The cursed part of the flesh burns itself without responding to any secular moral imperative. If we no longer make the condition of a purpose, an end, it seems to be a pure electrocution, an empty instrument, pure exuberance: "self-destruction without any other reason than the very desire to burn." The heart of darkness of the flesh – this "dazzling dissolution in totality" – is likened by Bataille to "an immense comic painful convulsion," to an "unmotivated feast" equal to the insubordination of laugh, dance, and orgy, which is unaware of the material and moral ends (Bataille, 1973, "Preface," sect. 10; my translation).

Bataille's description of the sheer flesh quite parallels Kimura's (1992) description of the *intra festum* temporality. Like in the atmosphere of the feast, in the intra festum temporality we find the irruption of spontaneity and ecstasy, oblivious of past and future. The intra festum is chaotic immediateness. The person is absorbed in an unmediated instantaneity – the pure or *absolute now* devoid of all relation with anteriority and posteriority, that is, with the past as the Self's retention of the bygone, and with the future as the Self's projection of the now in the forthcoming. Here, Kimura follows Husserl in defining "retention" as the past as intentionally contained in the present, and "protention" as the future as anticipated in the present, so that when both retention and protention are functioning, the present moment keeps in view past and future. This is not the case with the intra festum where the *nows* are pure presentification, lacking protention and retention. Giving themselves independently from past and future, one cannot measure the length of these nows, as one could do with a present that develops out of the past and toward the future. Each *now* thus becomes an infinity that in some sense "communicates with eternity" (Kimura, 1992, p. 150) – but it is also at the threshold of death because it is not projected into the future. The absolute now has no temporal delimitation, no historical determination and no linguistic-symbolic articulation. Thus, the absolute now of the *intra festum* is without any relation with a Self as a narrative Self.

In the sheer flesh as in the intra festum temporality, there is an *absorption in immediateness*. This profile of the flesh, therefore, is where life is closest to death because it is farther from the noetical, reasoning consciousness. In the flesh, we run the risk of experiencing life in the vicinity of death. Yet, it is the greatest proximity that can be reached to the source of life. And indeed, sometimes feeling my flesh is an experience that resembles intoxication, trance, frenzy; the flesh is the place not lit up by the light of reason, where the word is silent. It is, as it were, *unconscious consciousness* on the threshold of total unconsciousness.

Perhaps that is why, as Genet (2007) writes, one may dream with nostalgia of a universe in which man, instead of acting on the visible appearance, is committed to disentangle from it, to get rid of it, to discover that secret place in oneself from which it is possible to start a human adventure altogether different, and no doubt – Genet argues – more just. Nostalgia for the flesh as living body may drive me to dream of a world that makes me try to venture elsewhere from what is representable, expressible, and measurable, that is, away from the "object" and its false utilitarian appearance. In order to feel my flesh as living body, I have to get rid of any objectifying and reflexive representation of my body.

The Body as an Object

One of the anchors not to let my body go adrift in the shadow line of the sheer flesh is to let my body become an object among other objects in the world. The first body, it has been said, is the living flesh (which none the less has two sides: self-affection that enforces my feeling of belonging to myself and links me the world, and the sheer flesh that exceeds the bounds of comfortably dwelling in myself and in the world); the second is the lived body, the remembered-body posited at a distance in the past (although a very recent past), thus becoming an object of discourse. The third body is the flesh when it is tipped into its exterior. It is the body fully spatialized. It is said in various ways: "body-I-have," "object-body," or "body-object" (Husserl, 1952).

We have seen how the process of exteriorization or evagination of the body is already incipient in the body called "lived" with respect to the "living" body. This transition from immediacy to mediatedness, from pure impression to representation, from prereflective to reflective, from the background to the foreground, from the implicit to the explicit – and ultimately from within to without and from the invisible to the visible – becomes fully discernible in the body-object. The transit from the living body to the object body, through the lived body, is a journey of outsourcing and objectivization. It resembles a kind of hernia that makes visible what was internal, and therefore invisible, and locates it out there, where it can be seen as any object.

The flesh is under siege. Often the sufferings and anomalies of my flesh, such as feeling deprived of my vitality, my capacity to desire, excite and move, feeling isolated from myself, from others and from the world, push me toward experiencing my body as an inert object. Whereas before I was a living bodily being, now I realize I am nothing but *this* material, lifeless "corporealized" (Fuchs, 2000a, 2000b) body.

But quite the opposite may happen too: My flesh is at risk of falling into the object-body if my living body becomes a deafening noise, a pandemonium of raw sensations, a vertiginous chaos of impulses. Then, the only possible silencer to this uncanny feeling is to strip the living body of its spontaneity and relegate it to be an object among other objects, characterized by concreteness that is only suitable for objects. I have *that* body out there perceived as a kind of impersonal mechanism that is located, in part or totally, outside of my self-boundaries and works out of my control – thus out of my responsibility.

It may also happen that the third-person perspective toward my body is taken not from a weakening or from an excess of its vitality, but from the desire for enhancement. My body becomes my possession to take care of; an object to be subjected to some technique, that is, to be measured, manipulated, and improved. I am in front of my body like in front of *that image* in a mirror. I want to have a powerful, energetic, beautiful body. The body then becomes for me a reality to be built in the image and likeness of a representation of an ideal body – toned, muscular, strong; or thin, abstinent, ascetic.

Videor Ergo Sum

To recap: There are four ways to experience my body, thus to experience my Self. The first is to experience myself as a living body; this first mode is suspended between the shine of spontaneous self-affecting life and its

Dionysian dimension at the threshold of the darkness of death. The living body is the tacit guarantee that I am one with my Self, the source of my vitality and the hub of my sensations, as well as of my belonging to the world. But at the same time, it is always at risk of falling into the shapeless and vital chaoticity of pure effort and sensation. A little further, outward, lies the second body: It is experienced as a lived body, that is, the body in the first-person perspective but already subject to a retrospective look (if I am now "here," this experience of my body is already a little earlier and more *beyond* this "here") that gives the living body form, representation, history, and meaning. Already as a thing in the outside world there is then the third body – that one called object-body, which is given out there, in the sphere of things visible and ready to be manipulated.

In addition to these three bodies (living body, lived body, and object-body), there is a fourth that we could call being-a-body-for-the-other or *body-for-other*. Sartre (1986) speaks of this experiential dimension of the body with foresight showing that I can hire a further perspective on my body: *I can feel my body because it is watched by another person.*

The gaze of others, or rather, feeling the object of the gaze of others, is in this fourth dimension of bodily experience the necessary condition to feel my body. While in the living and lived body dimensions, the sense through which I am in contact with my bodily Self is coenaesthesia (although in the lived body is already incipient the action of the gaze), in the body-object and in the body-for-the other is the *eye* to be the master. But with a substantial difference: In the body-object, it is *my* gaze that objectifies my body and places it as an entity outside my Self, beyond the reach of the coenaesthesia. In the perspective that here we define body-for-other, it is *the gaze of others* that makes my body an object. But it is precisely this gaze that gives me back my body as part of my Self, that makes me *feel* my bodily Self, like the inside of a glove that, paraded, becomes visible on the outside.

With the appearance of the gaze of others – writes Sartre (1986) – I have the revelation of my being as object. My flesh is alienated by the gaze of the other, and as alienated, it makes me feel a body among other bodies. I realize that I am a body – that is what I am told when feeling watched by others. I have to know myself as I am known by others: as a body that can be seen from without.

Sartre tries to explain this way of experiencing one's body while looked at by the other through the example of shame. "I feel that I'm blushing" is an improper expression that when ashamed I use to describe my state: What I mean by this is that I become aware of my blushing body not *for me*, but *for others* – that is, from the others' perspective. I should say more correctly "I see myself blushing looking at myself with the eyes of others."

It is commonly said that the shy person is "embarrassed by his body." To be honest, even this expression is improper; I could not be embarrassed by my body – it is my body-for-others that embarrasses me. That is why I make an effort to hide my body from the other's gaze.

Although the shy person says that they no longer want to have a body, to disappear as a body, to become "invisible"; in reality, something paradoxical happens: Feeling clumsy and awkward because of one's body is still a way of feeling, and as such *more desirable than not feeling at all*. If the risk is not to feel at all, that is, the evanescence of the body; then the antidote, that is, feeling embarrassed – that is, feeling though at the price of feeling embarrassed – can be a relief, a comfort.

It is precisely the other's gaze that returns my body to me. In the impossibility of defining myself on the basis of the feeling that binds me to my own flesh, I know my Self from the others' vantage as the appearance of my body. When I experience my body through the others' gaze, I do not simply indulge in the logic of a *pornographic* vision of my own Self by letting others define my own Self by the way it appears as a visible body. For sure, I let the others define my Self as what appears in my visible body. But at the same time, the others' gaze returns my possibility to feel my body. We defined the flesh as feeling myself while experiencing something (Descartes' *sentio me videre*); the body-for-others is experiencing myself when perceived by the others, in the passivity of being perceived – *videor ergo sum* (*I am seen therefore I am*) (Stanghellini, 2020).

Of course, this is not a voluntary decision arising from some kind of reflection, rather an involuntary and, first and foremost, unconscious coping reaction.

The effect of this practice, which in the first place restores my capacity to experience my body in the first-person perspective, although with the mediation of the others' gaze, is none the less doubly alienating: first, because the fate of my Self is delivered into the hands (indeed in the eyes) of others. Second, because what the others return is a purely cognitive and linguistic construction, which increasingly distances me from an immediate experience of myself. Yet for those who cannot feel themselves, or do not feel at all (like Estella in Sartre's [1989] drama *No Exit*), feeling oneself with the eyes of the others' gaze is a resource of self-identification, rather than simply a source of alienation. Those who are subject to the evil of the evanescence of the living and lived body can try to feel and know their own body through the gaze of others.

A Synopsis of the Ways the Body Can Manifest Itself

Before passing to the analysis of body manifestations in psychopathology, I will provide a synopsis of what we have discussed in the previous paragraphs.

(1) Body-I-am
  (1.1) ***Lived body***: Proto-reflexive semi-experiential/semirepresentational manifestation of one's corporeality
  (1.2) ***Living body***: Immediately felt, pathic, purely impressive, pre-reflective, background, implicit, nonrepresentational, experiential and invisible manifestation of one's corporeality
    (1.2.1) **Self-affection**: Primordial bodily chiasm enforcing one's feeling of belonging to oneself and to the world
    (1.2.2) **Sheer flesh**: Chaotic plurality of invisible bodily forces immediately felt without the intercession of a representation
(2) **Body-object**: Mediated, representational, gnostic, reflective, foreground, explicit, and ultimately visible manifestation of one's corporeality
(3) **Body-for-others**: Felt, experiential manifestation of one's corporeality mediated by the other's gaze

Experts in clinical phenomenology may have recognized in some of these epiphanies of bodily experience the correlate of a specific psychopathological condition. This will be the topic of the following sections.

The Psychopathology of the Living Body

The living body insofar as it is deformed by a plurality of invisible forces is the catastrophic body, immediately felt without the intercession of a representation, a *cliché*, a story, language, or thought that can be found in the *borderline condition* (Stanghellini, 2016, 2018, 2020; Stanghellini & Mancini, 2017, 2019b). The living body is experienced by borderline persons as the headquarters of a destructive as well as exhilarating power. It is experienced as an energy that takes the representation of oneself to pieces, reducing it to a mere accumulation of disordered emotions and drives. Yet it is also the center of a vital power that expresses a boosting vitality, seducingly in touch with invigorating sensations. It is the glorification of a thrilled flesh, an intensive body vibrating at one with emotions, needs, desires, and all the powers of the involuntary. It is an intensive body, expressing an irrepressible and wild vitality, a brutal vitality entirely at the mercy of the basic biological values, a crude unmediated bodily vitality that does not accommodate to prereflective intentional structures or to reflective cognitive efforts – in short, as Pier Paolo Pasolini (2001) would put it: a "desperate vitality."

Under the pressure of this almost unlivable power, intentional structures (perception) and narrative structures (identity) crumple. Bodily reactions take dominance over bodily action, and the intimate sense of being an embodied Self is eclipsed by the sense of having an intimidating body. The borderline person feels the presence of a spontaneous energy without any clear direction or definite target. This chaotic vitality, being devoid of intentional structure and content, desperately seeks an object, mostly a person, at which to direct its surplus of energy. It is emotional energy that throws itself at the other with an overwhelming intensity.

The Psychopathology of the Object-Body

Persons with schizophrenia display a morbidly objectified body. The weakening of the basic sense of being an embodied Self, the emergence in the field of explicit awareness of the implicit bodily functioning that normally tacitly remains in the background, and the disruption of body-to-body attunement with others are the basic dimensions manifesting a fundamental disturbance of the bodily Self in schizophrenia (Stanghellini, 2009).

The most represented phenomena include *blurred demarcation*, that is, experiences of violation of bodily boundaries as for instance experiencing the intrusions of external entities into one's body or vice versa the externalization of bodily parts; *diminished bodily vitality*, that is, experiences of one's body or its parts as inert/lifeless morbidly objectivized things or impersonal mechanisms as in morbid objectivization and robotization; *disorders of bodily coherence*, that is, experiences of decomposition/fragmentation of the internal structure or *Gestalt* of one's body; *impairments of identity/sameness*, that is, experiences of transformations of one's body and dysmorphic phenomena; and finally *anomalies of activity*, that is, unpleasant or painful feelings in one's body passively suffered, including dysesthetic paroxysms and pain-like phenomena (Stanghellini et al., 2014).

In general, one's body – or more typically its fragmented parts or functions – are experienced as *out there*, in a place external to the Self, as impersonal objects or mechanisms imposing to the person to think, feel, experience, act in a given way out of the person's control.

The Psychopathology of the Body-for-Others

So-called eating disorders (EDs) are epiphenomena of a more profound disorder of bodily experience. ED persons feel extraneous from their own body (Stanghellini, Mancini, Castellini, & Ricca, 2018), their possibility to feel themselves is weakened, or threatened by coenaesthopathic and emotional paroxysms, their bodily feelings are discontinuous over time (Stanghellini & Mancini, 2019a). Their coenaesthetic apprehension of their own body as the more primitive and basic form of self-awareness (Stanghellini, 2019a, 2019b) is severely affected. This entails a fleeting feel of selfhood and an evanescent sense of identity.

In ED persons, the other's gaze may produce shame for one's body, but it may also imply a "positive" effect since they can feel their body only when they are looked at by another person. The other's look restores a feeling of unity and condensation. Since their experience of their body from within (the living and lived body) is flawed or inconsistent, they cope with this by apprehending their body *from without through the other's gaze*. The way they feel while looked at by other persons is the only possibility they have to feel themselves and define their identity.

Being a body-for-others is a peculiar feature of ED psychopathology. People with ED experience their body as an object being looked at by another, rather than coenaesthetically or from a first-person perspective (Stanghellini, Ballerini, & Mancini, 2019). Their body is principally given to them as an object to "be seen." Thus, their body is exposed and subjected to the other's gaze and thus reduced to its appearance.

Towards a Clinic of the Sheer Flesh: A List of Still Unanswered Questions

The living body is the implicit condition of possibility for the experience of appetite, vital energy, the point of orientation for my motivations, choices and actions, and the pivot of my experiential world as *my own* and the correlated pattern of meanings. And finally, and even more importantly, it is the condition of possibility of self-affection, which grounds these appetites, vital energies, motivations, choices, actions, experiences, and meanings in a coherent and significant Self that I experience as *my own Self*.

Yet the living body has a second face – the sheer flesh as the heart of darkness of my vitality – a chaotic, kaleidoscopic universe of raw feelings and conation in which the power of life is almost unlivable. The dark side of the living body can intrude at any time – although it may remain undetermined how many persons have ever experienced themselves as sheer flesh, how many times, and why. But the possibility is there for everybody – and what is called the "borderline" incarnates the pathological condition that typically falls prey to this kind of desperately vital bodily experience.

Is it legitimate to speculate that the origin of most (if not all) pathologies of the body (and thus of the Self) derives from the breakdown of the dialectic proportion between the bright side and the dark side of the living body – between the flesh as self-affection and as desperate vitality? Several other, still unanswered questions derive from this. Listing these questions may help to imagine the research agenda opened up by the clinic of the sheer flesh sketched in this chapter.

Is the sheer flesh – a mere body entirely at the mercy of fragmented and incoherent basic biological values – the original phenomenon, whereas other more disciplined forms of bodily experiences in which the *logos* can moderate the *pathos* of bodily feelings – the lived body being one of them – represent a domestication of this almost unlivable original experience?

Is the dynamic proportion between the sheer flesh as the product of nature, and the lived body as the product of culture – respectively the figures of *pathos* and *logos* – a guarantee of health and of the good life?

If the sheer flesh is the original (natural) phenomenon, which are the cultural apparatuses that can bind its power? Should we look for these moderating apparatuses in the phenomenon of intersubjectivity? Is the experience of being an embodied *self-with-others* – thus the experience of holding, attachment, attunement, synchronization, and mirroring, which take place in the infant's world thanks to the attention and recognition of its caregiver – what secures us from the unlivable intensity of the sheer flesh?

What happens if these apparatuses fail in their mitigating and integrating tasks? Can the sheer flesh become such an insupportable experience so that *other forms of bodily experiences arise as a shelter or defence*?

Can the experience of morbid objectification and robotization of the body (and its fragmented parts) that occurs in schizophrenia be considered a shelter protecting the schizophrenic person from feeling accountable for the sheer body's untamed and irrepressible forces and the terrible deeds that may derive from them? By putting the sheer body center stage, can alienation – the outsourcing (loss of agency and myness) of disorganized and uncontrollable impulses, emotions, desires, volitions, intentions coming from one's body – be considered a form of self-protection from intolerable responsibility?

Can the way people with EDs first and foremost experience their body as a body-for-others be considered a coping strategy, although involuntary, to achieve a sense of bodily Self, in the face of experiences of weak coenaesthetic apprehension of oneself, thus of unstable selfhood and precarious self-identity?

Is our common-sense and "normal" way to experience our body a movement of flight away from the threat of experiencing the living body as sheer flesh? What is the condition of possibility for experiencing our body as sheer flesh without falling into a psychopathological condition?

And, last but not least, can this limit-experience exposing a brutal vitality coming from within myself help me to understand more profoundly who I am, and the *conditio humana* in general?

References

Aristotle. (1957). *On the soul. Parva naturalia. On breath* (W. S. Hett, Trans.). Cambridge, MA: Harvard University Press.

Bataille, G. (1973). *Sur Nietzsche* [On Nietzsche]. Paris, France: Gallimard.

Bataille, G. (1988). *The accursed share: An essay on general economy.* Volume I: Consumption (R. Hurley, Trans.). New York, NY: Zone Books.

Deleuze, G. (2003). *Francis Bacon. The logic of sensation* (D. W. Smith, Trans.). Minneapolis, MN: University of Minnesota Press.

Fuchs, T. (2000a). *Leib, Raum, Person. Entwurf einer phänomenologischen Anthropologie* [Body, space, person. Outline of a phenomenological anthropology]. Stuttgart, Germany: Klett-Cotta.

Fuchs, T. (2000b). *Psychopathologie von Leib und Raum. Phänomenologisch-empirische Untersuchungen zu depressiven und paranoiden Erkrankungen* [Psychopathology of body and space. Phenomenological-empirical investigations in depressive and paranoid disorders]. Darmstadt, Germany: Steinkopff.

Genet, J. (2007). *L'atelier d'Alberto Giacometti* [The studio of Alberto Giacometti]. Paris, France: Gallimard.

Henry, M. (1965). *Philosophie et phénoménologie du corps* [Philosophy and phenomenology of the body]. Paris, France: Presses Universitaires de France.

Henry, M. (2000). *Incarnation.* Paris, France: Seuil.

Husserl, E. (1952). *Ideen zu einer reinen Phänomenologie und phänomenologische Philosophie. II. Phänomenologische Untersuchungen zur Konstitution* [Ideas pertaining to a pure phenomenology and to a phenomenological philosophy. II. Studies in the phenomenology of constitution]. The Hague, Netherlands: Martinus Nijhoff Publishers.

Kimura, B. (1992). *Écrits de psychopathologie phénoménologique* [Writings in phenomenological psychopathology]. Paris, France: Presses Universitaires de France.

Merleau-Ponty, M. (1962). *The phenomenology of perception* (C. Smith, Trans.). London, UK: Routledge & Kegan Paul.

Merleau-Ponty, M. (1968). *The visible and the invisible* (C. Lefort, Ed., A. Lingis, Trans.). Evanston, IL: Northwestern University Press.

Pasolini, P. P. (2001). Una disperata vitalità [A desperate vitality]. In *Poesie* (p. 133).Milan, Italy: Garzanti.

Sartre, J.-P. (1986). *Being and nothingness* (H. Barnes, Trans.). London, UK: Routledge.

Sartre, J.-P. (1989). *No exit and three other plays* (L. Abel, Trans.). New York, NY: Vintage International.

Stanghellini, G. (2009). Embodiment and schizophrenia. *World Psychiatry*, 8(1), 56–59. doi:10.1002/j.2051-5545.2009.tb00212.x

Stanghellini, G. (2016). *Lost in dialogue. Anthropology, psychopathology and care.* Oxford, UK: Oxford University Press.

Stanghellini, G. (2018). *L'amore che cura* [The love that cares]. Milan, Italy: Feltrinelli.

Stanghellini, G. (2019a). Embodiment and the Other's look in feeding and eating disorders. *World Psychiatry*, 18(3), 364–365. doi:10.1002/wps.20683

Stanghellini, G. (2019b). The optical-coenaesthetic disproportion in feeding and eating disorders. *European Psychiatry*, 58, 70–71. doi:10.1016/j.eurpsy.2019.02.005

Stanghellini, G. (2020). Selfie. Sentirsi attraverso lo sguardo dell'altro [Selfie. Feeling oneself through the gaze of the other]. Milan, Italy: Feltrinelli.

Stanghellini, G., Ballerini, M., Blasi, S., Mancini, M., Presenza, S., Raballo, A., & Cutting, J. (2014). The bodily self: A qualitative study of abnormal bodily phenomena in persons with schizophrenia. *Comprehensive Psychiatry*, 55, 1703–1711. doi:10.1016/j.comppsych.2014.06.013

Stanghellini, G., Ballerini, M., & Mancini, M. (2019). The optical-coenaesthetic disproportion hypothesis of feeding and eating disorders in the light of neuroscience. *Frontiers in Psychiatry*, 10, 1–7. doi:10.3389/fpsyt.2019.00630

Stanghellini, G., & Mancini, M. (2017). *The therapeutic interview in mental health. Emotions, values, and the life-world.* Cambridge, UK: Cambridge University Press.

Stanghellini, G., & Mancini, M. (2019a). Abnormal time experience in persons with feeding and eating disorders: A naturalistic explorative study. *Phenomenology and the Cognitive Sciences*, 18(4), 759–773. doi:10.1007/s11097-019-09618-5

Stanghellini, G., & Mancini, M. (2019b). The life-world of persons with borderline personality disorder. In G. Stanghellini, M. R. Broome, A. Raballo, A. V. Fernandez, P. Fusar-Poli, & R. Rosfort (Eds.), *The Oxford handbook of phenomenological psychopathology* (pp. 665–681). Oxford, UK: Oxford University Press.

Stanghellini, G., Mancini, M., Castellini, G., & Ricca, V. (2018). Eating disorders as disorders of embodiment and identity. Theoretical and empirical perspectives. In H. L. McBride & J. L. Kwee (Eds.), *Embodiment and eating disorders. Theory, research, preventions and treatment* (pp. 127–142). London, UK: Routledge.

Straus, E. (1963). *The primary world of senses: A vindication of sensory experience.* New York, NY: Free Press of Glencoe.

Tedder, R. (2013). Counting stars [Recorded by OneRepublic]. On *Native* [CD, MP3 file]. Los Angeles, CA: Mosley Music Group.

4.1

Commentary on "The Heart of Darkness of the Living Body"

The Epiphany of the Body: Some Remarks on the Translation of Leib *from German*

Lorenzo Gilardi

Introduction

In the previous chapter, Stanghellini argues for the necessity of distinguishing between the *living* and the *lived* body. Stanghellini's approach seems intended in a functional way to recognize a dimensional field for distinguishing the psychopathology of corporeality in certain mental disorders, mainly a borderline personality disorder. This foregrounding of the living body and the recognition of its double face is long overdue in the phenomenology of corporeality since it acknowledges the *Abgrund* from which consciousness arises as embodiment. This point is most evident in the Janus-faced epiphany of the living body: the chiasmus between myself and the world as it "touches itself seeing and touching the things" (Merleau-Ponty, 1968, p. 146), on the one hand, and on the other, the "sheer flesh," the un-form, a chaos of forces (precisely the *Abgrund*) that exists before the subject can appropriate it and give it a form, a structure, a purpose, a meaning.

The history of the phenomenology of corporeality (and, later, embodiment) starts with the founder of the phenomenological movement, Husserl, who first underlined the transcendental distinction between, on the one hand, the body-subject, the body-I-am (to retain the expressions used by Stanghellini), in German *Leib*, and, on the other, the body-object, the body-I-have (but also other people's bodies), in German *Körper*, or, indeed, *Körperding* (the "body-thing"). In the initial stages of phenomenological research, this remained the transcendental framework for understanding the phenomenology of corporeality. It is only with Sartre's introduction of the body-for-others (which Stanghellini refers to as the fourth epiphany of the body, essential for grasping the experiential nucleus of persons with eating disorders) and his acknowledgment that the body is the only true psychic object, and subsequently Merleau-Ponty's theorization of the body as the center of gravity of one's life with the notion of *chair*, "flesh" (the first epiphany and Stanghellini's main topic of discussion), that the phenomenology of embodiment springs into life and takes roots in psychopathology.

Here, I will argue that the intricacies of the epiphanies of the body parallel the translational difficulties in trying to render full justice to the polyvalence embedded in the body itself, and that a close semantic and etymological examination of the original German terminology (first used by phenomenology) can shed light on the constitutive ambivalence of the body and hence form the basis for Stanghellini's arguments. The first point I shall make, therefore, is that the original translations of the German word *Leib* in other languages with the past participle ("corps vécu" in French, "lived body" in English, and "corpo vissuto" in Italian) are inaccurate and misleading since they entail a *deflation* of the semantic pregnancy of the German term and possibly a subversion of its etymology.

Leib in German and Its Translations

Nothing in the semantics of *Leib* authorizes a univocal translation using the past participle as opposed to the present participle. In German, the semantic spectrum of the word in question makes it practically untranslatable into non-German languages, since no translation captures the fact that *Leib* encompasses, without mediation or distinction, both a past and a present participle. *Leib* is both the living and lived body referred to by Stanghellini: If it is related to any other word, it comes closest to *leben* ("to live"); indeed, middle-high German contained the variant **leiben*.

A closer look at the semantic field of the word *Leib* helps to shed light on the inaccuracy of the aforementioned translations. Some idiomatic expressions already indicate how *vibrant* is the semantic nucleus of the word: *Der Leib Christi* refers to the body of Christ in the Eucharist, emphasizing not only the living nature of the term but also its *enlivening* power, which gives access to an *authentic* form of life; *einer Sache zu Leibe gehen* ("to go to the heart of something") again displays the "warm" nucleus of the word; *etwas am eigenen Leibe erfahren* ("to experience something in the flesh") refers to the most visible dimension – the "flesh"(Merleau-Ponty, 1962, 1968; Stanghellini, 2018, 2021) – of the body; *sich jemanden vom Leib zu halten* ("to keep someone at arm's length") seems to point to an original co-belonging of *Leib* and *Raum* ("space"), to an original positioning of the *Leib* not so much as *occupying* a *quid* of space as *opening* a space that is living/lived. In such a space, every object is situated in proportion to the gestures of the *Leib*, because it is from the *Leib* that the coordinate system that renders geometric space *inhabitable* and so *liveable* originates. Here, we see a contrast with certain psychopathological conditions in which space is experienced as a homogeneous geometrical area lacking a coordinate system that could give it order, sense, and direction (schizophrenia) or as a place that has lost its perspective and is reduced to a two-dimensionality in which objects are only *transcendent* and never *immanent* (depression). Lastly, *die Leibeskraft* identifies the "vital force" that inhabits the *Leib*, its condition of possibility and the point from which it exerts itself, its vector of transmission into the world.

To summarize, *Leib* is the living *and* the lived body, my own body, the body alive (the first two epiphanies of Stanghellini's conceptualization of corporeality). It stands in opposition to *Körper*, the body-object (the third epiphany), comparable to the organism objectified by medicine (first analyzed anatomically and subsequently resynthesized physiologically; in so doing losing every vibrant and "warm" character) as to every other object encountered in the world.

The link between *Leib* and Merleau-Ponty's "flesh," as introduced in the previous chapter by Stanghellini, is further reinforced by certain other idiomatic expressions of German: *Beleibt sein* means "to be corpulent" (in Italian: "essere in carne" means "flesh"); *leibhaftig* means "in the flesh"; both expressions point to the embodied character of *Leib* (Fuchs, 2000a, 2000b).

Hermann Schmitz's (2002) translation "felt body" seems truer than other attempts but it does not exhaust the semantic arc of the German word and seems to have been introduced to delineate the different conceptualization of *Leib* in Schmitz's *Neue Phänomenologie* (with its emphasis on the prereflexive characteristics of the terminological/conceptual apparatus of classical phenomenology) in opposition to Husserl and his followers. In sum, probably the best way is to translate *Leib* with "body" and *Körper(ding)* with "organism."

Erlebnis and "Lived"

The issue, however, does not end there. The use of the past participle in non-German languages extends also to the "lived" term itself, taken as a noun.

Again, it is important to point out how German does not employ a substantivized past participle to render the concept, but chooses the noun *das Erlebnis*, derived from the verb *erleben* ("to live," but *in a deep sense of*, "to feel," "to experience," even "to live as long as/so much as"). As a noun, its gender is *neuter*.

Here, it is also worth noting a central feature of standard translations from German. When we talk in the past participle, we express an objectified, located, and finished modality of an action, and the use of *Erlebnis* tends in the same direction, but not quite enough to make German speakers use the past participles (*gelebt, erlebt)*, which are at their disposal.

In fact, the particle *er** identifies a form of distancing from the simple noun or verb, one that is situated in the middle between the experience lived momentarily and locally and the experience finished and remembered (and so is highly apt for capturing Stanghellini's distinction between the living and the lived body: Could we perhaps say that the living body is the body *gelebt*, whereas the lived one is the body *erlebt*?).

There are many instances in which the particle *er** serves to give color to a partial objectification and distance the actions expressed by some verbs: If *kennen* means "to know," *erkennen* means "to distinguish (from)"; if *klären* means "to clarify," *erklären* means "to explain"; if *kämpfen* means "to fight," *erkämpfen* means "to obtain something fighting"; if *geben* means "to give," *ergeben* means "to render, to result" and, in the reflexive mode, "to delineate oneself, to emerge," even "to be born" *sensu latu*.

The intermediate position that the particle *er** occupies in the German language also lets it express the ambivalent or even polyvalent character of the "lived" concept: *Das Erlebnis* finds itself suspended in an intermediate condition between active and passive, between the present and the past, in a temporal horizon of present perfect (hence still *acting on the present*), in a middle region from which it can simultaneously and immediately access the eternal instant of the present and the time just past but transcendentally still present in the modality of the Husserlian *retentio*.

This intermediate and ambivalent nature of the German word is further reinforced by its neuter gender, a fact that should not be underestimated.

Das Erlebnis des Leibes

What has been said earlier about the semantic pregnancy of the word *Leib*, on the one hand, and the neuter gender and the particle *er** in the word *Erlebnis*, on the other, allows us to see how in German the body is "experienced" ingenuously and simultaneously both as a subject and as an object, without the need to recover via philosophical analyses (see, e.g., Henry, Richir, Merleau-Ponty) the unity of this feeling (the first and second epiphany of corporeality). The original meanings of *Leib* and *Erlebnis* are nicely encapsulated in the following sentence by Umberto Galimberti:

> *Nature* and *culture* are not the poles of a journey that mankind has never travelled, but simply two names that we use here to designate the ambivalence with which the body expressed itself in archaic societies and the equivalence to which it has been reduced today in our societies by the codes that preside over them and by the set of their institutions. (Galimberti, 1983, p. 11; my translation)

What was said in the first paragraph about the *Leib* and its semantic domain can therefore be extended to the two polarities of "nature" and "culture" in human existence, because the wide spectrum thereby covered allows us to differentiate not only the discipline of the body into the various codes that history has imposed on it but also, and above all, that same ambivalence that persists, regardless, at the periphery of all codifications because, indeed, "indifferent to the principle of identity and difference through which every codification expresses its bivalent symmetry, [*der Leib*] says to be this, *but also* that" (Galimberti, 1983, p. 11; my translation).

This ambivalence of *Leib* is exactly what Stanghellini unfolds with his distinction between living and lived body and his recognition of the double nature of Merleau-Ponty's "flesh." He emphasizes how, in his view, classical phenomenology is badly equipped to handle such a prereflexive and precognitive dimension of corporeality, and points out how nonphenomenologists such as Deleuze and Bataille could enlighten the darkest aspects of the sheer flesh in an unintended phenomenological way. Phenomenology, in the end, can be done by anyone, as long as they let phenomena speak for themselves.

References

Fuchs, T. (2000a). *Leib, Raum, Person. Entwurf einer phänomenologischen Anthropologie* [Body, space, person. Outline of a phenomenological anthropology]. Stuttgart, Germany: Klett-Cotta.

Fuchs, T. (2000b). *Psychopathologie von Leib und Raum. Phänomenologisch-empirische Untersuchungen zu depressiven und paranoiden Erkrankungen* [Psychopathology of body and space. Phenomenological-empirical investigations in depressive and paranoid disorders]. Darmstadt, Germany: Steinkopff.

Galimberti, U. (1983). *Il corpo* [The body]. Milan, Italy: Feltrinelli.

Merleau-Ponty, M. (1962). *The phenomenology of perception* (C. Smith, Trans.). London, UK: Routledge & Kegan Paul.

Merleau-Ponty, M. (1968). *The visible and the invisible* (C. Lefort, Ed., A. Lingis, Trans.). Evanston, IL: Northwestern University Press.

Schmitz, H. (2002). Hermann Schmitz, the "Neue Phänomenologie". In A.-T. Tymieniecka (Ed.), *Phenomenology world-wide. Foundations – expanding dynamics – life engagements. A guide for research and study* (pp. 491–494). Dordrecht, Netherlands: Springer.

Stanghellini, G. (2018). *L'amore che cura* [The love that cares]. Milan, Italy: Feltrinelli.

Stanghellini, G. (2021). The heart of darkness of the living body. In C. Tewes & G. Stanghellini (Eds.), *Time and body: Phenomenological and psychopathological approaches* (pp. 60–75). Cambridge, UK: Cambridge University Press.

5

Microphenomenology of Chronicity in Psychosomatic Diseases

Diabetes, Anorexia, and Schizophrenia

Natalie Depraz

Introduction

I wish here to examine a few aspects of the peculiar temporality of this *chronic* time, which is considered as pathological for the subject. I will show how such a time also has intrinsic psycho-emotional-bodily and relational-intersubjective dimensions. This I will do in the light of three different diseases, either more somatic (diabetes), mental (schizophrenia), or narrowly interweaving the lived body and consciousness (anorexia).

We chose to study these diseases in our research program in collaboration with three adolescent psychiatric hospitals (in Rouen-Normandie, Sud-Yvelines Paris, and Lille-Armentières) where each of them is mainly dealt with. I will show how they involve specific intersubjective relational modalities, respectively: some forms of depressive solipsism in diabetes, a kind of maniac openness in schizophrenia, and of hostile otherness in anorexia.

Since the chronicity inherent in these perhaps misnamed, as we will come to see, "chronic" diseases is predominantly absent in the theoretical literature as a theme of study and is neither available as a concept in philosophy, I will also rely first on standard and well-known phenomenological views of time: namely, the Husserlian dynamic of the living present, and also the Husserlian passive time in genetic sedimentation. Then, I will also refer to the depressive melancholic past introversion, the maniac absent-minded all-openness in Ludwig Binswanger, and the traumatic repeated compulsion as it is dealt with early on by Freud and Ferenzci and later also by M. J. Larrabee (1995) in her pioneering article entitled "The Time of Trauma: Husserl's Phenomenology and Post-Traumatic Stress Disorder"; finally, I will rely on my own research project on trauma: "Trauma and

Phenomenology" (Depraz, 2018). These approaches to time offer interesting tools to get closer to the specificity of *chronic* temporality.

Last but not least, I will compare such phenomenological approaches of time with a few genuine first-person accounts of the chronic lived time gathered thanks to microphenomenological interviews. These I led (and still lead) in the very framework of the Adochroniq research program, which is based – and this is its originality – on qualitative semidirective existential and nondirective microphenomenological explicitation interviews. The latter in particular are meant to collect the very words of the patients and the medical staff in charge of them, the testimonies of the lived experiences they go through, and their idiosyncratic way of expressing them. By doing so, I suggest a qualitatively refined phenomenological description of this peculiar bodily and relationally disturbed time, which is how we may come to see chronic time.[1]

My aim here is not necessarily to find out which insights we gain for the understanding of psychiatric disorders by investigating the intertwinement of time, body, and intersubjectivity, which would amount to having philosophy play the dominating part of clarifying clinical, here chronic, experiences. Rather, I aim to find out how clinical experience crucially helps philosophers to refine their a priori categories into experienced embodied categories.

Is Chronicity a Transverse Societal Pathology?

Chronicity and chronic time (as well as diseases) refer in their etymology to the god Kronos, son of Ouranos and Gaïa. Kronos helped his mother Gaïa take revenge on his father Ouranos, who hated his children and planned to kill them. In turn, however, Kronos imprisoned his own brothers and devoured the children he had with his sister Rhea. Thus, Kronos is the symbol of an uncontrollable and repeated destruction, and he is therefore also associated with fate and destiny. The meaning of time he carries with him is characterized by duration, passivity, and negativity. It is distinct from at least two other concepts of time represented in the Greek mythology by Kairos (the timely instant) and Aiôn (a cyclical time).

Closer to us in history, "chronic" has definitively become a medical term. It qualifies a disease and is attested as early as the thirteenth century

[1] For the techniques of microphenomenological interviews, see the founding book by Vermersch (1994/2011); for an analysis of microphenomenological interviews, see Depraz, Gyemant, and Desmidt (2017); and for an application of the microphenomenological interview in the framework of neurophenomenology (especially cardiophenomenology), see Depraz and Desmidt (2018).

from the Latin *chronicus* by Master Henri de Mondeville in his book *La Chirurgie* (de Mondeville, 1897). For Mondeville, the symptoms of a chronic disease appear slowly, it lasts a very long time, and sometimes settles permanently, as opposed to an acute disease, which is quite brief and intense. In order to further contextualize the term in history and medicine, let us add that chronic diseases are increasingly mentioned in the second half of the nineteenth century: for example, by writers such as the naturalist Emile Zola, who writes of "chronic alcoholism" in his novel *Nana*, or again by Guy de Maupassant in his short stories *Le bûcher* and *Le Horla* or by George Sand in *Histoire de ma vie*, who both describe "chronic" affections of the throat. Chronic diseases thus seem to apply mainly to somatic or psychosomatic diseases. More recently in the second half of the twentieth century, the French *Encyclopédie Médicale Quillet* (Gaucher, 1965/1972, p. 365) also indicates how severe forms of facial nerve pain may "become chronic" (the expression being in French: *passer à la chronicité*) and make the patient's life unbearable. Again, chronicity seems to mainly apply to lived-bodily diseases.

Does this mean that it is only relevant in these cases and, if so, how does it apply to mental illness? When examining the clinical psychiatric literature, it appears that chronicity has been increasingly used and claimed in the last two or three decades in two different but possibly intermingling cases and contexts.

First, chronicity is said to characterize the peculiar time of major depressive disorders as a time of "recurrence." It is thematized as such by the French psychiatrist Frédéric Rouillon (2004) in his book *Les Troubles Dépressifs Récurrents* (Recurrent Depressive Disorders). "Recurrence" is first defined by the *persistence* of the diagnostic criteria of a depressive episode lasting at least two years; second, it is characterized by many *relapses* with residual symptoms between the episodes over at least two years (Rouillon, 2004). For example, the study by Hammen, Shih, Altman, and Brennan (2003) shows the enhanced "chronic social difficulties" of depressed teenagers aged 15 when living with a depressed mother.

Second, chronicity is now widespread as a "hospital psychiatric chronicity." Thirty years ago, it was already identified by the systemic family psychiatrists Wieviorka and Kannas (1989) in their pioneering article "Approche Systémique et Chronicité en Milieu Hospitalier Psychiatrique" (Systemic Approach and Chronicity in Psychiatric Hospitals), published in the well-known French journal *L'Evolution Psychiatrique* (*Psychiatric Evolution*). They show how the hospital is a place where chronic patients settle down and stay indefinitely with no longer apparent symptoms.

Furthermore, they demonstrate how hospitalization is even a process that may provoke the "chronicization" of their illness. Long before the work of the well-known French psychiatrist Georges Lantéri-Laura (1997) in his book *La Chronicité en Psychiatrie* (Chronicity in Psychiatry) and his leading motto "la chronicité [hospitalière] est une caractéristique essentielle de la psychiatrie" (hospital chronicity is an essential feature of psychiatry), Wieviorka and Kannas provide as early as 1989 a remarkable description of hospital chronicity and of hospitalized chronic patients:

> Anybody durably working in a psychiatric hospital cannot but notice the existence of a population that is quite stable though fluctuant in its composition. According to the history of the hospital, of the service or both, this population corresponds to about one to two thirds of hospitalized patients. They are chronically ill patients. In our field this expression has a dynamic meaning. They are patients who apparently do not change. In reality each of them taken separately show a remarkable capacity to metabolize the inputs of various changes that twenty or thirty years of hospital changes have undergone (ideological, organizational, medical, nursing staff changes, etc.), not to mention the changes related to the evolution of the patients themself and of their family during all these years. They are professional patients in psychiatry, in hospitalization and in homeostasy. The "chronically ill patients" can be defined as follows: 1) a continuous hospital stay, more than two years in general. The criterion is arbitrary, but accounts well enough for the fact that beyond a certain period of hospitalization the probability of exit diminishes and hospitalization itself causes effects that make social operativity even more problematic; 2) absence of disorganizing acute pathology. They are most of them chronic psychotic patients, schizophrenic or not, severe chronic depressive states, severe neurotic states, etc.; 3) absence of severe organic or psychiatric pathology, requiring the constant help of a third person. In other words, these are patients who behave in such a way that there is no intention of limiting their stay in the hospital, but who are capable of performing the basic acts of daily life, or for whom there is no direct relationship between the medical diagnosis and the restriction of their ability to leave the hospital. In fact, for such patients, whose psychiatric symptoms are often described as blunted, packed, the only true symptom gradually becomes chronic hospitalization itself, which they seem not to complain about. In a systemic view, in which we consider not only the meaning but also the function of the symptom in the context in which it appears, we can ask what is the meaning, the function of a symptom of which we do not complain. To ask such a question is to observe the frequent coupling of these patients with contexts of rejection, abandonment or betrayal. (Wieviorka & Kannas, 1989, pp. 595–596, my translation)

It is worth quoting Kannas' description and analysis at length because it helps better understand through the context of the hospital precisely what a chronically ill patient is. Thus, what Kannas calls "chronically ill patients" (*des malades chroniques*) – and also rather provocatively, with a light touch of humor, "professional patients" – are in fact chronicized patients, that is, patients whose illness is in a great part produced and at least reinforced by institutionalization in an asylum. In this context, psychic mechanisms are not solely and primarily intrapsychic mechanisms; they are relational, that is, they become stronger and may even be identified as fixed symptoms through the contextual institutional organization, which eventually forbids any possibility of change. In fact, it is this very definition of chronicization that was anticipated in the sixties by the French philosopher Michel Foucault and later on by the Scottish psychiatrist Ronald Laing in the frame of the radical political and social stream of "antipsychiatry."

To conclude our first step based on the review of the clinical literature on the subject, it seems that chronicity is less a property of a particular disease (diabetes, anorexia, and schizophrenia) than a pathology as such. So testifies Linda Normandin in Québec in her book *La Vie des Uns, le Mépris des Autres* (The Life of the Ones, the Despise of the Others) with her account of addictions at the Center of Specialized Care for Toxicomans (Normandin, 2013). Here, we can see that any disease may conversely end up becoming a property of chronicity. We would thus have a diabetic, an anorexic, and a schizophrenic chronicity as so many variations of this pathology, just to name the diseases we focus on in our research program. Chronicity would be the traverse, strongly relational–institutional, that is, social, political, and maybe even civilizational – pathology of any disease – whether somatic, psychosomatic, or mental (about such a relational component of chronicity, see [Œuvray, 2010]). Do we not live in a world where we do not seem to be ill, where we might have no symptom, but where we are so conditioned and absorbed by the daily dependency to our work that we do not even have the opportunity to wake up and deeply question its relevance for our human life? Are we not "chronic" human beings most of the time, with only a few and too rare flashes of lucidity, during which the becoming aware is so dizzy that we quickly close the door of our consciousness and move on with our daily routine, our daily chronicity?

What Resources for Conceptualizing Chronicity?

My second step will now explore some leading approaches of time in phenomenology and phenomenological psychiatry meant to gather descriptive resources for a finer conceptual understanding of chronicity. First and foremost, Husserl's approach toward time in his *On the Phenomenology of the Consciousness of Internal Time* (Husserl, 1991) and in his *Analyses Concerning Passive and Active Synthesis* (Husserl, 1966) is highly valuable. It offers a dynamic view of the self embedded in their lived-bodily and relational retentional and protentional lived time experience. The present time is thus a living present where we repeatedly open new possibilities on the basis of repeatedly self-reactivating past horizons. Thus, the passivity of the human subject facing the obvious entropy of time amounts to a dynamic passivity, even a receptivity to open possibilities and not a dead and closed sedimentation. In that respect, Husserl's view of time is a dynamic, lived-bodily, relational view of time, and it potentially offers the structural resources for a therapeutic time as a kind of antidote to chronicity, at least understood as it is so far as a negative, closed, unchanging, and motionless time. In short, the virtue of Husserl's cartography of embodied intersubjective living time paves the way for an a priori nonpathological time, here, for a counter-chronic temporality.

It is also interesting to look at Ludwig Binswanger's productive step in his pioneering book *Melancholie und Manie* (Melancholia and Mania) (1960), which is based on Husserl's positive, dynamic (therapeutic) view of time as I just presented it. Indeed, Binswanger explores the pathological structures of time and intersubjectivity at work in two interconnected and mirrored psychoses, melancholia and mania. As it is well known, Binswanger describes melancholic time as an immersive dwelling in the past and as an obstruction of horizons (along with a self-closed attitude). As a contrast, maniac time is seen by him as an anarchic opening to coming events in any directions and consequently as a complete absentmindedness of the self. The reasons for the promotion of the Binswangerian analysis of time are of two types here: first, the closely Husserlian-anchored analysis provided by Binswanger regarding the two main and mirror psychoses of melancholia and mania offers a helpful better characterization of some features of the specific time at work in chronicity; the second reason is a negative one: The analyses of schizophrenia available in Blankenburg's *Der Verlust der natürlichen Selbstverständlichkeit* (The Loss of Natural Self-Evidence) (1971) or in Kimura's *L'entre* (The Between) (1988/2000) do not focus on the temporal dimension of the psychosis but rather on the alteration of embodied space and intersubjectivity as being precisely "lost" in the sense of a disconnection of the self. In order to better understand the time at work in schizophrenia as a chronic psychosis, it is therefore fruitful to appeal to psychoses when investigated in the light of their altered temporality.

The time disorders Binswanger describes in *Melancholie und Manie* (1960) therefore provide us with useful resources to get closer to the chronic time, above all with the closed and obstructive attitude of the complaining self in melancholia. Why is it so? Because the closed attitude of the melancholic self is in fact one of the main properties of the chronic self, that is, a motionless and unchanging attitude. Another way to interpret such a closed attitude in melancholic depression would be to see it as a "de-synchronization," that is, as an uncoupling of the temporal relation of body and environment, by which the person falls out of communally tuned living time (Fuchs, 2005), although the stress is then more on the distortion of alterity spatially understood than on the distortion of time itself. Furthermore, as far as depression is concerned, it is of course necessary to be more specific. We need to distinguish between melancholia as a severe major depression and depression in general – there are today more than two hundred different known forms of depression – insofar as not all depression is chronic in the sense of the motionless dimension in the severe form at work in melancholia.

Let us now look more closely at the specificity of another kind of pathological time known as the traumatic time. We might hopefully be able to discover some other helpful properties in order to move closer to the chronic time.

The process of traumatization is based on a trauma often initially ignored. It is such an act of ignoring, such a nonconsciousness by the subject of what happened to themself (e.g., a rape that is "forgotten") that generates a looping setting made of repetitions (recurrences) and anarchic segmented unexpected reactivations in the course of which the initial event (the rape) will come back in a distorted and incomprehensible way. Such recurrences were notably described by Sigmund Freud (1920/1922) in his book *Beyond the Pleasure Principle* under the term "repetition compulsion." The description of the anarchic time of traumatization as made of segmented and unexpected reactivations was also very well described by the British philosopher Simon Critchley and the French philosopher Guy Félix Duportail in their accounts of trauma, both of which were based on the cross-account of the psychoanalyst Jacques Lacan and the philosopher Emmanuel Levinas. Regarding this matter, let me also refer to my own contribution entitled "Trauma and Phenomenology" (Depraz, 2018) in the Polish journal *Eidos* in Warsaw and, earlier, to Larrabee (1995) and Matthew Yaw's (2015) article "Husserl and PTSD." In this respect, Robert Stolorow's essay *Trauma and Human Existence* also remarkably shows how Heidegger's conception of time and the psychoanalytic conception of trauma mutually enriched each other (Stolorow, 2009; cf. Depraz, 2016; for a bodily based approach on traumatic memory, see Fuchs [2018, pp. 134–140]).

Unlike chronicity, traumatic time seems to be a dynamic time with multiple reactivations, but like chronicity it does not seem to bring any fundamental change for the subject, enabling them "to move on"; yet, unlike chronicity, it seems to be a time that may be overcome, thanks to different kinds of therapy, but, like chronicity, it also seems to make the self definitely vulnerable and to compel the subject to live with this vulnerability, rather than really recovering from it. Like chronic diseases, posttraumatic stress disorder seems to be a transverse pathology reinforcing or revealing standard categorized psychosomatic illnesses. For example, traumatization may take root in a first depressive episode or may reveal an emerging schizophrenic disorder.

Let us now conclude this second part. On the basis of the categories available in the above approaches, our cartography of chronic time as a pathological time for the self becomes refined and strengthened.

First, with Husserl and Binswanger, chronicity seems to be linked to an inner state of motionlessness and of absence of change, in contrast to the dynamic of the living present, of the receptive process of reactivation but similarly with the melancholic state of the closed complaining self. Second, along with the comparison with traumatic time, we may develop a finer view of chronicity. It clearly adopts features (recurrence, fragmentation, distortion), which do not merely point out deficiencies but end up as a possible structural concept: a transverse and trans nosographic time-quality of many (if not all) diseases.

The Refinement of the Phenomenal Experience and Description of Chronicity

In this third final part, I will directly confront diseases that are called "chronic diseases" as such (not diseases that may "become chronic" but that are chronic as such), like diabetes, anorexia, and schizophrenia (even if of course not all forms of them are intrinsically chronic). With such chronic diseases, does the emerging conception of chronicity as a transverse property of all diseases still stand? With such intrinsic chronic diseases, does, for example, the identification of chronicity as motionlessness and the absence of change still stand? Because of the lack of available descriptions and categories in the clinical and theoretical philosophical–phenomenological literature, I will let experiential categories emerge and build upon them, drawing material from first-person interviews and using a methodology that has now demonstrated its rigor, that is, microphenomenological explicitation interviews.

Unlike many qualitative methods that still remain far too exposed to the private particular subjectivist opinion of the subjects and are thus not able to provide sufficient scientific universalizable patterns, microphenomenology enables access to a concrete singular experience that may become a universal experiential pattern for many people.[2]

Before going into some results that could be revealed thanks to this specific technique of interview, let me say a bit more about this microphenomenological explicitation interview (see Depraz, 2020). Indeed, the birth of microphenomenology is a recent one. The term was coined four years ago, in the spring of 2016, during talks held by researchers belonging to the Husserl-Archives (Claire Petitmengin, Michel Bitbol, Dominique Pradelle, and myself), and the recently deceased Pierre Vermersch, a psychologist trained in Jean Piaget's teachings, and founder in the early 1980s of the technique of the explicitation interview (*entretien d'explicitation*), now called microphenomenological interview, within the frame of his research into organizational psychology as early as 1976 (Vermersch, 1994/2011).

Starting from everyday professional or personal activities and their distinction into time sequences, in which the subject performs successfully what they perform, and knows how they perform it (disassemble a microprocessor, go to the baker's to get some bread), Vermersch's question was the following: *How* does the subject do what they do? And as a corollary, are they capable of describing *the manner* in which they go about doing what they do? Indeed, if one asks somebody how they have done what they have done, most of the time one receives an answer that supplies their *representation* of what they have done, much more than *how they effectively went about* doing what they have done. I linger on the starting point of Vermersch's interrogation, since as a researcher in psychology, it underlines the core of what becomes his specific practice of describing a subject's preconscious experience, which he terms "pré-réflexive," or "implicite" and

[2] Let's mention that the choice of the microphenomenological interview-analysis as a qualitative first-person interview does not exclude semistructured interview-analysis (e.g., Blanchet, 2003; Smith, Jarman, & Osborn, 1999), in fact, the specificity of the Adochroniq research program is to combine and methodologically articulate these two types of qualitative approaches, that is, microphenomenological and semistructured (named here "existential") interviews. So in our research a first semistructured interview is meant to delineate, thanks to an interview guide, the relevant themes to be asked by the interviewer of the interviewee regarding the illness as it is lived by the patients in the course of their illness, then a microphenomenological interview focuses on a particular *hic et nunc* moment of the lived experience of illness and seeks to unveil preconscious bodily related experiences, feelings, perceptions, affections happening to the patient at this particular salient moment (it may be the initial moment of awareness of being ill, a moment of felt transitory recovery or, on the contrary, of worsening of the disease).

which leads him to set up an interview technique aimed at enabling this subject to "make explicit" (*expliciter*) their manner of doing what they do with a great degree of fineness and precision, a rarely achieved "granularity" (*granularité*), as he himself puts it.

Indeed through the technique of the microphenomenological explicitation interview, one enables the subject to have a more fine-tuned access to their singular lived experiences, which are often covered up by generic representations. Typically, if I ask *how* you woke up this morning, and you answer me that in general, the alarm clock wakes you up, you are describing the usual structure of your reality of waking up, or your own spontaneous representation of this morning's waking up. According to Vermersch, you would be describing a "class of lived experiences," but not your lived and unique experience of that particular morning: In other words, the formulation of this morning's experience is in fact the implicit and sedimented result of a multiplicity of experiences. This is the type of description one reads in the analyses of phenomenological philosophers when they refer to a situation, but also the kind of general lived experience we collect when leading a semistructured interview. For example, in §27 of his *Ideas I*, Husserl writes:

> I can let my attention wander away from the writing table which was just now seen and noticed, out through the unseen parts of the room which are behind my back, to the veranda, into the garden, to the children in the arbor, etc. (1983, p. 51)

In spite of the fact that the statement is in the present tense, contains a deictic ("this desk"), and is carried by an I situated in a concrete and familiar living space, all indicators of an embodied speech ("*prise de parole incarnée*," in Vermersch's words), the example remains generic and the description structural. In fact, the indicator of the structural generality of the experience consists in the mode of possibility, which begins in the description: "I *can* let my attention wander." Husserl might well have lived this experience dozens of times; he in fact reproduces for us a structural experience of attentional displacement, which we can enter, of course, and which we can even carry out for ourselves, in accordance with an imaginary mode of transposition of the phenomenological level of possibility inherent in the Husserlian proposition. Nevertheless, this attentional experience has nothing singular about it, and so as a consequence, the description remains general.

I suggest that you return to the precise moment when you woke up this morning and describe the micro-process of emerging into consciousness that was your awakening. By doing so, inviting you to go back to that moment precisely, I will receive a fine-tuned description of your experience of that moment. First describe the context: your lying position, what sort of room are you in (airy or close), the lighting, the heat, go back to the precise moment when the alarm clock rings, or whether you wake up before it rings, how you feel, what sort of emotional or cognitive state you are in, about your possible internal orientation movements in space, the speed (or absence of it) with which you recognize the environment, whether you are in a hotel room or anywhere that is not your usual environment.

In short, the explicitation interview, recently rebaptized microphenomenology, is a fine-tuned description technique of micro-processes both bodily (feelings, kinesthesis, proprioception, cardiac) and internal (cognitive, attentional, emotional, imaging) of a singular moment lived by a subject at a given time and in a given space. Placing themselves in the wake of the Husserlian discipline of the description of lived moments of consciousness, Pierre Vermersch (1999) and later Claire Petitmengin (2006, n.d.), whose specific purpose it was to situate the microphenomenological interview on a theoretical research scientific ground, chose a singular and fine-tuned description, which, compared with Husserl's approach, shifts the descriptive focus in two ways: (1) The lived experience is singular, content-laden, not generic and structural; (2) the granularity level of the description is reinforced, which gives rise to fine-tuned micro-sequences, to detailed emergence of lived processes and the highlighting of (quasi) synchronic moments of experience (Depraz, 2014, 2020).

In some interviews I led with health medical professionals in charge of patients with diabetes, eating disorders, and schizophrenic disorders, I was able to find out some specific features of chronicity in each of these so-called chronic diseases.[3]

Diabetes is a clearly somatic disease. Even though it has of course psychological effects for the patient, there is an objective irreducible reality of the sick physical body (of the *Körper* in Husserlian terms). Namely, there is a dysregulation of the blood sugar level, which implies a standard insulin therapy (above all with diabetes type 1). Here, the chronic dimension of the disease is obviously linked to a dependency, which goes hand in hand with immutability and permanency. Claire Gayet as a child psychiatrist at the Rouen Hospital (Normandie) expresses it clearly: "John is a patient with

[3] I was able to lead a microphenomenological interview with an anorexic teenager this year (April 2019), but I prefer to keep the data for a further article, where I will be able to gather other microphenomenological materials.

diabetes since he is 2 years old. He is now 15 years old"; "I meet him every two weeks to check his sugar level and give him his injection"; then she comes back to a specific moment during her last encounter with him: "I see you have trouble dealing with your disease, it is very compelling: you must live with it but you are frequently hospitalized because of acute complications of your diabetes." The time-properties of diabetes chronicity emerge from this first-person testimony: it is (1) physical bodily, (2) long term (permanent), (3) the condition deteriorates if treated with drugs, (4) it possibly stabilizes if constantly checked, (5) it restricts the subject's freedom, and it therefore often includes (6) relational difficulties and self-withdrawal attitudes.

At the other end of the spectrum of chronic diseases, schizophrenia is clearly a mental illness. Even though it may cause bodily disorders, there is an obvious and independent reality of the psychic endogenous disorders at play in it, and these express themselves in feelings of being persecuted, of losing the concrete and vital contact with daily reality, or in seeing hallucinated images or voices that other people do not see or hear. Unlike diabetes, which may be diagnosed very early during childhood, schizophrenic disorders typically appear with adolescence, at a moment where the body, the consciousness, and relational intersubjectivity grow and undergo intense transformations. Here, it becomes difficult to merely identify chronicity with motionlessness and an absence of change, since schizophrenic disorders often coincide with a crisis of delirium (also often linked with feelings of paranoiac persecutions). The emergency psychiatrist Frédéric Mauriac at the Charcot Hospital near Paris (Île-de-France) gives an acute account of the chronic schizophrenic disorders of a young man, 18 years old, while coming back to a specific moment within the discussion with his parents:

> I went again through all the components that seem to me were objectifying the disorders he had, that showed that he was in a delirium, that he was persecuted and that it was impossible to convince him, even though at different moments he seemed to be so "normal," and besides I said it to his parents: "you know, your son, he is really empathetic, you really feel he is quite normal, he has quite a standard behavior and at some points, when you start to enounce a limitation, then he breaks out."

Schizophrenic chronicity seems here to be rather linked to a kind of mobility made of patterns of reactivation of critical events in a quite similar form to how it occurs in traumatic time.

Halfway between diabetes and schizophrenia, eating disorders (mental anorexia) combine somatic uncontrollable expressions and feelings of self-control in quite a unique way. The objectified *Körper* symptom is the crucial weight loss, which often brings about hospitalization and needs to be medically treated like diabetes. But unlike diabetes, the *Körper* symptom is here the direct–indirect result of both a willful conscious and passive preconscious attitude of the subject who wants to control their body, so that the medical treatment becomes here a psychiatric therapy strongly dealing with relational disorders and which is also closely linked to body image, one's body and self-underestimation, itself directly connected to the underestimation of the others. Here, we typically have to do with an intersubjective *Leib-Körper*-disease, a relational disease of lived body consciousness.

Now, what is the specificity of the anorectic chronicity? It combines *Körper* (physical living body) and *Leib* (lived body) dimensions. For all that, does it combine the objectifying dimensions of diabetes (1) physical bodily, (2) long term namely permanent, (3) deterioration if not treated with drugs, (4) possible stabilization if constantly checked, and as lived effects: (5) restriction of the subject's freedom, and therefore often the inclusion of (6) relational difficulties and a self-withdrawal and the lived mental dimensions of schizophrenia (an apparent standard behavior that is suddenly and then recurrently broken by critical events, such as the pathological destructive reactivation process being typical of the mental ill-functioning)?

The teenager psychiatrist Amélie Robin at the Armentières-Lille Hospital in the north of France thus accounts for quite a specific moment when she meets the 16-year-old E., who has been hospitalized over and over during the last year. The specific moment corresponds to the moment when the doctor announces to her that she needs to be hospitalized again. The explicitation interview succeeds in bringing the doctor back to the very moment of the announcement, how she felt and how she saw E. felt:

> [S]he has a dull complexion, she hardly stands, I feel she needs to be hospitalized. I tell her it is important, she begins to cry and to show anger against me. Here I have this inner speech: she cries, she does not control anything any longer, her letting go is quite genuine. (A. Robin)

Thus, it seems to be that the specificity of this chronic disease lies in the intrinsic interplay between body and consciousness. But unlike diabetes and schizophrenia, which permanently lock up the subject in their disease, anorexia in some cases seems to have the possibility of evolving into recovery. In E.'s case indeed, her crying and her letting go, which are due to her second hospitalization, correspond to the first moment where she really began to feel better and to eventually recover after more than one year.

To sum up, all of the three chronic diseases we chose to explore in this research program include the hospital setting in their definition. Unlike neurosis, which may also be characterized as "chronic" due to its long-term and often incurable reality for the subject, the specific chronicity at play in our diseases seems to be linked to a "hospital chronicity": Indeed for the three patients we mentioned, hospital is a quasi-daily reality.

Conclusion

Let us draw now a few conclusive stances regarding the theme of chronicity on the one side, regarding the combined methodological dimensions I put to work on the other side.

With regard to "chronicity," we face an important question: Is there an invariant of chronicity given the heterogeneity of the chronic diseases? Beyond the negative content-connotation of chronicity, it rather corresponds to a long-term disease. Is the impossibility to change, that is, to heal, to recover, a characteristic feature of chronic diseases? I would say it is more a sort of stabilization than a sheer motionlessness, so there seems to be a kind of dynamic and possible evolution within chronicity, even though these patients remain "chronic" insofar as they will remain at least vulnerable and at most socially dependent. Another invariant structural feature would be its transverse meaning: Chronicity is not a property of many diseases, but the diseases are the properties of chronicity, which is as such a core pathology.

As far as the methodology is concerned, in this contribution I suggested combining different levels of experience and analysis in order to produce a refined concept of chronicity, experientially grounded: first, the clinical level, both psychopathological and systemic institutional; second, the phenomenological, philosophical, conceptual structural resources; third, the microphenomenological explicitation interviews and their specific analysis, of which I gave only a few segments. Such a combination articulates third-person philosophical categories, first-person existential clinical accounts, and genuine first-person microphenomenological accounts.

Even though I am well aware of the preliminary character of what is still a first sketch of a microphenomenology of chronicity,[4] I hope I was able with this modest contribution to open up a few aspects of what is intriguing and worth questioning in chronicity as a pathology as such.

[4] For a more extensive and systematic use of microphenomenological interviews correlated with physiological markers and philosophical categories, see Depraz and Desmidt (2018) and Depraz et al. (2017) in the framework of the ANR research project Emphiline *Surprise in Depression*.

Acknowledgment

This contribution relies on an ongoing research program (2016–2019) I am leading at the University of Rouen–Normandie called *Adochroniq: Les Adolescents face à la Maladie Chronique* (Adochroniq: Teenagers Facing Chronic Diseases) supported by the Normandy region, which I thank very much for its support.

References

Binswanger, L. (1960). *Melancholie und Manie* [Melancholy and mania]. Pfullingen, Germany: Neske.

Blanchet, A. (2003). *Dire et faire dire. L'entretien* [Saying and making say. The interview]. Paris, France: A. Colin.

Blankenburg, W. (1971). *Der Verlust der natürlichen Selbstverständlichkeit. Ein Beitrag zur Psychopathologie symptomarmer Schizophrenien* [The loss of natural self-evidence: A contribution to the study of symptom-poor schizophrenia]. Stuttgart, Germany: Enke.

de Mondeville, H. (1897). *La chirurgie* [The surgery] Vol. II. Paris, France: Librairie de Firmin Didot et Cie.

Depraz, N. (2014). *Husserl, psychologue?* [Husserl, a psychologist?]. In M. Gyemant (Ed.), *Psychologie et psychologisme* [Psychology and psychologism] (pp. 203–227). Paris, France: Vrin.

Depraz, N. (2016). De l'événement à la surprise: le trauma et son expression [From event to surprise: The trauma and its expression]. *Lectures du Monde Anglophone*, 2, 123–141.

Depraz, N. (2018). Trauma and phenomenology. *Eidos. A Journal for Philosophy of Culture*, 2(4), 53–74. doi: 10.26319/4716

Depraz, N. (2020). Husserlian phenomenology in the light of microphenomenology. In I. Apostolescu & C. Serban (Eds.), *Husserl, Kant and transcendental phenomenology*. Berlin, Germany: De Gruyter.

Depraz, N., & Desmidt, T. (2018). Cardiophenomenology: A refinement of neurophenomenology. *Phenomenology and the Cognitive Sciences*, 18(3), 493–507. doi: 10.1007/s11097-018-9590-y

Depraz, N., Gyemant, M., & Desmidt, T. (2017). A first-person analysis using third-person data as a generative method. A case study of surprise in depression. *Constructicvist Foundations*, 12(2), 190–203. Retrieved from http://constructivist.info/12/2/190.depraz

Freud, S. (1922). *Beyond the pleasure principle* (C. J. M. Hubback, Trans.). London, UK: The International Psychoanalytical Press. (Original work published 1920)

Fuchs, T. (2005). The phenomenology of body, space and time in depression. *Comprendre*, 15, 108–121.

Fuchs, T. (2018). La mémoire corporelle de la douleur et du traumatisme [The body memory of pain and trauma]. *Phanomenon*, 28, 127–145.

Gaucher, M. (Ed.). (1972). *Encyclopédie médicale Quillet. Nouvelle encyclopédie pratique de médecine et d'hygiène* [Quillet medical encyclopedia. New practical encyclopedia of medicine and hygiene]. Strasbourg, France: A. Quillet. (Original work published 1965)

Hammen, C., Shih, J., Altman, T., and Brennan, P. A. (2003). Interpersonal impairment and the prediction of depressive symptoms in adolescent children of depressed and nondepressed mothers. *Journal of the American Academy of Child & Adolescent Psychiatry*, 42(5), 571–577. doi: 10.1097/01.CHI.0000046829.95464.E5

Husserl, E. (1966). *Analyses concerning passive and active synthesis: Lectures on transcendental logic (1918-1926)* (A. J. Steinbock, Trans.). The Hague, Netherlands: Nijhoff.

Husserl, E. (1983). *Ideas pertaining to a pure phenomenology and to a phenomenological philosophy. First book: General introduction to a pure phenomenology* (F. Kersten, Trans.). The Hague, Netherlands: Martinus Nijhoff.

Husserl, E. (1991). *On the phenomenology of the consciousness of internal time (1893-1917)* (J. B. Brough, Trans.). Dordrecht, Netherlands: Kluwer Academic.

Kimura, B. (2000). *L'entre* [The between] (C. Vincent, Trans.). Grenoble, France: Jérôme Million. (Original work published 1988)

Lantéri-Laura, G. (1997). *La chronicité en psychiatrie* [Chronicity in psychiatry]. Paris, France: Empêcheurs de penser en rond.

Larrabee, M. J. (1995). The time of trauma: Husserl's phenomenology and post-traumatic stress disorder. *Human Studies*, 18(4), 351–366. doi: 10.1007/BF01318616

Normandin, L. (2013). *La vie des uns, le mépris des autres* [The life of the ones, the despise of the others]. Saint-Zénon, Canada: Louise Courteau.

Œuvray, K. (2010). *Rester dépendant des institutions médicosociales* [Remaining dependent on socio-medical institutions]. Paris, France: L'Harmattan.

Petitmengin, C. (2006). Describing one's subjective experience in the second person: An interview method for the science of consciousness. *Phenomenology and the Cognitive Sciences*, 5(3), 229–269. doi: 10.1007/s11097-006-9022-2

Petitmengin, C. (n.d.). *Micro-phenomenology*. Retrieved from www .microphenomenology.com/home

Rouillon, F. (Ed.). (2004). *Les troubles dépressifs récurrents* [Recurrent depressive disorders]. Nantes, France: John Libbey Eurotext.

Smith, J. A., Jarman, M., & Osborn, M. (1999). Doing interpretative phenomenological analysis. In M. Murray & K. Chamberlain (Eds.), *Qualitative health psychology* (pp. 219–240). Thousand Oaks, CA: Sage.

Stolorow, R. D. (2009). Trauma and human existence: The mutual enrichment of Heidegger's existential analytic and a psychoanalytic understanding of trauma. In R. Frei & D. M. Orange (Eds.), *Beyond postmodernism: New dimensions in theory and practice* (pp. 155–173). London, UK: Routledge.

Vermersch, P. (1999). Introspection as practice. *Journal of Consciousness Studies*, 6(2–3), 17–43.

Vermersch, P. (2011). *L'entretien d'explicitation* [The explicitation interview]. Paris, France: ESF. (Original work published 1994)

Wieviorka, S., & Kannas, S. (1989). Approche systémique et chronicité en milieu hospitalier psychiatrique [Systemic approach and chronicity in psychiatric hospitals]. *Evolution psychiatrique*, 54(3), 595–614.

Yaw, M. (2015). Husserl and PTSD: The traumatic correlate. *Journal of Phenomenological Psychology*, 46(2), 206–226. doi: 10.1163/15691624-12341293

5.1

Commentary on "Microphenomenology of Chronicity in Psychosomatic Diseases: Diabetes, Anorexia, and Schizophrenia"

Chronicity as Stigma

Samuel Thoma

In her article, "Microphenomenology of Chronicity in Psychosomatic Diseases: Diabetes, Anorexia, and Schizophrenia," the renowned French phenomenologist Natalie Depraz reflects upon chronicity as a category that might be common to different forms of chronic diseases. In my comment I will first summarize Depraz's analysis, which will then allow me to elaborate on some open questions that her chapter seems to leave us with.

Given the high relevance and prevalence of chronic diseases in medicine and society, Depraz tries to understand what we actually mean by chronicity in its different forms. Are we actually referring to one and the same chronicity when we speak of chronic diseases such as arterial hypertension, arthritis, or recurrent depression? Could chronicity maybe even be a disease category of its own, expressing itself in all these different disorders? To tackle this complex issue, Depraz opts for an interdisciplinary approach: On the one hand, she is pursuing a historically informed approach by investigating the evolution of the concept of chronicity in Western medicine, on the other hand, she looks at chronicity through a phenomenological lens. The core of her analysis, however, is empirical and consists in the analysis of semistructured interviews by the means of a qualitative phenomenological method (so-called *microphenomenological explicitation*), thus allowing us to grasp the factual experience of chronicity in its different forms. Moreover, it should be noted that Depraz's research project mainly focuses on chronic diseases in adolescents.

To begin with, Depraz notes that until now the concept of chronicity has been poorly studied, which seems baffling given the high prevalence of chronic diseases in Western societies. When focusing on the history of the concept of chronicity in Western medicine, she then focuses especially on the effects of long-term institutional treatment, especially on mental diseases and their chronification. What Depraz has in mind are patients living in a psychiatric clinic for many years without suffering from any acute disorder and who are both dependent on the institutional setting and cut off from the social world, in short: "patients whose illness is in a great part produced and at least reinforced by institutionalization in an asylum" (Depraz, 2021, p. 86).

Next, Depraz goes looking for a philosophical definition of chronicity. With reference to the epistemological origins of the concept in ancient Greek mythology, she defines chronicity as a particular form of lived time that can be observed in various chronic diseases. To specify this lived time, Depraz falls back on Husserl's analyses of temporal constitution in the realm of transcendental consciousness and Binswanger's adaptation of these analyses of lived time in depression and mania. Depraz's fundamental idea is that in the state of chronicity, the subject is sealed off from the eventfulness of the world. Chronicity thus would equal a stagnation of the subject in time and hence a stagnation of the unfolding of the subject's life.

The strength of Depraz's approach lies in her critical empirical examination of this hypothesis. She undertakes this examination in relation to three different disorders: diabetes, anorexia, and schizophrenia. Depraz justifies this selection by noting that diabetes is a bodily condition, schizophrenia a psychological one, and anorexia a psychosomatic one (Depraz, 2021).

In order to understand the different experiences of time connected with these three chronic illnesses, Depraz then analyses interviews with medical practitioners. Here, she brings *microphenomenological analysis* to bear, a newly developed qualitative methodology for the analysis of experiential sequences on the basis of phenomenological concepts. Through these interviews, Depraz comes to the conclusion that chronicity reveals itself in a variety of disorders across a kind of spectrum. Although Depraz believes that the analysis confirms, at least with some qualifications, her hypothesis that chronicity is a structure that encompasses a variety of illnesses, she also challenges the assumption that one might be inclined to make that chronic illnesses lead to a complete loss of temporal and existential dynamics. Depraz emphasizes that it is possible to observe the subject developing and adapting even while subject to chronic illnesses like anorexia.

The way the text ends by weighing these arguments is characteristic of Depraz's open style of argumentation in general. It is more important to her to pose questions than to provide answers. Her approach invites the reader to question their own preconceptions and to join in with her search.

However, Depraz's analysis can itself be challenged on a few points, and it is these that I would like to focus on now. For the further development of the research project, it would in my view be advisable to elaborate more on Depraz's initial remarks on the institutional production and reinforcement of chronicity and on the extent to which our common sense picture of chronicity might be formed by this institutional framework. I will henceforth restrict myself to the case of schizophrenia to give an example of what such an elaboration could look like.

The image of schizophrenia as a chronic disease accompanied by acute phases is first and foremost a historically rooted product of institutional perception and treatment practice. Hence, Depraz's definition of the *eidos* of chronicity that the author mainly elaborates at the level of the lived time of the individual subject is deemed to be insufficient since it brackets out this institutional and clinical framework. An almost classical critique of this pitfall of phenomenological psychiatry made by the German social psychiatrist Erich Wulff (1972, p. 5; my translation) seems to apply here, according to which "a seeming essence obscures social and natural reality." This, Wulff argues, leads to phenomenological approaches to psychiatry withdrawing from "the conflict with possible pathogenic factors in the familial or social environment, but also from that with institutions that reproduce illness, such as large psychiatric wards" (Wulff, 1972, p. 4; my translation).

If, however, one were to take such pathogenic factors into account, one would have to acknowledge that schizophrenia is in fact not a chronic disease. After many long-term studies on people with schizophrenia, we know today that about two-thirds of schizophrenic disorders ebb into states with no or only slight ongoing psychotic symptoms (cf. for instance Huber, 2005, pp. 322–336). If we add to this finding a consideration of contemporary concepts from recovery-oriented research, the actual number of chronic cases of schizophrenia would, in my view, turn out to be even lower. As is generally known, the recovery approach asserts that it is not the cessation of symptoms (e.g., no longer hearing voices or having delusions), but the experience of coherence and sense in life despite (or even because of) having symptoms that are decisive for recovery (cf. Davidson, 2003). Moreover and from an ethical point of view, it seems problematic in the case of adolescents to even frame schizophrenia as a chronic disease since only a few young subjects diagnosed with schizophrenia will ever become chronic, whereas all of them will have to deal with significant distress on account of such a categorical medical verdict.

As a result, I have the impression that the author herself is not reflecting on her own (institutionally framed) premises on the issue of schizophrenia. This seems problematic since she herself claims not to describe her own experience or her premises but to actually describe the experience of a schizophrenic subject. This problem becomes even more virulent when instead of interviewing people diagnosed with schizophrenia (or another apparently chronic disease) Depraz in fact interviews the professionals diagnosing these people. She thereby risks again reproducing institutional and professional premises about chronicity instead of letting us see the subject's own experience of chronicity.[1]

To avoid this risk, I would strongly recommend to integrate people diagnosed with schizophrenia into the research process in terms of a user-involved or even user-controlled approach (Rose, 2003). Proactively including psychiatry's users in the research process would in my view lead to a stronger focus both on recovery theory (see above) and on the stigmatizing power of the medical concept of chronicity in terms of *epistemic violence* (cf. Spivak, 1988). Moreover, for a more comprehensive perspective on the issue, ethnographic analyses on the institutional construction of chronicity (von Peter, 2016) could be equally useful as a phenomenology of stigma that I would like to sketch out in the following passage.

Before I do so, let me clarify that I don't mean to reduce chronic diseases to a mere mirage produced by psychiatric institutions and their knowledges. *There is such a thing as chronicity* in terms of an ongoing individual, familial, and social suffering, and we know that for instance in the case of chronic schizophrenia this suffering leads to a high suicide rate, mostly linked to the experience of solitude and feelings of inferiority (Škodlar, Tomori, & Parnas, 2008). But chronicity also takes the form of a social stigma that might aggravate or even co-constitute chronic suffering, especially through the mediation of an internalized stigma. This is why we also need a phenomenology of stigma to actually understand the (inter-)subjective constitution of chronicity.

"I'm afraid you won't make it without life-long medication." This is what a colleague of mine once said to one of my patients diagnosed with schizophrenia. This patient, who despite hearing voices from time to time, has in fact lived without medication for the last few years. He told me that retrospectively this professional assessment was for him no less violent than the compulsory measures he had undergone in psychiatric clinics in acute moments of his psychosis. My colleague's assessment felt to him like an omen, like a shadow that would haunt him for the rest of his life: Would my colleague have turned out to be right if, by not taking medication, my patient somehow ended up "failing" in his life? What would "not making it" mean? As a psychiatrist, this makes me wonder: Did we, did psychiatry maybe turn this man into one of the chronics that Depraz is referring to (p. 83–85), by in fact offering him only two possibilities, both equally desperate: not

[1] Hence, what Depraz so far seems to deliver is in fact not an analysis of the subjective experience of chronicity but of its institutional construction (or constitution).

"making it" without medication or "making it" with medication – thereby forcing him to undergo medical side effects (e.g., being constantly sedated, or feeling stiff), side effects that in return we as professionals would all too often interpret as another proof of his chronicity?

Phenomenology could help us to understand how the medical diagnosis of a chronic disease, such as the one I have just given an example of, inscribes itself into the embodied experience of a person and how it might transform a person's sense of self. A good starting point might be Sartre's theory of the objectifying gaze of the other, whose impact on a person's self-understanding Sartre famously exemplified in his studies on anti-Semitism and Jewish identity, and on Jean Genet (Sartre, 1971, 1995). Fanon applied Sartre's theory of the gaze to his experience of being racialized as a black person: In *Black Skin, White Masks*, Fanon (1967, p. 111) reports being stared at by a child, who commented "Tiens, un nègre!"("Look, a Negro!"). He then continues to analyze how this racializing gaze inscribes itself into his body schema, structuring his being-in-the-world. Although one should not confuse the social category of race with mental illness, we could nonetheless look for analogous situations experienced by patients in clinical encounters, for instance when being hospitalized and being considered as "another one of these chronic schizophrenics (or addicts or anorectics, etc.)."

In line with Depraz's approach, the effects of such a stigma could be taken into account in terms of lived time: The interpretative eidos of "the chronic" expressed within institutional framework and applied to a patient seems to be *already there* and *already valid*, obliterating the patients' own intimate experience of their states of mind hitherto (e.g., "I'm just going through a crisis and I don't feel chronically ill."). They get the sense that their personal experience arrives "too late," that it is invalid vis-à-vis the medical knowledge that claims to have already understood them.[2] But of course, these hypotheses need further empirical investigation and should also be verified with regard to the other examples given by Depraz.[3] In any case, Depraz's method of microphenomenological analysis could prove very fruitful for this purpose if applied to interviews with psychiatry users/patients.

Depraz's research project has laid the grounds for a comprehensive understanding of chronicity. With my theses here, I tried to suggest a way to supplement this project. This could allow us to grasp chronicity as a

[2] In a similar vein, Al-Saji (2016) analyzes the experience of the racializing look (as in the case of Fanon) as a feeling of "lateness."

[3] For an analysis of anorexia combining phenomenology and social science, see for instance Marcinski (2014).

phenomenon that is both experienced by the subject and constituted by medical institutions and our society. Last but not least, such an approach could help us not only to understand chronicity but also to avoid the suffering it may cause.

References

Al-Saji, A. (2016). A phenomenology of racialized lateness. In I. Marcinski & H. Landweer (Eds.), *Dem Erleben auf der Spur: Feminismus und Phänomenologie* [Following the trail of experience: Feminism and phenomenology] (pp. 303–318). Bielefeld, Germany: Transcript.

Davidson, L. (2003). *Living outside mental illness: Qualitative studies of recovery in schizophrenia*. New York, NY: New York University Press.

Depraz, N. (2021). Microphenomenology of chronicity in psychosomatic diseases: Diabetes, anorexia, schizophrenia. In C. Tewes & G. Stanghellini (Eds.), *Time and body: Phenomenological and psychopathological approaches* (pp. 82–97). Cambridge, UK: Cambridge University Press.

Fanon, F. (1967). *Black skin, white masks* (C. L. Markmann, Trans.). New York, NY: Grove Press.

Huber, G. (2005). *Psychiatrie: Lehrbuch für Studium und Weiterbildung* [Textbook of psychiatry] (7th ed.). Stuttgart, Germany: Schattauer.

Marcinski, I. (2014). *Anorexie – Phänomenologische Betrachtung einer Essstörung* [Anorexia – Phenomenological analysis of an eating disorder]. Freiburg, Germany: Alber.

Rose, D. (2003). Collaborative research between users and professionals: Peaks and pitfalls. *The Psychiatric Bulletin*, 27(11), 404–406. doi:10.1192/pb.27.11.404

Sartre, J.-P. (1971). *Saint Genet: Actor and martyr* (B. Frechtman, Trans.). New York, NY: New American Library.

Sartre, J.-P. (1995). *Anti-Semite and Jew: An exploration of the etiology of hate* (G. J. Becker, Trans.). New York, NY: Schocken.

Škodlar, B., Tomori, M., & Parnas, J. (2008). Subjective experience and suicidal ideation in schizophrenia. *Comprehensive Psychiatry*, 49(5), 482–488. doi: 10.1016/j.comppsych.2008.02.008

Spivak, G. C. (1988). Can the subaltern speak? In C. Nelson & L. Grossberg (Eds.), *Marxism and the interpretation of culture* (pp. 271–316). London, UK: Macmillan Education.

von Peter, S. (2016). *Die Aktualisierung von "Chronizität" in der institutionellen Praxis* [The actualization of "chronicity" in institutional practice] (Doctoral dissertation, Free University of Berlin). Retrieved from http://dx.doi.org/10.17169/refubium-4996

Wulff, E. (1972). *Psychiatrie und Klassengesellschaft: Zur Begriffs- und Sozialkritik der Psychiatrie und Medizin* [Psychiatry and class society: A conceptual and social critique of psychiatry and medicine]. Frankfurt am Main, Germany: Fischer-Athenäum.

6

Time and Embodiment in the Process of Psychotherapy: A Dynamical Systems Perspective

Wolfgang Tschacher

Introduction

The goal of this chapter is to develop a quantitative approach to the exploration of psychotherapy. I will sketch a dynamical modeling method with a focus on high-resolution time series. These time series allow mapping therapy processes at the timescale of seconds, namely, the exact timescale of consciousness, which resides in the here-and-now, in the present moment. Such nowness therefore constitutes the core of the social exchange between therapist and client. In short, I am emphasizing the significance of time and of the body for this specific type of social interaction, psychotherapy.

Time in Psychotherapy

At the risk of arguing for the obvious and self-evident, my general claim is that time is the core of psychotherapy. Let me briefly list reasons that speak for a time-based, that is, dynamical, approach to psychotherapy. Some reasons simply derive from the definition of psychotherapy: Psychotherapy is defined as a social interaction, most often between one therapist and his or her client, where the interaction induces a client's learning (and sometimes also learning on the side of the therapist). Learning can come in the guise of adopting new behaviors, new emotional responses, and cognitive insights, or in the guise of unlearning problematic behaviors, emotions, and cognitions. Thus, psychotherapy is all about dynamics and change, and it must therefore be described and explored as a process, that is, generally by how variables are changing along the time dimension (Tschacher & Haken, 2019). In line with this proposed dynamical understanding of psychotherapy, therapeutic change is achieved by the application of interventions, be they specific interventions, that is, therapy techniques (Tschacher, Junghan, & Pfammatter, 2014), or non-specific interventions, that is, contextual common factors (*Wirkmechanismen*: Grawe, 1998; Wampold, 2015).

Further reasons come from first-person accounts of therapeutic change: Dynamics is also at the heart of the phenomenological aspects of therapeutic interactions, that is, the therapist's and client's experiences. The temporal perspective is particularly crucial for an understanding of consciousness – people can only be fully conscious *now*, that is, during the present moment (Stern, 2004). The living person and the psychological self exist in the now. The experience of this present time has some duration; it is unlike the knife's edge of clock time in physics, but rather extended. Any kind of experience, perception, or emotionality occurs at a specific timescale at the range of few seconds, which represents "a strict correlate of present-time consciousness" (Varela, 1999). The psychotherapy session is the node in space and time where therapist and client create and share their mutual therapeutic presence (Geller & Porges, 2014). We have claimed that experiencing this shared nowness is essential for psychotherapy to be efficient (Tschacher, Ramseyer, & Pfammatter, 2020). Nowness can be defined not only for psychotherapy but also for any social interaction. This has led to the measure of the "social present" (Tschacher, Ramseyer, & Koole, 2018), the temporal interval during which two persons are significantly coupled. Thus, the first-person dynamics of experiencing can be derived and modeled by third-person durational measures. The procedure to define the social present will be introduced technically later in this chapter.

A research prerequisite of a dynamical approach in psychotherapy is that one develops the means for modeling that behavioral and experiential dynamics. In other words, we need to model and operationalize them. In Tschacher and Haken (2019), we have described the explicit steps of a dynamical modeling approach (Figure 6.1).

- We first have to describe the processes of interest, for example, by repeated measurements of observables such as movement behavior, physiological signals, or verbal expressions. This means acquisition of time series, preferably dense and high-resolution data, which address the delicate phenomena of interest occurring at a timescale of seconds.
- Second, a process model must be chosen. There is a large choice of process models, which may be linear or nonlinear. For principal reasons, all models should include a stochastic and a deterministic term to account for the perennial mix of chance and causation in the observable world. All models must be grounded in observation.
- Third, dynamical modeling on the basis of observations allows predicting changes.

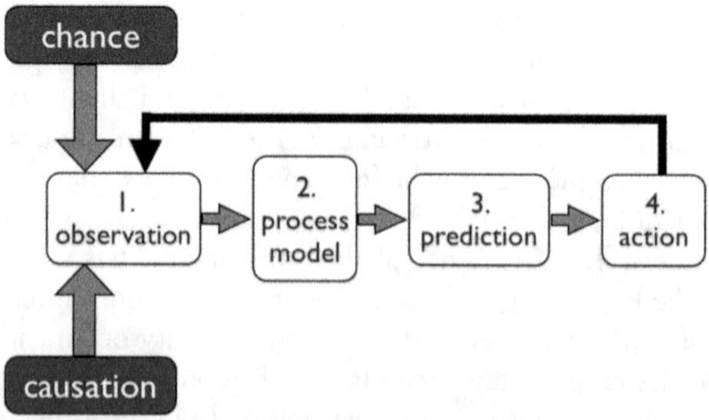

Figure 6.1 A dynamical model of psychotherapy is based on observation, which by way of modeling generates predictions and allows actions based on predictions (after Tschacher & Haken, 2019).

- Fourth and on the basis of prediction, goal-directed actions may be performed. To close the loop, action changes the observations that can be made, thereby initiating new cycles of the process model.

The loops connecting description and prediction, and the role of causation and chance in these loops, are an adequate starting point for modeling the dynamics of psychotherapy scientifically. At a different timescale and level, such circular processes at the same time provide a principle for understanding what sentient beings continuously do in their everyday environments – the respective principle of cognition is called "active inference" or "predictive coding" (Hobson & Friston, 2014). Similar ideas were previously introduced as the reafference principle by von Holst and Mittelstaedt (1950). In the words of enactive cognitive science, action–perception loops are the cornerstone of adaptive functioning and of intelligent cognition. With each loop, better models lead to more precise prediction and more adequate actions. The general goal of cognition via action-perception loops is thus to minimize the error of prediction. Friston (2011) further advanced this idea in the context of his free-energy principle of the brain.

Why emphasize the interplay of causation and chance in the context of the dynamical approach in psychotherapy? Addressing causation, that is, causal-deterministic effects in and of psychotherapy, is part of the conventional picture of psychotherapy because the goal of therapeutic interventions is to facilitate beneficial changes of experiencing and/or behavior in the client, and the therapist's task is to become instrumental in alleviating symptoms and problems. Thus, the application of interventions with such goals obviously constitutes the deterministic effect in any kind of therapeutic

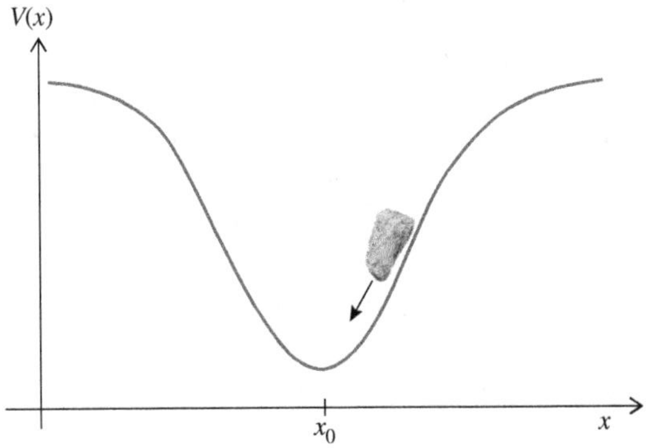

Figure 6.2 An attractor ("valley") is a dynamical deterministic structure that exerts forces on a variable x. The present state of x is metaphorically denoted by the "stone" on the slope of the "valley." The forces make the system state change until it reaches the minimum of the potential $V(x)$, which is located at x_0.

setting. In the dynamical approach, deterministic effects are represented by the so-called attractors (Figure 6.2), attractor being an abstract concept of dynamical systems theory that describes the forces that act on the states of some variable x (Tschacher & Haken, 2019). One may equate x with a client's depression value – then the effect of the attractor describes a client's dynamics where depression values of x_0 are stable even in the face of external perturbations. If x_0 is high, Figure 6.2 stands for a psychopathological problem, and the therapist's task is to shift or destruct the attractor through appropriate interventions. The effect of attractor dynamics is to exert forces to a system that are always directed toward the minimum of the potential. The potential function $V(x)$ is a direct equivalent to Friston's free energy.

Deterministic causation is, however, only one side of the coin of psychotherapy. The other side is chance, that is, the randomness and stochasticity of processes relevant for therapy. Chance has much less been a topic of theories and models of psychotherapy. Yet chance enters psychotherapy processes inevitably and in many different ways, for example, as extratherapeutic variables – according to Lambert (2013), extratherapeutic "Client/Life" variables explain 40 percent of treatment outcome. All states of an individual client can be subject to environmental fluctuations, that is, to unpredictable, random events. By their nature, random events have a destructive impact on all structures and all ordered patterns of system dynamics, such as corrosion destroys metal surfaces and the shuffling of a deck of cards destroys the initial sequence of the cards. Yet the effects of chance inputs on treatment outcome need not always be negative

– destruction of a psychopathological attractor, which keeps a client at an unfortunate x_0 of depression, would on the contrary be considered beneficial. Thus, next to the deterministic interventions, we must be aware of "stochastic interventions" (Tschacher & Haken, 2019). One example of such an intervention is boundary regulation, that is, procedures that can shield sensitive clients from being perturbed by chance events. In other cases, the loosening of boundary regulation may help expose clients to random new stimuli and thus destabilize preexisting attractors.

A dynamical approach that integrates both causation and chance in a comprehensive dynamical model is the Fokker–Planck equation, which was extensively discussed in Tschacher and Haken (2019). Applications derived from this equation allow detecting and visualizing the attractors by their potential functions (as shown in an idealized form in Figure 6.2); the potential function of an attractor can be computed on the basis of the observed empirical time series data.

The Body in Psychotherapy

In recent decades, researchers and theorists have increasingly claimed that cognition cannot be fully conceived without addressing the body of a cognitive agent. The embodiment turn took place in different fields of science, sometimes quite independently. Embodiment became a new trend in the field of artificial intelligence and computer science as a result of the field's failure to build and program intelligent machines (Pfeifer & Scheier, 1999) – consequently leading to a focus on robotics (i.e., embodied artificial agents) and a renewed interest in neural networks and deep learning. In cognitive science, the emphasis on embodied cognition signaled a renunciation of the symbol systems hypothesis of the mind (Newell, 1980). At about the same time, embodied cognition also appeared on the agenda of social psychology (Cacioppo, Priester, & Berntson, 1993; Niedenthal, Barsalou, Winkielman, Krauth-Gruber, & Ric, 2005) and, with some delay, clinical psychology (Koole & Tschacher, 2016). Aspects of embodiment have even begun playing an increasing role in various disciplines of the humanities (Alloa, Bedorf, Grüny, & Klass, 2012; Tröndle et al., 2020), notwithstanding the fact that the bodily corporeal constitution of the mind was proposed already by phenomenological philosophers such as Husserl, Heidegger, and Merleau-Ponty in the early twentieth century (Fuchs, 2016).

Embodiment is commonly defined as the bidirectional (reciprocal) interaction between mind and body. Bidirectionality means that, first, motor behavior, nonverbal body expressions, and physiology are results of mental and emotional processes, as is common wisdom; but second and in addition to this, mental processes are also shaped by bodily behavior, which is often less evident. The first direction of influences, from mind to body, commonly occurs with full awareness of the individual, whereas the second type of direction, from body to mind, often happens implicitly and outside the agent's awareness.

"Implications of embodiment" (Tschacher & Bergomi, 2011) are that these bidirectional influences between mental states and bodily states are found throughout psychology, especially also in psychotherapy. Hence, psychotherapy encompasses not only Sigmund Freud's "talking cure" nor only the cognitive-behavioral restructuring of beliefs, but the process of psychotherapy importantly also involves exchanges at the nonverbal level of participants in therapy. The same is true for psychopathological diseases: Schizophrenia spectrum disorder, for instance, is characterized by certain psychomotor abnormalities (Tschacher, Giersch, & Friston, 2017), so that schizophrenia may constitute a disembodiment disorder (Fuchs & Schlimme, 2009; Martin, Koch, Hirjak, & Fuchs, 2016). The longstanding focus on the cognitive deficits found in psychopathological diseases today appears one-sided.

Recently, the concept of nonverbal synchrony has entered psychotherapy research (Ramseyer & Tschacher, 2011), and this is where the dynamical approach and the embodiment turn become intrinsically connected. Synchronization is observed ubiquitously in a large number of dynamical systems, be they physical (Nicolis & Prigogine, 1977), biological (Rodriguez et al., 1999), or social (Grammer, Kruck, & Magnusson, 1998). Synchronization means that previously independent components of a complex dynamical system can become "entrained," that is, increasingly coupled. "Components" may be the participants in a social interaction system. Synchronization events are typically found in contexts, where patterns of a complex system spontaneously emerge by a process of self-organization (Haken, 1977). Such self-organized synchrony presents the signs of a stable dynamics – synchrony has all the properties of an attractor.

Nonverbal Synchrony and the Social Present

In psychotherapy, synchrony is commonly seen in behavioral time series of therapist and client monitored during sessions. Many studies have used time series of body movement (Ramseyer & Tschacher, 2011; Tschacher, Rees, & Ramseyer, 2014) or physiological recordings (Tschacher & Meier,

2020) to study nonverbal synchrony. Body movement and physiology provide measures that can be continuously acquired with high sampling rates in the range of 20 Hz and more, from both participants of a social interaction. Based on such "big" datasets, the synchrony of patient and therapist can be estimated using the cross-correlation function (windowed cross-correlation [WCC]: Boker, Xu, Rotondo, & King, 2002). Surrogate tests can be applied to determine the statistical significance of the WCC correlations (Moulder, Boker, Ramseyer, & Tschacher, 2018). Such computations are "big data" applications and rather complex. The various signatures of synchrony obtained by the apps surrogate synchrony (SUSY) and surrogate concordance (SUCO) and the corresponding computational steps are detailed in Tschacher and Meier (2020).

A recent extension of this methodology is to quantify the social present based on SUSY – how long, in seconds, are interacting people significantly coordinated and synchronized? To derive the average social present of an interaction (such as a session of psychotherapy), the cross-correlations are computed across the therapist's and client's time series, and plotted within a window of 10-second extension, from lag −5 seconds through to +5 seconds (Figure 6.3). The time series data in Figure 6.3 consisted of both individuals' respiration activity measured by breathing belts throughout a psychotherapy session. Then, the cross-correlations of shuffled surrogates were obtained. Surrogates are time series that consist of the same data that were actually measured, but their temporal sequence is randomly generated by a permutation procedure called shuffling, like the shuffling of a deck of cards. As the shuffling procedure can be performed many times, the surrogate cross-correlations are aggregated across many surrogate time series (in Figure 6.3 obtained from $n = 920$ surrogates). In the example of Figure 6.3, the social present had a duration of approximately 4.3 seconds.

What does a result such as the one presented in Figure 6.3 mean? First, it indicates that the therapist's and client's breathing in this specific therapy session (session code: vreme2) was synchronized because the area under the peaked curve was higher than the curve of surrogates. Surrogate data can be considered as a control condition because surrogates consist of the actual empirical data, which were however randomized with respect to their temporal sequences. In this case, surrogate cross-correlations varied around a mean of zero on the ordinate axis. The social present had over 4-second duration – thus, on average, the therapist's and client's breathing was synchronized for 4 seconds throughout this session. And finally, the peak of this synchronized breathing was not centered in zero but shifted

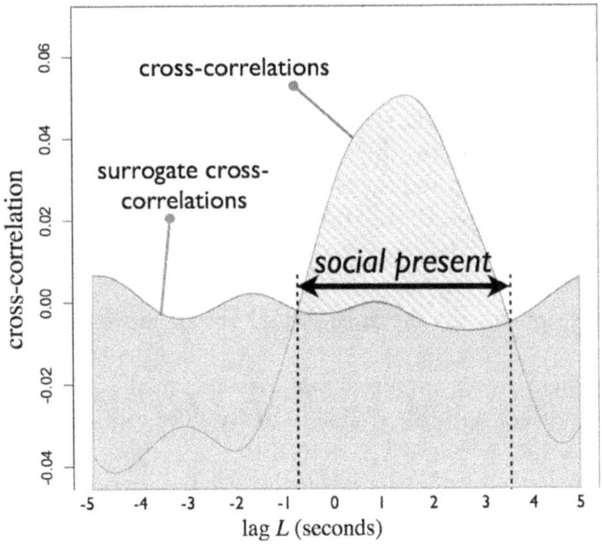

Figure 6.3 Cross-correlation function of therapist's and client's respiration time series (denoted "cross-correlations"). The aggregated cross-correlations of randomly permutated ("surrogate cross-correlations") are printed as a smooth curve with values of about zero. The social present is defined as the duration of cross-correlations exceeding surrogate cross-correlations.

to the right, which suggests that the therapist tended to lead, whereas her client followed her with an average time delay of approximately 1.5 seconds.

A Quantification of the Social Present in a Sample of Therapy Sessions

The dataset of the complete sample consists of two psychotherapy courses conducted by a female psychologist with two different female clients in a day-hospital setting at a university psychiatric hospital in Switzerland. Figure 6.3 displays an example taken from this sample. The therapist administered psychodynamic psychotherapy in seated position. Sessions were held at weekly intervals and had total durations of up to 60 minutes. Forty-seven sessions were monitored (37 sessions vreni, 10 vreme). Respiratory behavior was registered by a strain-sensitive belt attached over the diaphragm above the clothing. The breathing data of both therapist and client were recorded using the Vitaport-4 ambulatory-measurement device (Mutz & Becker, 2006) at a sampling rate of 16 Hz. Additionally, after each session, session report questionnaires were filled out by the therapist and the client independently, which yielded six scales (Flückiger, Regli, Zwahlen, Hostettler, & Caspar, 2010). These self-report scales concerned the therapist's evaluation of the quality of therapeutic relationship (Alliance_th), of the patient's cooperation (Cooperation_th), and of progress in therapy (Progress_th). Three other scales captured the client's assessment of the therapy session: the quality of therapeutic relationship (Alliance_cl), own well-being (Well-being_cl), and therapy progress (Progress_cl). For example, items loading on the scale Alliance_cl are these: "Today I felt comfortable in the relationship with the therapist," and "The therapist and I understand each other."

The complete study analyzed four physiological signals of therapist and client to detect signs of physiological synchrony (Tschacher & Meier, 2020). We found, among other results, that breathing behavior in these therapy sessions was significantly synchronized in-phase. This means that inhalation and exhalation of therapist and client were coordinated with an effect size of ES = 0.62. This respiratory synchrony likely occurred outside the awareness of therapist and clients, who were not instructed to observe or even imitate each other's breathing. We may assume that this synchrony was a signature of embodied cognition in the therapy session. In the present chapter, however, I am interested in the social present that can be derived from the breathing synchrony we found. The mean duration of the social present across the 47 sessions was 5.3 seconds (SD = 1.87 seconds). This value was yielded with SUSY default parameter settings of window size 10 seconds; the segment size for the segment-wise shuffling of surrogates was 30 seconds; and the number of surrogates generated for the analysis of each session was fixed at a maximum of 1,000.

I additionally conducted a hierarchical regression analysis with "therapy" (codes: vreme, vreni) as a random effect and the six scales of session report questionnaires as fixed effects in order to predict the respiratory "social present," which served as the dependent variable. I found that Alliance_cl was a significant predictor ($t = 3.00$, $p < 0.01$) of the social present. This indicates that a longer duration of breathing synchrony, that is, longer social present, was associated with a better therapeutic relationship as rated by the client.

This result may show that the dynamical approach in connection with embodied process measures can yield promising insights – the quality of the therapeutic alliance is one of the most effective change mechanisms recognized by psychotherapy research. I used this result, however, only for the purpose of illustration, not for claiming evidence of a general association between the social present and alliance quality.

Discussion

Time is the key to an understanding of psychotherapy. This is true for obvious reasons because psychotherapy is about changing the behavior, cognitions, and emotions of a client in a relatively short time. With this minimal description of psychotherapy in mind, a minimal dynamical approach may consider time by simply comparing attributes of a client at the initiation of therapy to the attributes at the end of therapy. This is of course the approach of conventional effectiveness and outcome studies of psychotherapy research. I am arguing, however, for a more rigorous dynamical and time-related approach, one that addresses the very moment of therapeutic changes, at the timescale of few seconds.

Why study the dynamics of client and therapist at this high-resolution timescale? The most important reason is that consciousness resides exclusively in the here-and-now, with nowness consisting of a short moment extended over just a few seconds (Pöppel, 2009; Varela, 1999). When we wish to monitor and explore these fleeting but essential moments in a continuous fashion and with quantitative methods, the usual questionnaire-based methods of psychology are largely inadequate. What is needed instead is a big-data time-series approach. Whenever this approach can be implemented, a direct empirical access to the relevant phenomena can come within reach. In support of this dynamical endeavor, we can make use of the introduced concepts of dynamical systems theory, such as attractor and coupling. This will allow studying relevant psychological phenomena such as the stability of mental and psychopathological states as attractors. The concept of coupling unlocks the social phenomenon of interpersonal synchronization, which is known to be essential for psychotherapy to work. From measures of synchronization one may even derive the social present, as a signature of nowness and, possibly, consciousness.

All of these research goals depend on just two prerequisites. First, I consider as essential and necessary that we make use of a dynamical modeling approach with time as an explicit dimension. Second, we need to rely on monitoring with high sampling rates as can be achieved with movement and physiological variables. In this respect, the embodiment stance in psychology is an indispensable second prerequisite. In a nutshell, what is required for this research approach to unfold is time and the body.

References

Alloa, E., Bedorf, T., Grüny, C., & Klass, T. N. (Eds.). (2012). *Leiblichkeit: Geschichte und Aktualität eines Konzepts* [Corporeality: History and actuality of a concept]. Tübingen, Germany: Mohr Siebeck.

Boker, S. M., Xu, M., Rotondo, J. L., & King, K. (2002). Windowed cross-correlation and peak picking for the analysis of variability in the association between behavioral time series. *Psychological Methods*, 7(3), 338–355. doi:10.1037/1082-989X.7.3.338

Cacioppo, J. T., Priester, J. R., & Berntson, G. G. (1993). Rudimentary determinants of attitudes. II: Arm flexion and extension have differential effects on attitudes. *Journal of Personality and Social Psychology*, 65(1), 5–17. doi:10.1037/0022-3514.65.1.5

Flückiger, C., Regli, D., Zwahlen, D., Hostettler, S., & Caspar, F. (2010). Der Berner Patienten- und Therapeutenstundenbogen 2000 [The Bern patient and therapist session report 2000]. *Zeitschrift für Klinische Psychologie und Psychotherapie: Forschung und Praxis*, 39(2), 71–79. doi:10.1026/1616-3443/a000015

Friston, K. J. (2011). Embodied inference: or "I think therefore I am, if I am what I think". In W. Tschacher & C. Bergomi (Eds.), *The implications of embodiment – Cognition and communication* (pp. 89–125). Exeter, UK: Imprint Academic.

Fuchs, T. (2016). *Das Gehirn - ein Beziehungsorgan. Eine phänomenologisch-ökologische Konzeption* [The brain – A mediating organ. A phenomenological-ecological conception] (5th ed.). Stuttgart, Germany: Kohlhammer.

Fuchs, T., & Schlimme, J. E. (2009). Embodiment and psychopathology: A phenomenological perspective. *Current Opinion in Psychiatry*, 22(6), 570–575. doi:10.1097/YCO.0b013e3283318e5c

Geller, S. M., & Porges, S. W. (2014). Therapeutic presence: Neurophysiological mechanisms mediating feeling safe in therapeutic relationships. *Journal of Psychotherapy Integration*, 24(3), 178–192. doi:10.1037/a0037511

Grammer, K., Kruck, K. B., & Magnusson, M. S. (1998). The courtship dance: Patterns of nonverbal synchronization in opposite-sex encounters. *Journal of Nonverbal Behavior*, 22(1), 3–29. doi:10.1023/A:1022986608835

Grawe, K. (1998). *Psychologische Therapie* [Psychological therapy]. Göttingen, Germany: Hogrefe.

Haken, H. (1977). *Synergetics – An introduction. Nonequilibrium phase-transitions and self-organization in physics, chemistry and biology.* Berlin, Germany: Springer.

Hobson, J. A., & Friston, K. J. (2014). Consciousness, dreams, and inference. The Cartesian theatre revisited. *Journal of Consciousness Studies*, 21(1), 6–32.

Koole, S. L., & Tschacher, W. (2016). Synchrony in psychotherapy: A review and an integrative framework for the therapeutic alliance. *Frontiers in Psychology*, 7, 1–17. doi:10.3389/fpsyg.2016.00862

Lambert, M. J. (2013). The efficacy and effectiveness of psychotherapy. In M. J. Lambert (Ed.), *Bergin and Garfield's handbook of psychotherapy and behavior change* (pp. 169–218). New York, NY: Wiley.

Martin, L. A., Koch, S. C., Hirjak, D., & Fuchs, T. (2016). Overcoming disembodiment: The effect of movement therapy on negative symptoms in schizophrenia – A multicenter randomized controlled trial. *Frontiers in Psychology*, 7, 1–14. doi:10.3389/fpsyg.2016.00483

Moulder, R. G., Boker, S. M., Ramseyer, F., & Tschacher, W. (2018). Determining synchrony between behavioral time series: An application of surrogate data generation for establishing falsifiable null-hypotheses. *Psychological Methods*, 23(4), 757–773. doi:10.1037/met0000172

Mutz, G., & Becker, K. (2006). Ambulante physiologische Messgeräte – Entwicklung und Stand der Technik am Beispiel von Vitaport und Varioport [Ambulatory physiological measurement devices – Development and state of the art exemplified by Vitaport and Varioport]. In U. W. Ebner-Priemer (Ed.), *Ambulantes psychophysiologisches Monitoring – neue Perspektiven und Anwendungen* [Ambulatory psychophysiological monitoring – New perspectives and applications] (pp. 137–147). Frankfurt am Main, Germany: Peter Lang.

Newell, A. (1980). Physical symbol systems. *Cognitive Science*, 4, 135–183.

Nicolis, G., & Prigogine, I. (1977). *Self-Organization in nonequilibrium systems: From dissipative structures to order through fluctuations*. New York, NY: Wiley-Interscience.

Niedenthal, P. M., Barsalou, L. W., Winkielman, P., Krauth-Gruber, S., & Ric, F. (2005). Embodiment in attitudes, social perception, and emotion. *Personality and Social Psychology Review*, 9(3), 184–211. doi:10.1207/s15327957pspr0903_1

Pfeifer, R., & Scheier, C. (1999). *Understanding intelligence*. Cambridge, MA: Massachusetts Institute of Technology Press.

Pöppel, E. (2009). Pre-semantically defined temporal windows for cognitive processing. *Philosophical Transactions of the Royal Society of London B: Biological Sciences*, 364(1525), 1887–1896. doi:10.1098/rstb.2009.0015

Ramseyer, F., & Tschacher, W. (2011). Nonverbal synchrony in psychotherapy: Coordinated body-movement reflects relationship quality and outcome. *Journal of Consulting and Clinical Psychology*, 79(3), 284–295. doi:10.1037/a0023419

Rodriguez, E., George, N., Lachaux, J. P., Martinerie, J., Renault, B., & Varela, F. J. (1999). Perception's shadow: Long-distance synchronization of human brain activity. *Nature*, 397(6718), 430–433. doi:10.1038/17120

Stern, D. N. (2004). *The present moment in psychotherapy and everyday life*. New York, NY: Norton.

Tröndle, M., Greenwood, S., Ramakrishnan, C., Uhde, F., Egermann, H., & Tschacher, W. (2020). Integrated methods: A call for integrative and interdisciplinary aesthetics research. In O. Vartanian (Ed.), *Oxford handbook of empirical aesthetics*. Oxford, UK: Oxford University Press. doi:10.1093/oxfordhb/9780198824350.001.0001

Tschacher, W., & Bergomi, C. (Eds.). (2011). *The implications of embodiment: Cognition and communication*. Exeter, UK: Imprint Academic.

Tschacher, W., Giersch, A., & Friston, K. J. (2017). Embodiment and schizophrenia: A review of implications and applications. *Schizophrenia Bulletin*, 43(4), 745–753. doi:10.1093/schbul/sbw220

Tschacher, W., & Haken, H. (2019). *The process of psychotherapy: Causation and chance*. Cham, Switzerland: Springer. doi:10.1007/978-3-030-12748-0

Tschacher, W., Junghan, U., & Pfammatter, M. (2014). Towards a taxonomy of common factors in psychotherapy – Results of an expert survey. *Clinical Psychology & Psychotherapy*, 21(1), 82–96. doi:10.1002/cpp.1822

Tschacher, W., & Meier, D. (2020). Physiological synchrony in psychotherapy sessions. *Psychotherapy Research* 30, 558–573. doi:10.1080/10503307.2019.1612114

Tschacher, W., Ramseyer, F., & Koole, S. L. (2018). Sharing the now in the social present: Duration of nonverbal synchrony is linked with personality. *Journal of Personality*, 86(2), 129–138. doi:10.1111/jopy.12298

Tschacher, W., Ramseyer, F., & Pfammatter, M. (2020). The social present in psychotherapy: Duration of nowness in therapeutic interaction. In M. Ochs, M. Borcsa, & J. Schweitzer (Eds.), *Systemic Research in Individual, Couple, and Family Therapy and Counseling* (pp. 39–53). Cham, Switzerland: Springer Nature. doi:10.1007/978-3-030-36560-8_3.

Tschacher, W., Rees, G. M., & Ramseyer, F. (2014). Nonverbal synchrony and affect in dyadic interactions. *Frontiers in Psychology*, 5, 1–13. doi:10.3389/fpsyg.2014.01323

Varela, F. J. (1999). Present-Time consciousness. In F. J. Varela & J. Shear (Eds.), *The view from within: First-Person methodologies* (pp. 111–140). Exeter, UK: Imprint Academic.

von Holst, E., & Mittelstaedt, H. (1950). Das Reafferenzprinzip. Wechselwirkung zwischen Zentralnervensystem und Peripherie [The reafference principle. Reciprocity between central nervous system and periphery]. *Naturwissenschaften*, 37, 464–476.

Wampold, B. E. (2015). How important are the common factors in psychotherapy? An update. *World Psychiatry*, 14(3), 270–277. doi:10.1002/wps.20238

6.1

Commentary on "Time and Embodiment in the Process of Psychotherapy: A Dynamical Systems Perspective"

The Musicality of Human Interaction

Valeria Bizzari

Minkowski described the therapeutic relationship in terms of "two melodies being played simultaneously" (Minkowski, 1933/1970, p. 182). The final aim of therapy, in his view, was to establish a certain balance between these two melodies and grasp the patient's psyche. Accordingly, the therapeutic process should be conceived as a participatory experience, a dialogical, intercorporeal space (Fuchs, 2007) where the primary components are prereflective elements that converge into a participatory "we-subject."

This phenomenological description of the therapeutic setting finds its empirical corroboration in Tschacher's analysis, which introduces a dynamic time-based modeling method that is able to map the psychotherapeutic interaction. Tschacher claims that the very core of the social exchange between therapist and client can be identified in what he calls "newness," that is to say, the node in space and time where therapist and client create and share their mutual therapeutic presence. By using a quantitative perspective on this specific kind of social interaction, Tschacher is able to measure the "social present," the temporal interval during which two persons are significantly coupled. In fact, according to him, consciousness resides in the "here and now," that is to say, the present moment, and any kind of experience occurs at a specific timescale at the range of few seconds. More specifically, the study focuses on measuring a series of respiratory activities sampled from psychotherapy sessions. The entire analysis sheds light on the centrality of two components that appear necessary for the occurrence of a fulfilling and effective encounter: *time* and *embodiment*.

Temporality is a basic structure of the human self: According to Zahavi, "every experience is a temporally extended lived presence" (Zahavi, 2014, p. 67). In other words, self-awareness implies the sense of the lived duration of experience.[1] On the other hand, embodiment is the means by which we are able to live and act in the world, "the primordial form of subjectivity, but it is at the same time spatiality, situatedness, directedness to a horizon of possibilities which offer themselves to the body" (Fuchs, 2016, p. 217). By emphasizing these two features of subjectivity, Tschacher follows the "embodiment turn" trend and seems to be influenced by both the phenomenological tradition and the enactivist approach. In fact, he emphasizes that there is a bidirectional, reciprocal interaction between mind and body: Motor behavior, nonverbal communication, and bodily expressions shape mental and emotional processes that, in turn, cause further nonverbal, motor reactions.

The process of psychotherapy is described as a social interaction aimed at the client's learning (and sometimes also learning at the side of the therapist). It appears to be shaped and characterized by the intertwining and "balance" (using Minkowski's words) of two embodied and temporal subjects.[2] In particular, this process involves exchange at the nonverbal level, a mechanism that Tschacher identifies with *synchronization*. In his view, this happens when "previously independent components of a complex dynamical system can become 'entrained', i.e., increasingly coupled" (Tschacher, 2021, p. 109). The dynamic modeling approach allows us to consider psychotherapy as an activity in comprising three elements: observation, predictions,[3] and actions. Nonetheless, this activity is influenced by the interplay of causation and chance: The clinician can grasp specific attractors (forces that act on the states of some variable), but they should also be aware of the presence of unpredictable events. Accordingly, the clinician should also consider "stochastic interventions," such as boundary regulation that can shield the client from being perturbed by chance events. All of these decisions and actions seem to be engrained in the "shared nowness": In other words, according to Tschacher's analysis, the synchronization is an *attractor*, an element necessary for the efficacy of psychotherapy itself, for the threefold process of observation–prediction–action. The analysis of breathing behavior (which is read as a "signature of

[1] This explains why mental pathologies usually involve a fragmentation or the weakening of the temporal experience (Binswanger, 1960; Fuchs & Pallagrosi, 2018; Jaspers, 1913; Minkowski, 1933/1970; Tatossian, 1979).

[2] Nonetheless, we should underline that being embodied and temporally shaped are features common to every kind of interaction. In fact, especially, for a phenomenological perspective, being a temporal and embodied being is essential from face-to-face encounters to more complex social interactions (like we-actions or group-based tasks). See, for instance, Fuchs (2017b).

[3] Tschacher adopts the "predictive coding approach" (Hobson & Friston, 2014) according to which the general aim of cognition is to minimize the error of prediction. In the specific case of psychotherapy, the aim of the therapist should be to perform actions directed at the client's change.

embodied cognition in the therapy session) (Tschacher, 2021, p. 112) in therapy sessions sheds light on the fact that the therapist's and client's breathing is synchronized on average for 4 seconds throughout the session. Furthermore, the collected data identify a longer duration of breathing synchrony (i.e., a longer "social present") with a better therapeutic relationship (as rated by the client). In other words, we can affirm that being synchronized is synonymous with a good intersubjective relationship able to allow communication and perform action (cf. Ramseyer & Tschacher, 2011).

It is interesting to notice that Tschacher's *quantitative* analysis is coherent with a *qualitative* approach on synchrony. In the philosophical debate regarding joint action (e.g., Bratman, 2013; Gilbert, 1989; Searle, 1995; Tuomela, 2013), where the focus is usually on the higher levels of cognition, such as the processes of action planning, commitments, and goals, we can find the theory (Tollefsen & Dale, 2012) according to which there is an "alignment system" that involves lower-level coordinative structures that help to implement higher-level goals. When individuals engage in a joint activity such as a conversation (for instance, the one between therapist and client) or joint problem solving, they become aligned at a variety of different levels, which include coordinated eye movements, similar speech patterns, and *synchronized bodily movements*. Richardson and Dale (2005) have shown that *the better the alignment, the better the participants are understanding each other*, and they fulfill the shared goal of communicating with one another (Tollefsen & Dale, 2012, p. 393). In other words, the presence of an alignment system (where we can also include nonverbal synchrony) explains how we-intentions can be formed without prior planning and agreement. Tschacher's quantitative analysis and philosophical, qualitative studies seem to converge into a multilayered account of interactive processes (such as the therapeutic one) where lower-level components are necessary for higher-level mechanisms (such as prediction and action).

This can explain why people who suffer from intersubjective disorders, such as high-functioning autistic subjects, seem to register impairments at the level of synchronization with other individuals.[4] First-person reports of social interaction in these cases include descriptions of "being flooded," having the "inability to keep up," and not knowing "when and how" to respond to what others do, whereas observing others (as distinguished from interacting with them) allows for thinking through the situation, albeit in an effortful way (Schilbach et al., 2013, p. 411). Being in the presence of

[4] This deficit has been linked to a deficit in cognitive empathy (Koehne, Hatri, Cacioppo, & Dziobek, 2016).

others normally changes the perception of the environment, but individuals with high-functioning autism seem "immune" to interpersonal motor alignment, despite their competent and explicit social cognitive capacities (Schilbach, Eickhoff, Cieslik, Kuzmanovic, & Vogeley, 2012, p. 159).

A phenomenologically informed study (Bizzari & Guareschi, 2017) conducted on patients who attend music therapy sessions whose goal is "playing together" (an activity requiring the ability to "tune in" and "synchronize with" the other) sheds light on the importance of nonverbal, bodily, and prereflective components, such as rhythm and synchrony, for the development of joint intentional skills.

In this sense, the use of the word *rhythm* here is to refer to the pattern of temporal intervals and the specific and quantifiable relationships between them. In the development of the selfhood, rhythm plays a central function. We can argue that body and brain are rhythmically coordinated through the processes of interoception and proprioception (see Fuchs, 2018) that result in a homeodynamic regulation and a basic bodily sense of self. We can describe this level as an "internal musicality," which allows the subject to develop cognitive and perceptual abilities correctly and to have a diachronic awareness of oneself as an agent. Then, we have seen how *synchrony* (or synchronized rhythm with an external being) corresponds to a form of bodily alignment that, in phenomenological terms, we can also define as "intercorporeality." That is the prereflective intertwining of lived and living bodies that mutually resonate with one another without requiring inferential capacities; it is the mutual bodily synchrony that allows two subjects to experience subjective and objective qualities through their lived bodies (see Fuchs, 2017a).

As Tschacher's study emphasizes the importance of the temporal dimension and of bodily, nonverbal synchrony in the therapeutic relationship, Bizzari and Guareschi's analysis suggests that subjects who register impairments at the level of rhythm (and accordingly, in their diachronic sense of time) and individuals with impairments at the level of synchrony (which involves synchronic sense of time and the ability to be bodily aligned with others) are unable to perform joint actions. The quality of the intersubjective activities and the intersubjective meeting is therefore influenced by these prereflective and bodily components. By pushing Tschacher's theory beyond the boundaries of the psychotherapeutic environment, we can propose that *interpersonal synchronization* sits at the very core of each significant relationship. It influences the central moment of interactions that take place in the "shared nowness" between two embodied "melodies."

Acknowledgment

Dr. Valeria Bizzari is grateful to the Fritz Thyssen Foundation, which supports her project "Asperger's Syndrome: A Philosophical and Empirical Investigation of Intersubjectivity and its Disruptions" (Az. 40.18.0.033PH), and to the Center of Psychosocial Medicine, Clinic University of Heidelberg.

References

Binswanger, L. (1960). *Melancholie und Manie* [Melancholy and mania]. Pfullingen, Germany: Neske.

Bizzari, V., & Guareschi, C. (2017). Bodily memory and joint action in music practice and therapy. *Quaderni della Ginestra*, 3, 114–121.

Bratman, M. (2013). *Shared agency: A planning theory of acting together*. Oxford, UK: Oxford University Press.

Fuchs, T. (2007). Psychotherapy of the lived space: A phenomenological and ecological concept. *American Journal of Psychotherapy*, 61(4), 423–439. doi:10.1176/appi.psychotherapy.2007.61.4.423

Fuchs, T. (2016). Embodied knowledge – Embodied memory. In S. Rinofner-Kreidl & H. A. Wiltsche (Eds.), *Analytic and continental philosophy: Methods and perspectives. Proceedings of the 37th international Wittgenstein symposium* (pp. 215–230). Berlin, Germany: De Gruyter.

Fuchs, T. (2017a). Intercorporeality and interaffectivity. In C. Meyer, J. Streeck, & S. Jordan (Eds.), *Intercorporeality: Emerging socialities in interaction* (pp. 3–24). Oxford, UK: Oxford University Press.

Fuchs, T. (2017b). Self across time: The diachronic unity of bodily existence. *Phenomenology and the Cognitive Sciences*, 16(2), 291–315. doi:10.1007/s11097-015-9449-4

Fuchs, T. (2018). *Ecology of the brain: The phenomenology and biology of the embodied mind*. Oxford, UK: Oxford University Press.

Fuchs, T., & Pallagrosi, M. (2018). Phenomenology of temporality and dimensional psychopathology. In M. Biondi, M. Pasquini, & A. Picardi (Eds.), *Dimensional psychopathology* (pp. 287–300). New York, NY: Springer.

Gilbert, M. (1989). *On social facts*. Princeton, NJ: Princeton University Press.

Hobson, J. A., & Friston, K. J. (2014). Consciousness, dreams, and inference. The Cartesian theatre revisited. *Journal of Consciousness Studies*, 21(1–2), 6–32.

Jaspers, K. (1913). *Allgemeine Psychopathologie* [General psychopathology]. Berlin, Germany: Springer.

Koehne, S., Hatri, A., Cacioppo, J. T., & Dziobek, I. (2016). Perceived interpersonal synchrony increases empathy: Insights from autism spectrum disorder. *Cognition*, 146, 8–15. doi:10.1016/j.cognition.2015.09.007

Minkowski, E. (1970). *Lived time: Phenomenological and psychopathological studies* (N. Metzel, Trans.). Evanston, IL: Northwestern University Press. (Original work published 1933)

Ramseyer, F., & Tschacher, W. (2011). Nonverbal synchrony in psychotherapy: Coordinated body movement reflects relationship quality and outcome. *Journal of Consulting and Clinical Psychology*, 79(3), 284–295. doi:10.1037/a0023419

Richardson, D. C., & Dale, R. (2005). Looking to understand: The coupling between speakers' and listeners' eye movements and its relationship to discourse comprehension. *Cognitive Science*, 29(6), 1045–1060. doi:10.1207/s15516709cog0000_29

Schilbach, L., Eickhoff, S., Cieslik, E., Kuzmanovic, B., & Vogeley, K. (2012). Shall we do this together? Social gaze influences action control in a comparison group, but not in individuals with high-functioning autism. *Autism*, 16(2), 151–162. doi:10.1177/1362361311409258

Schilbach, L., Timmermans, B., Reddy, V., Costall, A., Bente, G., Schlicht, T., & Vogeley, K. (2013). Toward a second-person neuroscience. *Behavioral and Brain Sciences*, 36(4), 393–414. doi:10.1017/S0140525X12000660

Searle, J. (1995). *The construction of social reality*. New York, NY: The Free Press.

Tatossian, A. (1979). *La Phénoménologie des psychoses* [The phenomenology of psychosis]. Paris, France: Masson.

Tollefsen, D., & Dale, R. (2012). Naturalizing joint action: A process-based approach, *Philosophical Psychology*, 25(3), 385–407. doi:10.1080/09515089.2011.579418

Tschacher, W. (2021). Time and embodiment in the process of psychotherapy – A dynamical systems perspective. In C. Tewes & G. Stanghellini (Eds.), *Time and body: Phenomenological and psychopathological approaches* (pp. 104–116). Cambridge, UK: Cambridge University Press.

Tuomela, R. (2013). *Social ontology: Collective intentionality and group agents*. Oxford, UK: Oxford University Press.

Zahavi, D. (2014). *Self and other: Exploring subjectivity, empathy and shame*. Oxford, UK: Oxford University Press.

Part II
Grief and Anxiety

7

Bereavement and the Meaning of Profound Feelings of Emptiness

An Existential-phenomenological Analysis

Allan Køster

Introduction

Losing an intimate other to death is one of the most profound and encompassing existential events in a human life. If you were especially close to the person you have been bereaved of, it is a life-altering event that saturates every aspect of your being. It is, therefore, not surprising that people who have suffered such a loss sometimes define their entire life with this event as their principal peripeteia. Keeping this in mind, the simple identification of grief with a singular emotion is obviously problematic. Rather, bereavement constitutes an existential event that inflicts a profound disruption of my entire being, and consequently, initiates a complex and open-ended process of adaptation to an altered life situation. That this complex process cannot be reduced to one well-defined emotional component has long been recognized in contemporary empirical grief research. Here, influential researchers, such as George Bonanno (2001), emphasize that the appropriate conceptualization of grief is one that recognizes grief as "a complex molar experience that generates various molecular components" (p. 494). This process is, of course, profoundly affective in nature. But as any empirically sensitive account will acknowledge, it involves a broad pallete of affects ranging from emotions such as sadness, longing, anger, resentment, hostility, hopelessness, fear, and guilt to alterations in moods such as depression and existential feelings of being altogether disconnected from the world (Fernandez & Køster, 2019). In this respect, I propose it makes more sense to say that grief manifests through a comprehensive *affective register* than through a well-defined emotion. Importantly, this is not to suggest that grief does not have a unified and distinct experiential quality, but rather that what unifies grief as an experience should be found at the intersection of several existential categories and not through its emotional distinctness.[1]

Attention to this complex nature of bereavement experiences should, of course, be reflected in phenomenological analysis. With this in mind, I believe we should aim to build an encompassing understanding of the integrated nature of bereavement experiences through piecemeal investigations of its various and specific components; that is, starting out by doing phenomenologies of grief, in the plural.

In this chapter, I contribute to this task by providing an existential-phenomenological analysis of the *meaning of postbereavement feelings of emptiness*. Feelings of emptiness are among the sources of suffering that are most consistently reported by persons who have been bereaved of an intimate other. However, since bereavement experiences vary in nature depending on the type of loss, that is, whether it is the loss of a life partner, a parent, a child, an idol, or even what is now referred to as ecological grief, I will specify my focus to what I call the *intimate other*. By an intimate other, I refer to a person with whom I share the most fundamental structures of my daily life. Since the paradigm example of an intimate other probably is that of a life partner, this will also be my guiding example throughout the chapter. However, this does not preclude that important aspects of the analysis equally apply to experiences of losing a parent or a child. What is important in this respect is the shared daily life.[2]

My main claim in this chapter is that postbereavement feelings of emptiness are an expression of a radical constriction in what I shall refer to as the *existential texture* of my sense of self-familiarity as a *being-with*. As an embodied creature, my sense of self and self-familiarity cannot be separated from my broader habituation to an ontogenetically specific world. When sharing a life with an intimate other, this world becomes a shared world, and when losing that person, it is not only the world that is emptied, but quite literally also my being.

In unfolding this perspective, I will proceed as follows: First, I address the problem that feelings of emptiness are inherently fuzzy and found across a range of dissimilar conditions. To lay a foundation for my analysis, I point out that feelings of emptiness are not expressions of an abstract nothingness, but admit of a differentiated intentional structure. However, this intentional

[1] For a philosophical discussion of the difficulties in construing grief as an emotion, see Goldie (2011, 2012) and Ingerslev (2018). For an interesting and well-argued phenomenological defense for viewing grief as an emotion by pushing our understanding of the concept of emotion, see Ratcliffe (2017).

[2] An example of this could be Roland Barthes' reflections on losing his mother in his *Mourning Diaries* (Barthes, 2009). The rather profound experiences he expresses here must be read in light of the fact that he, despite being sixty-two years old, still lived with her at the time of her demise. Barthes himself died only three years later.

structure cannot meaningfully be separated from the context of what they express an emptiness from. Second, I direct this line of questioning to the phenomenon of bereavement. Here, I emphasize that the Freudian proposal that grief-related feelings of emptiness exclusively emanate from the world, leaving the self otherwise untouched, is phenomenologically inadequate. Third, I argue that my sense of self-familiarity is a distributed phenomenon and that the existential texture of my self-familiarity can be inseparable from a sense of being-with. The fourth section exemplifies this by pointing to five modalities that tend to be sources of emptiness in bereavement. Fourth, and finally, I provide some concluding remarks and call attention to the ambiguity that what may initially have been a source for feelings of emptiness often is a vital source for the ability to stay connected to the deceased, which in the literature is called a continued bond (Klass, Silverman, & Nickman, 1996).

The Variety and Meaning of Feelings of Emptiness

A significant challenge in approaching any analysis of feelings of emptiness is navigating their fuzzy and ambiguous nature. Someone experiencing feelings of emptiness will tend to complain that "Everything feels empty"; "I feel so empty inside"; "The world feels empty"; or "Nothing makes sense, because of this emptiness," etc. However, when asked to elaborate on the nature of this experience the lay person, that is, a patient or a research informant, will usually tend to refer to a rudimentary bodily location of the feeling[3] and otherwise return to circular statements like: "I don't know, it just feels empty." Hence, feelings of emptiness exhibit a kind of language resistance. This is not to say that feelings of emptiness altogether evade expression. Rather, this language resistance makes empirical investigations of this phenomenon inherently difficult without a prior phenomenological clarification.

But why is this so? Why are feelings of emptiness so difficult to express? A tempting answer might be that there literally is nothing to describe; feelings of emptiness are exactly feelings of nothingness, and hence there is no referent, no intentional structure to be described. This conclusion is, however, too hasty. The fact that the intentional structures of feelings of emptiness are fuzzy and difficult to identify does not mean that they are not there. As already evident in the examples of statements given above, they imply the presence of structure insofar as they vary in pointing to emptiness as emanating from the world, the self, or meaning, respectively.

[3] In psychoanalysis, feelings of emptiness are most often traced back to the primordial physiological experiences of hunger (e.g., Greenson, 1949; Rado, 1928).

That there is an underlying structure to feelings of emptiness becomes even more specific if we turn to psychopathology. In psychopathology, feelings of emptiness are reported across a host of conditions ranging from psychosis and depression to personality disorders such as schizoid, narcissistic, and borderline (Zandersen & Parnas, 2019). In some instances, feelings of emptiness even count as a specific diagnostic criterion, as is the case in borderline personality disorder (BDP). Likewise, feelings of emptiness were part of the inventory for the early 2009 criteria for prolonged grief disorder (American Psychiatric Association [APA], 2016; Killikelly & Maercker, 2018).[4] Whereas this diversity surely tells of the widespread presence of the phenomenon, it also suggests that feelings of emptiness must admit of significant structural differentiation. For are we really to expect that feelings of emptiness refer to the same experiential structure and quality across variegated states such as psychosis, personality disorders, and grief? I feel very sure this is not the case. A glance at the research literature will support this. Here feelings of emptiness are associated with different states such as boredom (Greenson, 1953; Klonsky, 2008); a lack of a feeling of interest, values, and direction in life (Zandersen & Parnas, 2019); the loss of an overall sense of meaning (May, 1975); consumerism (Cushman, 1990); social loneliness; and concrete embodied feelings of having a hole inside after having suffered a miscarriage (Adolfsson, Larsson, Wijma, & Bertero, 2004).

In each of these cases, the experiential structure admits of differentiation. This is, I submit, because feelings of emptiness are not an experience of an abstract and meaningless nothingness, but rather an experience of a profound vacancy in the absence of a concrete presence. And this gives the experience specificity. Hence, although we probably should not entirely rule out the possibility of an experience of void or lack in existence itself, it is folly to demand a general definition of feelings of emptiness that is supposed to capture all of its meanings. Instead, *feelings of emptiness need to be analyzed specifically within the context of what they are experienced as an emptiness from.* Hence, we need to ask for the meaning of feelings of emptiness and, for each case, aim for a discerning phenomenological analysis.

Bereavement: A First Approximation

In light of this framing, what should guide a phenomenological analysis of postbereavement feeling of emptiness? What kind of emptiness is produced by the loss of an intimate other?

[4] Feelings of emptiness have since fallen out of the current International Classification of Diseases (ICD)-11 inventory for prolonged grief disorder.

In a sense, the answer does seem fairly straightforward: Postbereavement feelings of emptiness follow from the fact that a specific person has been lost, leaving a profound vacancy in the world. This kind of logic seems to be what guides Freud in his "Mourning and Melancholia." Here, Freud explicitly distinguishes grief from melancholia through reference to feelings of emptiness by suggesting that "In grief, the world becomes poor and empty; in melancholia it is the ego itself" (Freud, 1917/1957, p. 155). Although there surely is an intuitive appeal to this claim, my intention is to argue that it is, in fact, a far too categorical and phenomenologically inadequate proposition. Postbereavement feelings of emptiness cannot be understood as emanating exclusively from the world, leaving the self intact.

The problem with this account is that it assumes too strong a separation between self and world and self and other, respectively. That these cannot be strictly separated, are, of cause, basic phenomenological insights and expressed in fundamental phenomenological concepts and frameworks such as Husserl's analysis of intentionality (Husserl, 1982), Heidegger's (1927/2001) notion of being-in-the-world, and Merleau-Ponty's concepts of intercorporeality and being-toward-the-world (1964, 2012). Although I shall have more to say about certain aspects of this idea in the sections to come, it would digress from the focus of this chapter to engage in a detailed discussion of these frameworks here. Instead, I will exemplify this point by referring to a description of postbereavement feelings of emptiness that specifically emphasize how emptiness permeates the boundaries between the world and the self.

In her book *Time Lived, Without Its Flow*, Denise Riley (2012) reflects on what she calls the altered nature of experience after losing her son. In regards to feelings of emptiness, she tells us that this is like

> Wandering around in an empty plain, as if an enormous drained landscape lying behind your eyes had turned itself outward. Or you find yourself camped on a threshold between inside and out. The slight contact of your senses with the outer world and your interior only thinly separated from it, like a membrane resonating on the verge between silence and noise. If it were to tear through, there's so little behind your skin that you would fall out towards the side of sheer exteriority. Far from taking refuge deeply inside yourself, there is no longer any inside, and you have become only outwardness. As a friend, who'd experienced the suicide of a person closest to her, says: "I was my two eyes set burning in my skull. Behind them there is only vacancy." (Riley, 2012, p. 19)

This visceral description shows how postbereavement feelings of emptiness are not exclusively emanating from the world, but that embodied selfhood is itself experienced as a "vacancy" where the boundaries between interiority and exteriority have become fragile. And exceedingly so. Yet how do we make sense of this experience? If feelings of emptiness are to be analyzed specifically within the context of what they express an emptiness from, where does this scenario take us? Or, more specifically: How can the loss of another person cause an emptying of the multifaceted existential texture of the self?

Broadly stated, my suggestion is that postbereavement feelings of emptiness are rooted in the fact that the *existential texture* that makes up our daily sense of self-familiarity may be inextricably intertwined with intimate others. Hence, feelings of emptiness after losing an intimate other are not only an expression of the absence of that person, but equally an experience of a constriction in my own sense of self-familiarity. In effect, it is a kind of self-alienation. This is what is signified in phrases like: "Without her, I no longer know who I am" or "Losing him is like losing part of my self." It is this experience I will unpack in the following sections, and through that specify the meaning of postbereavement feelings of emptiness.

The Existential Texture of Self-Familiarity and *Being-With*

In approaching this question, we need to begin by reminding ourselves that from a phenomenological point of view, our sense of self-familiarity – that is, feeling at ease and at home with ourselves – is not something that is self-reliant and self-contained. It is not something static and given, but a temporal structure relying on daily experiences of confirmation. What does this mean? To avoid misunderstandings, I should start by emphasizing that the notion of self-familiarity I am referring to here is not the kind of basic self-awareness that may be said to be built into consciousness itself as a property of the stream of consciousness itself (Husserl, 1966; Zahavi, 1999). Claiming that this kind of basic self-awareness is in need of recollection would not only be phenomenologically inadequate, but it would also constitute an infinite regress (Zahavi, 1999). What I am referring to is rather my sense of self-familiarity as a *concretely* individuated embodied subject. As an embodied creature, this kind of self-familiarity is acquired through our ontogenetically specific habituation to a world; what Merleau-Ponty called our mode of "being-toward-the-world" (Merleau-Ponty, 2012). Self-familiarity, in this respect, is a distributed phenomenon which cannot meaningfully be separated from my broader world-entanglement. Hence, contrary to the notion of basic self-awareness, which is inherent to embodied subjectivity and not context-dependent, my concretely individuated sense of self-familiarity is an acquisition inseparable from my contextual embeddedness. Each day I am brought back to myself through a complicated set of contextual affordances and habitual practices. Because it is an acquisition, self-familiarity may also be lost in the absence of these affordances, as is manifest in certain experiences of self-alienation and feelings of estrangement.

This should be taken quite literally: The daily process of returning to a feeling of self-acquaintance begins the moment I wake up in the familiarity of my bed, the room, and (perhaps) the specific felt presence of my partner lying next to me. Through these rudimentary existential coordinates, I start to get my bearings and know not only where I am, but also acquire a sense of familiarity with who I am. From here, I follow my morning routines; I go through my habituated practices such as brushing teeth and making coffee, and, throughout, using my familiar things in a most habituated manner. I travel to work by my usual means of transportation and arrive at my office; I seek out my designated office space with my familiar chair, adjusted to my bodily comportments, my desk, my books, my piles of papers, etc. All of these elements reflect my habituated presence, and my acquaintance with them contributes to me feeling familiar and at home – to having a consolidated feeling of being myself. To see the relative importance of all of this, consider the contrasting case: Waking up in a foreign bed in an unfamiliar room that I do not immediately recognize, with the characteristic type of disorientation sometimes involved in the brief seconds after opening my eyes. Or, waking up in the absence or presence of a person who is either usually part of or alien to my bed. And, consider what it might feel like to arrive at work and sit at a colleague's office space, rather than my own desk, surrounded by that person's things and materially structured habits that all point to an entirely different history and style of habituation. Obviously, these are hardly devastating experiences. This is because they do not imply a complete uprooting of the various sources of self-familiarity, which at the broadest level includes the fundamental familiarity with a biological and cultural niche (Tewes, Durt, & Fuchs, 2017). But they nevertheless do point to a significant kind of estrangement – of not feeling quite settled and at home with myself. As rightly pointed out by John Sallis (2006), this state of being unsettled or uprooted is exactly what is amplified in, and the ground for feeling of, the homesickness that we might experience when traveling in a foreign country without companions, daily practices, or possessions to help us collect our sense of self-familiarity.

Hence, in a nontrivial sense, self-familiarity is a mediated phenomenon. Although directly experienced, it is not a direct possession, but sustained by and inseparable from the integrated web of constituents I daily use to recollect a sense of myself. I shall refer to this integrated web as the *existential texture of my self-familiarity*. This existential texture makes up my ontogenetically specific world relation, with the complex sets of modalities this involves. I know myself through my specific habituated embeddedness.

Yet how is this relevant to postbereavement feelings of emptiness? As already indicated, the distributed nature of my sense of self-familiarity also extends to my relations to other people, who may take up varying roles and degrees of import in this process. However, one type of relation stands out by not merely being a constituent among others, but rather integral to the entire existential texture of self-familiarity, namely, that of an intimate other. When we share our lives with intimate others, the invisible threads of intentionality that integrate us with our habituated world will tend to be inextricably interwoven with that specific person. In such cases, the very practices, places, things, etc. that constitute my habituated world retain their meaningfulness only through a reference to that person. Hence, my sense of self-familiarity becomes inseparable from a profound sense of *being-with* – of living a shared life.

When bereaved of this person, a devastating constriction in the overall existential texture of my self-familiarity is generated. Myriads of intentional threads are severed from the referent that sustains them with meaning, leaving me without the tether that anchors me to a stable sense of myself. Postbereavement feelings of emptiness are, I suggest, the affective expression of this sudden contraction of my being resulting from the loss of an intimate other. If this is true, then the model proposed by Freud is, of course, wrong. Feelings of emptiness resulting from the loss of an intimate other cannot be reduced to a unilateral emptiness emanating from the world, but must equally be seen as an emptying of the self – of my integrated sense of being me. In a variation of Thomas Attig's (1996) acclaimed notion that grief involves a "relearning of the world," we are hence equally justified in saying that bereavement demands the need for a profound *relearning of myself* – of who I am without my intimate other.

Bereavement and the Sources of Feeling Empty

My aim in this section is to demonstrate the phenomenological validity of this claim through providing a detailed analysis of how being bereaved of an intimate other causes a constriction in the existential texture of my self-familiarity. To do so, I will focus on five modalities: (1) intercorporeal integration, (2) habituated practices, (3) things and belongings, (4) sense of home, and (5) temporal horizon. The intention of pointing to these specific modalities is merely illustrative of the general point and does not strive toward completeness. Furthermore, I want to emphasize that the segregation of the experience of emptiness into various modalities, of course, is artificial and only serves an analytical purpose. From an experiential point of view, it is most often not possible to draw sharp boundaries between the modalities that will rather tend to permeate each other.

(1) Intercorporeal Integration

The possibility of grief arises from the depth of our interconnectedness with others. Although this statement might seem trivial, it is not. From a phenomenological perspective, the point is not the simple fact that we stand in external relations to others, but rather that this interconnectedness is internal in nature. This is expressed in the phenomenological concept of intercorporeality, which emphasizes that because we are embodied beings, we are always intertwined with others (Merleau-Ponty, 1964, 2012). This holds true as a general experiential structure and has been well-charted in the phenomenological literature. However, what is interesting in the present context is how my intercorporeal integration with intimate others becomes a constitutive part of my sense of self and self-familiarity. To begin with, it should be noted that the concept of intercorporeality is not pointing to an emphatic fusion that amounts to something like a liquidation of the boundaries with self and other, but rather that self and other can establish an internal relation to complete a unified system (Merleau-Ponty, 2012, p. 368). However, intercorporeal integration is not restricted to real-time interactions, but sediments in habituated structures of intercorporeal body memory (Fuchs, 2012). That is, our intercorporeal integration with intimate others establishes a fundamental felt sense of that person, which is retained in her absence. With intimate others, this felt sense is integral to my sense of self-familiarity.

To see this, consider the example of sharing a bed with a partner. While this cohabitancy initially required coordination and significant adjustments, intimate others gradually integrate into our habitual body to such an extent that the body scheme that constitutes this particular setting appears as incomplete in the absence of that person. This kind of intercorporeal integration applies more broadly, and is not restricted to a particular setting. Rather, the intercorporeal *reaching out* for an intimate other becomes a kind of habitual readiness embedded in the body. In her *Blue Nights*, Joan Didion (2011) describes the ambiguous experiences that occur when the body of the other is not to be reached:

> I know that I can no longer reach her. I know that, should I try to reach her—should I take her hand as if she were again sitting next to me in the upstairs cabin on the evening Pan Am from Honolulu to LAX, should I lull her to sleep against my shoulder, should I sing her the song about Daddy gone to get the rabbit skin to wrap his baby bunny in—she will fade from my touch. Disappear. (Didion, 2011, p. 187)

However, this kind of intercorporeal integration does not stop at touch, but may be said to cover a habituation to the entire sensory presence of a person – to what I have elsewhere called the felt sense or sensorium of the other (Køster, 2020). I may, for instance, gradually become habituated to my partner's soundscape – not only to the sound and melody of her voice, but just as much to all that which I am continuously "overhearing"[5] – the distinctly personal, yet ineffable sound of her presence, like the sounds of her pottering about in the kitchen. Or it could be her so familiar olfactory presence, like the traces of her distinctive smell that usually saturates our shared bed sheets or emanates from her coat hanging in the entrance hall. The French have a word for this: "sillage." Or the specific feel of her touch, the feeling of her embrace. When sharing a life with an intimate other, all of these sensory features are not only pointing to the felt sense of that person's presence, but they are equally significant elements in constituting my sense of self-familiarity. I find this familiarity in the sense of being at home in the tacitly felt sense of her presence: her soundscape, her olfactory manifestation, in being met by her embrace, etc.[6]

When bereaved of an intimate other this intercorporeality is not only disrupted, but permanently severed. This leaves a range of intentional threads, vital to my sense of self-familiarity, fluttering, and open-ended. The bed I usually share with her is not only experienced as empty due to the unoccupied space next to me, but equally through an embodied feeling of incompleteness or vacancy. Her characteristic soundscape, usually overheard in the background of everyday experience, suddenly becomes

[5] For an interesting analysis of the phenomenon of "overhearing," see Højlund, Kirkegaard, and Riis (in press).

[6] I have provided a detailed analysis of this phenomenon of a *felt sense of the other* in Køster (2020).

salient in the deafening silence of its absence. The absence of her particular touch, her embrace; or the familiar look in her eyes that has become a daily source for feeling enrooted, no longer meets me. These experiences not only point to a deprivation of the world, but equally importantly, to the embodied feeling of being me. I feel empty because my intercorporeal integration with this person has been amputated.

(2) Habituated Practices

The habitual practices that daily help in returning me to a sense of self-familiarity consist of a coherent system of actions, a referential web that is often integrated with and carries implicit and explicit reference to significant others. This might be in the most minute details, like how I start the day with a shower, which I implicitly time in consideration to the needs of my partner. I prepare morning coffee and set the table for two. When heading off to work, I may commute with my partner and once again time my day in accordance with her needs. When grocery shopping, I shop for two and anticipate cooking for her, considering her preferences and dislikes, etc. However, the habitual practices significant to the sense of self might, of course, also be more elaborate in nature and include hobbies that may be inextricably connected with our significant others, like playing golf, hiking, or going bird-watching together.

When bereaved, this coherent system of habituated practices remains active in all the structured anticipations and implied references to the deceased (Ratcliffe, 2017). Only now this referential unity is no longer intact, but left unsaturated. It is bereaved of a constitutive source that provides vitality and meaning to these references. I may still prepare coffee and set the table for two, only now this practice doesn't provide me with the usual comfort of familiarity, but rather echoes the emptiness of the seat from where she used to sit.[7] Similarly, practices like playing golf or hiking, which may be a strong source of identity, become meaningless and only point to a vacancy in my being: "Golf was something I played with her, it makes no sense doing it alone." Since these habitual patterns of practices constitute a significant part of my everyday process of returning to myself, being bereaved of a person integral to this structure leaves me with feelings of emptiness. I feel empty not only because of the de facto absence of a

[7] As has often been pointed out in the literature on grief, there seems to be a structural similarity between the continued anticipation of the presence of the other, and the experience of the phantom limb (e.g., Christine, 2008; Merleau-Ponty, 2012; Parkes, 1975; Waldenfels, 2000). For a critical engagement with this claim, see Ratcliffe (2019).

person, but because the entire system of practices that return me to my sense of myself has been disrupted and exposed to a profound emptying of significance.

(3) Things and Belongings

As pointed out in the previous section, things and belongings also play, with varying valences of import, a significant role in the existential texture of my sense of self-familiarity. However, when sharing a life with an intimate other, not all things that have significance in this respect need belong to me. The plants and flowers kept by my partner may, for instance, be a great source of comfort and familiarity to me in my daily life, but without in any way being under my jurisdiction of care. Similarly, when sharing a home with an intimate other, I may be habituated to being surrounded by a host of things, such as clothes, vases, and paintings, whose meaning is entirely dependent on that person. When bereaved, these things are exposed to a profound emptying of significance. In his novel *The Invention of Solitude*, Paul Auster (1992) gives the following description of the experience of being confronted with a dead person's objects:

> There is nothing more terrible, I learned, than having to face the objects of a dead man. Things are inert: they have meaning only in function of the life that makes use of them. When that life ends, the things change, even though they remain the same. They are there yet not there: tangible ghosts, condemned to survive in a world they no longer belong to. What is one to think, for example, of a closetful of clothes waiting silently to be worn again by a man who is not coming back to open the door? … Or an electric razor sitting in the bathroom, still clogged with the whisker dust of the last shave? … There is a poignancy to it, and also a kind of horror. In themselves, the things mean nothing … And yet they say something to us, standing there not as objects, but as remnants of thought, of consciousness … And the futility of it all once there is death. (Auster, 1992, p. 11)

Life is solidified in things, Simone de Beauvoir (1985) tells us, and when the person they belong to dies, they become orphaned and lose their identity (p. 98). This passage illustrates the swiftness of this process, and points to how things that may have once been an inextricable part of my existential texture as being-with may be emptied of significance, because the referential unity that provides them with vitality is gone.

(4) Sense of Home

Places, specifically those places we consider as home, are perhaps among the most important constituents of the existential texture that grounds our sense of self-familiarity. Home is, Bachelard (1994) tells us, "the non-I that protects the I" (p. 5). It is a vital space that daily enroots me in a sense of familiarity. Kirsten Jacobson (2009) has taken up this motif and points to how home is "a place of and for the self" and describes this connection in the following way:

> Whether by serving as an outer skin of sorts, by being specifically responsive to the body and its needs, or by serving as a regular base by means of which we engage the world our home is a second body for us. At the most basic level, home is like the body insofar as it is, as I have just been describing, a place of initial stability and a foundation for the self.... The experience of being-at-home and the bodily sense of self are thus inseparable; without home, there would be constant dispersion in the always retreating "there." (Jacobson, 2009, p. 361)

When sharing a life with an intimate other, this person becomes constitutive to our home as this intimate space. This means that when bereaved of that person, this vital space is not only deprived of the presence of a particular person, but its function as a foundational source of self-familiarity is also radically disrupted. Instead of being a space of comfort, it is now a scene of uncanniness. The following passage, provided by a young woman who lost her father as a young girl, describes her experiences of being in her childhood home after losing her father:

> It was so scary. I remember this period where my childhood home became very uncanny; I didn't like to stay there. And then again, I liked being with the animals. But I removed myself from it all. My mum said I should enjoy it while we still had the farm, but it felt so empty and uncanny to be there. So, I started staying at my grandmother's. Actually, I spent a lot of time at my grandmother's. The whole situation made me feel so empty inside.[8]

Again, the feelings of emptiness reported here are not exclusively expressions of an experienced absence of a loved person, but just as much a profound emptying of home as a significant constituent of the existential texture that carries my continued sense of self.

(5) Temporal Horizons

The last modality I will address is how self-familiarity is enrooted in a temporal horizon and how this may be integrated with an intimate other.

[8] This passage is taken from a qualitative interview conducted with persons who suffered early parental bereavement (between the age 5 and 18).

I know myself through having a past – a personal history – and through my anticipated and projected futures. Sometimes this temporal horizon is exposed to explicit and thematic structuring through narrative accounts, sometimes this is rather a tacit underlying structure.[9] In any case, this temporal horizon remains a lived reality that is significant to my continued sense of who I am.

When sharing my life with an intimate other, this temporal horizon stops being exclusively mine, and becomes entangled in a shared past and a shared projected future. I no longer say "when I get old" or "when I go to France on vacation this summer," but rather "when *we* get old" and "when *we* go to France on vacation this summer," etc. Drawing on Eugène Minkowski's (1970) concept of a "lived synchronism," Fuchs (2018, p. 50) has suggested the concept of "contemporality" as specifically designating the dyadic time of living together. Importantly, this is to be understood as lived time, as a kind of background temporality that structures a joint attention toward a shared past and a shared future.

When bereaved of this significant other, the shared temporal horizon of our contemporality is exposed to profound emptying of significance. While emptiness undoubtedly springs from the loss of a constitutive witness to a shared past, the emptiness of the loss of a shared future is arguably even stronger felt, since this no longer is allowed to manifest and attain reality. Denise Riley (2012) describes this feeling as a "sensation of having been lifted clean out of habitual time." As a person you have stopped, leading to a profound sense of emptiness. As she explains,

> Do you now say that *you* have stopped? Admittedly something still goes on; you walk about, you sleep a bit, you do your best to work, you get older. Yet in essence you have stopped. You're held in a crystalline suspension. Your impression of your own interiority has utterly drained away, and you are pure skin stretched tightly out over *vacancy*. You abide. (Riley, 2012, pp. 66–67)

This emptiness or vacancy emanates from a loss of temporal horizons; particularly a loss of a habituated sense of temporality as a *dyadic futurity*. This forces you, as Riley states, to exclusively inhabit the present, with no plans made for the future. Although such living in the moment might

[9] I have provided a detailed analysis of the relation between the temporal horizon of embodied selfhood and narrative (Køster, 2017a, 2017b; Køster & Winther-Lindqvist, 2018).

not prima facie appear as problematic it is in fact, according to Riley, a profound source of feelings of emptiness:

> Only in the present moment is our happiness: the stoics' pronouncement. The irony is that now you've succeeded brilliantly in living exclusively in the present, but only as the result of death. To endure, yes, but when the usual passage of time is in shards? What does your old philosophy of endurance mean, when there's no longer any temporality left in which to wait it out? (Riley, 2012, p. 26)

Since the death of an intimate other quite literally annuls dyadic time, the bereaved is left in a state of profoundly emptied temporal horizons. I am no longer familiar with who I am as a person existing toward a projected future and I lack a co-witness to a shared past. This emptying of temporal horizon pertains to the temporality of the self, to lived time, and not objective time.

Emptiness and Beyond: Some Concluding Remarks

My aim in this chapter has been to provide a phenomenological-existential analysis of postbereavement feelings of emptiness. I started out by emphasizing that feelings of emptiness are not expressions of an abstract nothingness, but experiences of a vacancy in the absence of a concrete presence. Hence, feelings of emptiness must be analyzed specifically within the context of what they express an emptiness from. In respect to postbereavement feelings of emptiness, I argued that Freud's suggestion that feelings of emptiness can exclusively be traced back to an impoverishment of the world is too simplistic and phenomenologically inadequate. This perspective neglects how my embodied sense of self cannot be separated from its broader appropriation of and habituation to an ontogenetically specific world. This means that my sense of self-familiarity and belonging in the world is a distributed and integrated web with multiple constituents ranging from things, habituated practices, to a sense of home, etc. I have referred to this integrated web as the existential texture of self-familiarity. When I share my life with an intimate other, this person becomes integral to the overall meaning and referential integrity of this web. In light of this, postbereavement feelings of emptiness can be seen as the affective expression of a profound constriction in my overall existential texture. Hence, postbereavement feelings of emptiness can be seen as an affective response to a quite literal *emptying of my being*.

It is a kind of self-alienation or state of *Unheimlichkeit* that points to the existential task of relearning myself and who I am in the absence of the intimate other. Understood in this way, postbereavement feelings of emptiness may, arguably, be considered as falling under the category of what Matthew Ratcliffe (2005) has called existential feelings. This is because, insofar as feelings of emptiness express a constriction in the existential texture of my being, they are not exclusively intentional in nature – that is, directed toward the lost person. Rather, they express an altered feeling of my being as such.

In closing, I need to point to a significant paradoxicality in the existential constitution of feelings of emptiness, namely, that the various sources of emptiness outlined above may simultaneously be the condition of possibility for the deceased's continued presence. Contemporary grief research has to a large degree been defined by a break with what is referred to as the "grief work hypothesis," namely, the premise that an adaptive process of grieving is one characterized by a detachment from the deceased. Instead, contemporary grief research has emphasized the premise that adaptive grief processes often involve maintaining a "continued bond" with the deceased (e.g., Klass, 2006; Klass & Steffen, 2017). However, preserving such a continued bond is not unproblematic, but requires perpetual maintenance and the utilization of a vast array of embodied practices, material objects, sociocultural practices, and symbolic resources. As I have argued in detail elsewhere, a particular challenge in this respect is maintaining a *felt sense of the deceased*; that is, an embodied sense of familiarity with the presence of the deceased as a concrete person (Køster, 2019, 2020). In this process, many of the elements I have referred to as sources of emptiness invert and rather become sources for a retention of the felt sense of the deceased. This could be how particular *things* that used to belong to the deceased now act as a *trace carrier* for his or her presence. An example could be how wearing a sweater that belonged to the deceased might help reestablish a sense of feeling near to them. Similarly, particular places or significant habitual practices like playing golf might serve the same function of being evocative of a felt sense of connection with the deceased.[10] In this way, the sources of emptiness are paradoxically also the sources of presence of the person who has passed away. Navigating this ambiguity between emptiness and presence is an inherent part of the existential reality of the grief process (see also Fuchs, 2018).

[10] I have explored this phenomenon in detail (Køster, 2019).

References

Adolfsson, A., Larsson, P. G., Wijma, B., & Bertero, C. (2004). Guilt and emptiness: Women's experiences of miscarriage. *Health Care for Women International*, 25(6), 543–560. doi:10.1080/07399330490444821

American Psychiatric Association. (2016). *Diagnostic and statistical manual of mental disorders* (5th ed.). Arlington, VA: Author.

Attig, T. (1996). *How we grieve: Relearning the world.* New York, NY: Oxford University Press.

Auster, P. (1992). *The invention of solitude.* London, UK: Faber and Faber.

Bachelard, G. (1994). *The poetics of space* (M. Jolas, Trans.). Boston, MA: Beacon Press.

Barthes, R. (2009). *Mourning diaries* (R. Howard, Trans.). New York, NY: Hill and Wang.

Bonanno, G. A. (2001). Grief and emotion: A social-functional perspective. In M. S. Stroebe, R. O. Hansson, W. Stroebe, & H. Schut (Eds.), *Handbook of bereavement research: Consequences, coping, and care* (pp. 493–515). Washington, DC: American Psychological Association. doi:10.1037/10436-021

Christine, V. (2008). *Bereavement narratives: Continuing bonds in the twenty-first century.* London, UK: Routledge.

Cushman, P. (1990). Why the self is empty: Toward a historically situated psychology. *The American Psychologist*, 45(5), 599–611. doi:10.1037//0003-066x.45.5.599

de Beauvoir, S. (1985). *A very easy death.* New York, NY: Pantheon Books.

Didion, J. (2011). *Blue nights.* London, UK: Fourth Estate.

Fernandez, A., & Køster, A. (2019). On the subject matter of phenomenological psychopathology. In G. Stanghellini, M. Broome, A. Raballo, A. V. Fernandez, P. Fusar-Poli, & R. Rosfort (Eds.), *The Oxford handbook of phenomenological psychopathology* (pp. 191–205). Oxford, UK: Oxford University Press.

Freud, S. (1957). Mourning and melancholia. In J. Strachey (Ed.), *The standard edition of the complete psychological works of Sigmund Freud* (Vol. XIV. 1914–1916. On the history of the psychoanalytic movement. Papers on metapsychology and other works, pp. 243–258). London, UK: The Hogarth Press and the Institute of Psycho-Analysis. (Original work published 1917)

Fuchs, T. (2012). The phenomenology of body memory. In S. C. Koch, T. Fuchs, M. Summa, & C. Müller (Eds.), *Body memory, metaphor and movement* (pp. 9–22). Amsterdam, Netherlands: John Benjamins Publishing Company.

Fuchs, T. (2018). Presence in absence: The ambiguous phenomenology of grief. *Phenomenology and the Cognitive Sciences*, 17(1), 43–63. doi:10.1007/s11097-017-9506-2

Goldie, P. (2011). Grief: A narrative account. *Ratio*, 24(2), 119–137. doi:10.1111/j.1467-9329.2011.00488.x

Goldie, P. (2012). *The mess inside: Narrative, emotion, and the mind.* Oxford, UK: Oxford University Press.

Greenson, R. R. (1949). The psychology of apathy. *Psychoanalytic Quarterly*, 18, 290–302. doi:10.1080/21674086.1949.11925763

Greenson, R. R. (1953). On boredom. *Journal of the American Psychoanalytic Association*, 1(1), 7–21. doi:10.1177/000306515300100102

Heidegger, M. (2001). *Sein und Zeit* [Being and time]. Tübingen, Germany: Niemeyer. (Original work published 1927)

Højlund, M., Kirkegaard, J. R., & Riis, M. S. (in press). The overheard – An attuning approach to sound art and design in public spaces. In M. Bull & M. Cobussen (Eds.), *The Bloomsbury handbook of sonic methodologies*. New York, NY: Bloomsbury.

Husserl, E. (1966). *Zur Phänomenologie des inneren Zeitbewusstseins* [On the phenomenology of inner time consciousness]. The Hague, Netherlands: Nijhoff.

Husserl, E. (1982). *Ideas pertaining to a pure phenomenology and to a phenomenological philosophy. First book: General introduction to a pure phenomenology* (L. Kersten, Trans.). Dordrecht, Netherlands: Kluwer Academic.

Ingerslev, L. (2018). Ongoing: On grief's open-ended rehearsal. *Continental Philosophy Review*, 51(3), 343–360. doi:10.1007/s11007-017-9423-7

Jacobson, K. (2009). A developed nature: A phenomenological account of the experience of home. *Continental Philosophy Review*, 42(3), 355–373. doi:10.1007/s11007-009-9113-1

Killikelly, C., & Maercker, A. (2018). Prolonged grief disorder for ICD-11: The primacy of clinical utility and international applicability. *European Journal of Psychotraumatology*, 8(Suppl. 6), 1–9. doi:10.1080/20008198.2018.1476441

Klass, D. (2006). Continuing conversation about continuing bonds. *Death Studies*, 30(9), 843–858. doi:10.1080/07481180600886959

Klass, D., Silverman, P. R., & Nickman, S. L. (Eds.). (1996). *Continuing bonds: New understandings of grief.* Washington, DC: Taylor & Francis.

Klass, D., & Steffen, E. M. (Eds.). (2017). *Continuing bonds in bereavement: New directions for research and practice.* New York, NY: Routledge.

Klonsky, E. D. (2008). What is emptiness? Clarifying the 7th criterion for borderline personality disorder. *Journal of Personality Disorders*, 22(4), 418–426. doi:10.1521/pedi.2008.22.4.41

Køster, A. (2017a). Narrative and embodiment – A scalar approach. *Phenomenology and the Cognitive Sciences*, 16(5), 893–908. doi:10.1007/s11097-016-9485-8

Køster, A. (2017b). Narrative self-appropriation: Embodiment, alienness, and personal responsibility in the context of borderline personality disorder. *Philosophy of Medical Research and Practice*, 38(6), 465–482. doi:10.1007/s11017-017-9422-z

Køster, A. (2019). Longing for concreteness: How body memory matters to continuing bonds. *Mortality*. Advance online publication. doi:10.1080/13576275.2019.1632277

Køster, A. (2020). The felt sense of the other: Contours of a sensorium. *Phenomenology and the Cognitive Sciences*. Advance online publication. doi:10.1007/s11097-020-09657-3

Køster, A., & Winther-Lindqvist, D. (2018). Personal history and historical selfhood – The embodied and pre-reflective dimension. In R. Alberto &

J. Valsiner (Eds.), *Cambridge handbook of sociocultural psychology* (pp. 538–555). Cambridge, UK: Cambridge University Press.
May, R. (1975). *Man's search for himself.* London, UK: Souvenir Press.
Merleau-Ponty, M. (1964). The philosopher and his shadow. In *Signs* (R. McCleary, Trans.) (pp. 159–181). Evanston, IL: Northwestern University Press.
Merleau-Ponty, M. (2012). *Phenomenology of perception* (D. A. Landes, Trans.). Abingdon, UK: Routledge.
Minkowski, E. (1970). *Lived time: Phenomenological and psychopathological studies.* Evanston, IL: Northwestern University Press.
Parkes, C. M. (1975). Psycho-social transitions: Comparison between reactions to loss of a limb and loss of a spouse. *The British Journal of Psychiatry: The Journal of Mental Science*, 127, 204–210. doi:10.1192/bjp.127.3.204
Rado, S. (1928). The problem of melancholia. *International Journal of Psycho-Analysis*, 9, 420–438.
Ratcliffe, M. (2005). The feeling of being. *Journal of Consciousness Studies*, 12(8–10), 43–60.
Ratcliffe, M. (2017). Grief and the unity of emotion. *Midwest Studies in Philosophy*, 41(1), 154–174. doi:10.1111/misp.12071
Ratcliffe, M. (2019). Grief and phantom limbs: A phenomenological comparison. In T. Burns, T. Szanto, A. Salice, M. Doyon, & A. A. Dumont (Eds.), *The new yearbook for phenomenology and phenomenological philosophy* (Vol. XVII, pp. 77–96). London, UK: Routledge.
Riley, D. (2012). *Time lived, without its flow.* London, UK: Capsule Editions.
Sallis, J. (2006). *Topographies.* Bloomington, IN: Indiana University Press.
Tewes, C., Durt, C., & Fuchs, T. (2017). Introduction: The interplay of embodiment, enaction and culture. In C. Tewes, C. Durt, & T. Fuchs (Eds.), *Embodiment, enaction, and culture: Investigating the constitution of the shared world* (pp. 1–22). Cambridge, MA: Massachusetts Institute of Technology Press.
Waldenfels, B. (2000). *Das leibliche Selbst. Vorlesungen zur Phänomenologie des Leibes* [The bodily self: Lectures on the phenomenology of the lived body]. Frankfurt am Main, Germany: Suhrkamp.
Zahavi, D. (1999). *Self-awareness and alterity: A phenomenological investigation.* Evanston, IL: Northwestern University Press.
Zandersen, M., & Parnas, J. (2019). Identity disturbance, feelings of emptiness, and the boundaries of the schizophrenia spectrum. *Schizophrenia Bulletin*, 45(1), 106–113. doi:10.1093/schbul/sbx183

7.1

Commentary on "Bereavement and the Meaning of Profound Feelings of Emptiness: An Existential-Phenomenological Analysis"

Relearning the Self among Intimate Others

Ditte Winther-Lindqvist

As a bereavement researcher rooted in developmental psychology (trained in a sociocultural and cultural–historical tradition) and with a keen eye to applied phenomenology, Allan Køster's idea of investigating bereavement responses in their particular aspects is appealing (Køster, 2021; Winther-Lindqvist, 2017). In Køster's persuasive analysis of the distributed self intertwined with intimate others, bereavement of an intimate other is described as a loss of self-familiarity. "I don't know who I am without you" is the paradigmatic statement; as a result, bereavement requires a *relearning of the self.* Along these lines, Køster suggests that the experiences of emptiness involved in bereavement relate to the "existential texture" of the self here and now and to its dyadic futurity, both of which are literally experienced as empty without the intimate other. Køster connects ideas of a distributed sense of self with the notion of being as always being-with, arguing that emptiness necessarily follows the loss of a partner, and it makes me wonder if this applies equally well to other kinds of losses? In this commentary, I will reflect upon this question. In the first part, I explore if and how it matters who the intimate other is who has been lost, and I conclude that a factor in the prevalence of experiences of emptiness is whether the dynamics of the relationship are mainly dyadic or triadic. I then illustrate this point with examples from an empirical study of adolescents who have lost a parent. I argue that the emptiness stemming from the absent parent is often filled with a doubled presence by the remaining parent. Finally, I reflect on the effect of time in ontogeny, as an open question concerning the process of grief and emptiness, as it evolves after bereavement. I suggest that the prevalence of experiences of emptiness varies as a function of the relational dynamic and particular context of the loss. This refining and specifying of Køster's argument follows the logic of his thinking and draws specifically on my work as an empirical researcher into the phenomenon of losing a parent during adolescence, and on my own experiences with losing a parent when I was a teenager.

Specifying the Loss of an Intimate Other in a Dyadic or a Triadic Relational Dynamic

Køster uses the paradigmatic case of loss of a partner to investigate emptiness in postbereavement existence; and through this choice, he focuses on a dyadic structure of adaptation, where the bereaved partner asks: Who am I now without you? This is a valid and insightful phenomenological analysis of the profound alteration of the existential texture of the self, which is at the core of the loss of a partner. However, in most other cases of bereavement of intimate others, the bereaved are not left *alone* but exist in a *family* that suffers loss, and whose members grieve alongside one another: In those cases, the question is rather: *Who am I and who are you and what are we now without X?* My proposal is that this *triadic* constellation is consequential for the grieving process, especially concerning the prevalence of experiences of emptiness in bereavement. The careful phenomenological analysis provided by Køster reveals that the loss of an intimate other profoundly changes the existential texture of one's self-familiarity, and he argues that feelings of emptiness follow from this alteration. Bereavement requires a relearning of the self – as Køster rephrases Attig's point (1996). Køster makes clear how comprehensive this task of relearning the self is, when the self was so intimately intertwined with the deceased party and in the case of the loss of a partner the bereaved is literally left home alone, experiencing the absent–present void of the loved one. The analysis builds on fundamental phenomenological ideas of the distributed self (Merleau-Ponty, 2012) and of the social ontology of being as always "being-with" (Heidegger, 2014). Along the same lines, I argue that in other cases of bereavement too this being-with continues after a loved one dies. Most bereaved people remain embedded in other relationships with intimate others (with parents, children, siblings, spouses) and this is a crucial part of the constitution of the grieving process (Nadeau, 1998). How the bereavement situation affects these ongoing relationships is of utmost importance, not least for bereaved children, who are so dependent upon the care and attention of their parents for their well-being and future development (Bowlby, 1980). Let us explore what this triadic situation may mean to the experiences of emptiness in grief. I will argue (as a developmental psychologist) that it matters a great deal who the bereaved is, and who the intimate other is – to the bereaved – in terms of the developmental situation and relational dynamic, because we typically enjoy different relationship roles, responsibilities, and caring tasks depending on our position as spouse, child, sibling, or parent. The alteration and relearning of the self is a process mediated by our relationship to the dead, as well as to those who live on. If it does indeed matter whether the grieving process plays out in a dyadic dynamics or a more complex triadic constellation, my suggestion is that feelings of emptiness are more prevalent in dyadic dynamics, as Køster has described it, when the bereaved party is precisely left behind – to be alone.[1]

The Absent Father and the Intensified Presence of the Mother

In my empirical work, I look into postbereaved existence among adolescents who have lost a parent. These adolescents are not left behind to be alone – but left behind to continue their life in a grief-struck family with ongoing relationships to the remaining parent and, in some cases, siblings living at home too. In these cases, the bereaved child has not only to navigate a new life situation without, for example, the father, but also has to adapt to a "new" self-absorbed mother, who for a long time is a more-or-less devastated widow. It is my impression that the emptiness stemming from the absence of the father often manifests itself in perceptions of the mother's *disproportionate presence*. In some instances, this even reaches a point where the adolescents feel that their mother is "sitting on them" and leaving them no room to mourn their father and to really feel his absence. During the illness, or in the first months after death, the adolescents tend to grow apart from their remaining parent, and in some dramatic cases, the adolescent sadly remarks that they somehow lost both their parents when their father died/became ill, whereas others just feel a new alienation between themselves and the remaining parent. In each circumstance, the emptiness at least includes both parents, albeit in different ways. Summing up, adolescents who are bereaved of a parent have to become part of new relationships where roles and caring responsibilities are often profoundly changed due to the bereavement situation, and where the relationship with the remaining parent seems to play as important a part as that with the deceased parent.

> I miss the three of us … because back then it was all different … she was different, and I was different. (Girl 16, a year after her father died)

In this quote, the adolescent girl misses not only her lost father, but also her mother as she used to be, and herself – in what we could call an existential texture constituted by a triadic dynamic. The absent parent is often perceived as absent through the doubled or contaminated presence of the remaining

[1] Being alone for most people is a temporary situation; even among elderly widow(er)s, many remarry or at least find a new partner, sometimes quite early after their loss (Hansson & Stroebe, 2007).

parent. As a result, rather than a pure sense of emptiness, there might be a contaminated sense of preoccupation with the *wrong* figure, so that for instance the mother takes on the empty placeholder of the father, leading to an increased distancing and conflictual dynamic between the parties: "Oh, it's you again (and not X…)."[2] This more hostile and angry side of adjusting to bereavement in the family is interwoven in complex ways with family members' deep concern and care for one another, often combined with a lessened ability to show compassion and to be actually caring toward one another. And this might be the main difference between the dyadic dynamic Køster describes and the more triadic one: that the emptiness becomes conflictual, contested, and guilt-ridden between equally grief-struck parties, who tend to mourn apart rather than together. This I find to be peculiar to families with teenage children and is not necessarily the case with younger children. The adolescent who is occupied with issues of identity and identification compares their lost parent with the remaining parent, often in ways where they tend to identify more with and idealize the dead parent. In the absence of the more desired parent, the newly altered and less appealing aspects of the remaining parent grow in prominence. In the absence of the father, the mother becomes annoyingly present everywhere. Even in instances where the bereaved manage to remain caring and open in their relationship after bereavement, and may even grow closer in the process, death seems to reverberate into and change the dynamics among those who live on. So, not only do the bereaved need to relearn the self in light of loss, they also encounter altered ongoing relationships in the midst of this process. In my own case, I lost my mother as an adolescent, but the experience is more that *we* lost her, and the most profound relearning of myself had to do with quickly becoming the best possible substitute for her in order to meet new and urgent needs for care and attention from my younger siblings. If I felt an emptiness in bereavement, it was in small cracks between a fullness of their needs, of constant conflicts and worries regarding the just-as-grief-stricken extended family, and of spending time with my friends and boyfriends, trying to get the most out of my youth in spite of the sadness.

Feelings of Emptiness across Time and Position in Ontogeny

I find it an open question in Køster's account whether emptiness *remains* a central part of the bereaved persons' subsequent development. In one

[2] I believe that this dynamic can also be found in examples where it is a child who dies and the siblings grow up in the shadow of the deceased. In some sad cases, the parents see in the remaining children only their lack of resemblance with the dead child (Oh, you again, and not X).

sense, it would follow logically from Køster's analysis that emptiness is particularly profound in acute grief, and thus most strongly connected to the first painful experiences of relearning oneself without the other. On the other hand, perhaps a sense of emptiness might actually grow in significance rather than diminish over time, because we gradually yet persistently lose a concrete sense of the intimate other in the postbereavement years (Køster, 2019). Having only experienced bereavement myself during adolescence, and only in the constellation of the loss of my mother, which is now decades ago, I am amazed at how little I remember, not only of her but also of how I was before we lost her. According to Køster, the existential texture of the self is sustained by everyday practices in the concrete world of particular places (the home, the school, the workplace) and particular habituated practices with other people and artefacts in these places. All those changes that relate to the death of the other add up to a new everyday life, and thus also to a new sense of stability and self-familiarity, now without the deceased person intertwined with it all. Following this line of thinking, the sense of emptiness as a continued experience must therefore reflect the developmental situation of the bereaved (time and position in ontogeny) as well as the specific nature of the loss of the intimate other. For the old widow(er) who loses a life-long spouse, it is more likely that the emptiness and emptied sense of self remain with them than for the bereaved child or adolescent who can reorient themselves toward a shared past with a deceased parent in the many years ahead of them. After all, a child's past is so short and their future so long. The pertinent issues in the lifeworld of the adolescent are the ongoing projects, engagements, and relationships with family, friends, partners, and peers. Among adolescents, this future orientation and the rapidly changing circumstances can, I suggest, lead to a quite rapid formation of a new sense of self-familiarity, which does not necessarily involve the deceased parent. The participants in my study are puzzled and surprised by how quickly they become absorbed by the hurly-burly of everyday life and become occupied with adjusting to the reconfigurations and changes in their ongoing relationships. They feel that they forget about their deceased parent too quickly. This paradoxical nature of our relations to the dead in grief is underscored in phenomenological accounts (Fuchs, 2018), and in my experience the paradoxical presence–absence of the deceased persists across time, although its character has somehow turned around. The disbelief connected to the gradual realization that my own existence and that of the others continued without my mother has, over the years, turned into an equally perplexing experience of disbelief and sense of emptiness connected to the fact that she was ever once among us. I would have been devastated had I been told: There will come a day when the world without her, and yourself without her, will be the only existence you know. Yet that is how it is, and I think this is true for bereaved children generally, though not for adults bereaved of a life-long partner.

References

Attig, T. (1996). *How we grieve: Relearning the world.* New York, NY: Oxford University Press.

Bowlby, J. (1980). *Attachment and loss: Vol. III. Loss sadness and depression.* New York, NY: Basic Books.

Fuchs, T. (2018). Presence in absence. The ambiguous phenomenology of grief. *Phenomenology and the Cognitive Sciences*, 17(1), 43–63. doi:10.1007/s11097-017-9506-2

Hansson, R. O., & Stroebe, M. (2007). *Bereavement in late life. Coping, adaptation, and development influences.* Washington, DC: American Psychological Association.

Heidegger, M. (2014). *Væren og Tid* [Being and time] (C. R. Skovgaard, Trans.). Aarhus, Denmark: Forlaget Klim.

Køster, A. (2019). Longing for concreteness: How body memory matters to continuing bonds. *Mortality.* Advance online publication. doi:10.1080/13576275.2019.1632277

Køster, A. (2021). Bereavement and the meaning of profound feelings of emptiness: An existential-phenomenological analysis. In C. Tewes & G. Stanghellini (Eds.), *Time and body: Phenomenological and psychopathological approaches* (pp. 125–143). Cambridge, UK: Cambridge University Press.

Merleau-Ponty, M. (2012). *Phenomenology of perception* (D. A. Landes, Trans.). New York, NY: Routledge.

Nadeau, J. W. (1998). *Families making sense of death.* Thousand Oaks, CA: Sage.

Winther-Lindqvist, D. (2017). Hope as fantasy: An existential phenomenology of hoping in light of parental illness. In B. Wagoner, S. H. Awad, & I. Bresco de Luna (Eds.), *The psychology of imagination: History, theory and new research horizons* (pp. 151–173). Charlotte, NC: Information Age Publishing.

8

Body-as-Object in Social Situations
Toward a Phenomenology of Social Anxiety

Shogo Tanaka

Introduction

The symptoms of social anxiety are often explained as "more than shyness" (e.g., National Health Service [NHS], 2017). Although everyone is shy to a certain extent, people with social anxiety disorder (SAD) suffer from an overwhelming feeling of fear in social situations. As might be imagined, symptoms are caused to occur in situations where one can be perceived and evaluated negatively by others. Decades before the concept of *social phobia* (i.e., the former name of SAD) was first established in the *Diagnostic and Statistical Manual of Mental Disorders (DSM)-III* (American Psychiatric Association, 1980), the psychiatrist Paul Schilder (1950), who left a pioneering work on body image, described the same symptom as "social neurosis." He described one patient as follows:

> The 31-year-old S. L. complains of blushing and sweating when he is in the presence of others. If he does not actually blush and perspire he is afraid of doing so. This fear hinders him in all his social contacts and makes him afraid of meeting anyone. His self-consciousness goes back to his very early childhood. He was very tall for his age and was always afraid that other people would look at him and wonder why he played with children so much smaller than himself. (Schilder, 1950, p. 227)

The patient is afraid that his own body (being tall) or bodily reactions (blushing and sweating) would be perceived and evaluated negatively by others. And the anticipatory anxiety related to social situations leads him to avoid interpersonal contacts. From this description, we notice that the experience of one's own body being perceived by others constitutes the origin of social anxiety and, in this sense, is continuous to shyness. In both cases, one would experience acute self-consciousness through one's own body perceived by others in social situations. In this chapter, I would like to explicate the relationship among social anxiety, bodily experiences, and interpersonal contact with others. In so doing, I will first revisit the phenomenology of bodily experiences and confirm the difference between the body-as-subject and the body-as-object. Next, I will describe the experiences of one's *body-as-object for others*, distinguishing them from those of one's body-as-object for oneself. Among phenomenologists, it was Sartre (1943/1956) who emphasized this aspect of bodily experiences as the "third ontological dimension of the body." On the basis of this notion, I will try to develop a phenomenology of social anxiety as well as its disorder.

From Body-as-Subject to Body-as-Object

In considering the body, the traditional phenomenological approach has a common tendency to emphasize the subjective aspect of the body. In contrast to the natural sciences, such as physiology, which objectifies the body, phenomenology starts with the body that makes possible very subjective experiences. Without the body, it would be impossible for me to perceive the world or to act in the world. Though my conscious attention is not directed to the body but to the world during my perception and action, the body operates smoothly in the background; I perceive the world through and from my body and I act in the world through and with my body. It was Merleau-Ponty (1945/2012) who emphasized the implicit subjective aspect of the body. He writes, "I can only understand the function of the living body by accomplishing it and to the extent that I am a body that rises up toward the world" (Merleau-Ponty, 1945/2012, p. 78). The body constitutes the "I" as a subject of perception and action. *Body-as-subject* is the proper name for this fundamental aspect of the body (e.g., Ichikawa, 1992; Zahavi, 2003).

However, what I need to focus on in the following is not the body that appears as a subject but as an object, which has been somewhat underestimated in past phenomenological discussion on embodiment (Ingerslev, 2013). Different from the manner in which the natural sciences analyze the body as an object from the third-person perspective, my body appears to me as an intentional object in diverse experiences. For example, I look at my body when I wear clothes, touch a certain spot when I feel pain at that point, or listen to my own voice when I speak. In all cases, the same body appears as the body-as-subject, on the one hand, and the *body-as-object*, on the other hand. Using the term body-as-object, I focus on the objective aspect of the body, which appears as an object of perception and action within the context of our ordinary experiences in the lifeworld.

First of all, for its opacity, my body appears to me as an object of visual perception. The body-as-object has a surface that prevents me from seeing through, so it stands out from the ground as a visual figure. For example, I see my own hands located "there" among many other objects on the desk, but at the same time, I feel it "here" through proprioception. The capacity of mirror-self cognition is based on this spatial split between the proprioceptively felt body and the visually perceived body (Tanaka, 2019). When I act in a self-directed manner such as when grooming in front of a mirror, I presuppose that the mirror image is the visual representation of my body viewed from the opposite end (visual-there), even though it is felt through proprioception as being located here (proprioceptive-here). When I look at myself in the mirror, my body-as-subject recognizes my body-as-object in a self-reflective manner.

Second, due to its shape and volume, I can touch, seize, stroke, scratch, and tap my body as an object. Though I do not become aware of it normally, in a conscious experience of self-touching, my body appears in an ambiguous manner; the same body appears as the touching subject as well as the touched object, and the double sensation occurs as Merleau-Ponty (1945/2012) describes. If I touch my left hand with the right, the left hand reversely appears as the touching subject while being touched. This reversibility embedded in self-touching is a sort of self-reflection that clearly distinguishes the body from other material things as "a thing of a particular type" (Husserl, 1952/1989, pp. 165–168). In terms of subjectivity, the touching hand that appears as "I" could be converted into the touched ("me"), as occurs in self-reflection when thinking "I" is objectified as "me" by a higher cognitive process. Following Merleau-Ponty (1945/2012), Ichikawa (1992) also states that "the double sensation is, so to speak, an externalized self-reflection" (p. 89). The experience of corporeal dissociation between the touching and the touched developmentally precedes and prepares the internal experience that "I" think of "me."

Third, the voice also appears as an object of perception. During speech, I can listen to my own voice as an auditory object. In relation to reflective thought, it is important to note that I can do so even if I do not speak aloud. I listen to my inner speech as a monologue, through which "I think." As Vygotsky (1934/1987) showed, in its developmental origin thinking is realized through internalized conversation with the self. If I were not the body-as-object that can be listened to, I would not be able to appear as a thinking subject. Regarding this point, Merleau-Ponty (1945/2012) states that "The Cogito that we obtain by reading Descartes and even the one that Descartes performs … is thus a spoken Cogito, put into words and understood through words" (p. 423). In other words, the thinking "I" requires "me" and its spoken words as audible objects. Because my body-as-object is embodied as an inner voice, "I" am able to think of "me" in a reflective manner.

Thus, my body appears to me as an object through multiple modalities of sensation. The body functions in a reflexive manner inasmuch as the body-as-subject perceives as the body-as-object. This reflexivity makes possible the body image, that is, "the mental picture one forms of one's body as a whole" (American Psychological Association, 2007, p. 128). As is well shown in the capacity of mirror-self cognition, one has either an implicit or explicit mental picture of one's own body and recognizes it in the mirror when grooming. Although it is sometimes confused in the related literature, the concept of body image should be distinguished from that of body schema (Gallagher, 2005). Both concepts refer to one's cognition of the body, but body schema is more closely related to the body-as-subject. The body schema is "a system of sensory-motor capacities that function without awareness or the necessity of perceptual monitoring" (Gallagher, 2005, p. 24). It underpins one's implicit cognition of ongoing bodily postures as well as how to organize body parts into a unified action (Tanaka, 2013). In contrast, the body image is rather related to the body-as-object. The body image "consists of a system of perceptions, attitudes, and beliefs pertaining to one's own body" (Gallagher, 2005, p. 24). Basically, not only is it a mental image based on the visual perception of one's own body but it also contains one's emotional attitude toward it (e.g., dissatisfaction, vanity, shame) and conceptual understanding of it (e.g., medical knowledge of one's symptoms). The point is that the body image is a reflexive system in which one perceives, feels, and thinks of one's own body as an intentional object, different from the body schema. And this reflexivity derives from the experiences of one's body itself.

In addition, this reflexive function within the body is the bodily basis of the distinction of the self that William James (1890/1950, pp. 291–401) proposed: "I" and "me." "I" is the self as the knowing subject and "me" is the self as the known object. In contrast to modern philosophers such as Descartes or Kant, James did not identify the "I" as the transcendental ego but simply as a thought. As such, the "I" cannot exist if it loses its connection with the empirical "me." One can also point out that there is a developmental process of the dialogue between "I" and "me," as is seen in the case of the inner voice. Though we do not know the order among modalities, the bodily dialogue between body-as-subject and body-as-object, such as *I look at my body*, *I touch my body*, and *I listen to my voice*, gradually achieves its abstract dimension until it culminates in the self-reflection of *I think of me*. Here, it is important to confirm that the subjective experience of self-reflection has its bodily basis even though it seems purely an abstract cognitive process (Tanaka, 2019).

The Body-as-Object for Others

One knows that the same body that appears as an object of perception and action for oneself also appears as an object for *others*. For example, while giving a lecture in an auditorium, I am fully aware that I am looked at and listened to by the students. When I see a doctor with a bad cold, the doctor checks my body by listening through a stethoscope, visually examining the tonsils and palpating the forehead and neck.

To articulate a further question involved here, let me examine the problem of body image once again. Developmentally speaking, it takes eighteen to twenty-four months after birth for humans to be able to recognize themselves in the mirror (Amsterdam, 1972; Butterworth, 1995). Most infants under twelve months perceive a mirror self-image as another person. After twenty months, they show increasingly self-directed behaviors such as hairdressing, in which one can act effectively on one's own body part only through a mirror image. At this stage, infants might be aware that the body they visually perceive in the mirror reflects their own body. Finally, at around two years of age, the image of the whole body seems to be formed in infants' minds, and they come to know explicitly the correspondence between the body in the mirror and their real body.

From a phenomenological perspective, however, the problem of visual perspective should be further explicated. To achieve mirror self-recognition, one must know how one's body looks from the external perspective, but this is actually impossible (Tanaka, 2017, pp. 50–71). As an example, consider the self-portrait drawn by the philosopher Ernst Mach (1906/1959, p. 59) and compare it with an ordinary body image drawn by a student (Tanaka, 2017, p. 52). If we insist on the precise visual perspective from which one can look at one's own body, there would be no other way for Mach to illustrate himself than the one he used (in Figure 8.1). Although one is not able to achieve an actual viewpoint that allows one to illustrate one's body as shown in Figure 8.2, one somehow holds the image of the whole body in the mind and is able to match it with the body reflected in the mirror. In other words, one has a visual representation of one's body-as-object that is perceived virtually from the external perspective.

Then, how does one form the image of one's whole body? By looking in the mirror repeatedly? This answer is not plausible. There are two empirical studies that allow us to consider this point. First, according to Priel and de Schonen (1986), infants without any prior experience with mirrors do not show a significant difference in their capacity for mirror-self cognition when compared with a group with habitual mirror familiarity. It does not

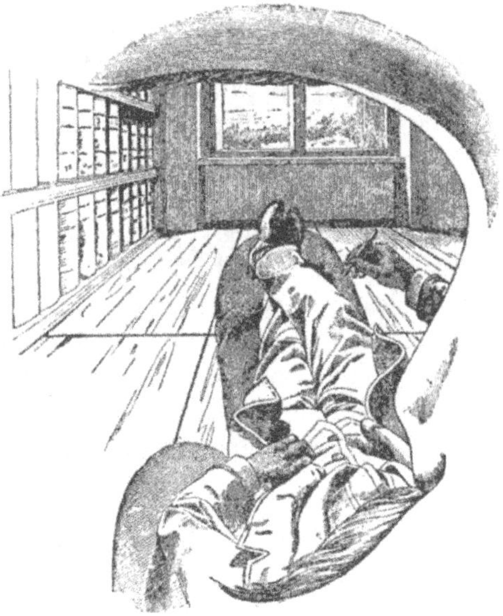

Figure 8.1 Ernst Mach's self-portrait (from Mach, 1959, p. 19).

seem necessary to look at one's own body reflected in the mirror during the process of forming the image of one's whole body in the mind. Second, chimpanzees reared in isolation are not able to recognize themselves in a mirror, whereas others reared normally in groups have this ability (Gallup, 1977). Social interactions with other individuals have a crucial impact on the capacity for mirror self-recognition in its developmental process.

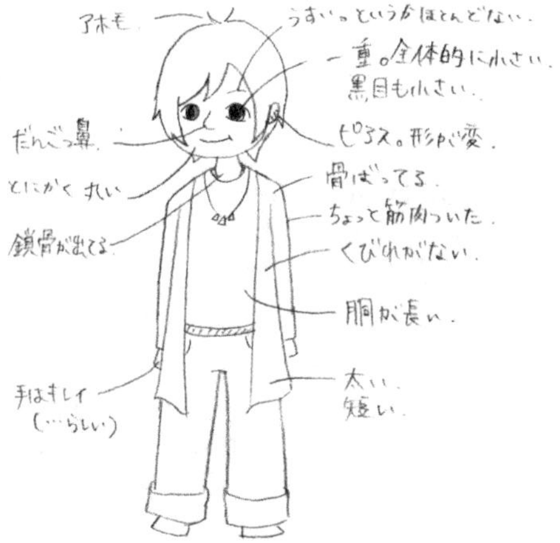

Figure 8.2 Example of a body image (from Tanaka, 2017, p. 52).

Based on these empirical facts, it is reasonable to think that one learns to view one's own body from another person's external perspective through social interactions. One's body appears as an intentional object for the gaze of others in diverse ways: it is glanced at, stared at, watched over, and so on. Reddy (2008, pp. 120–149) reports that seven-month-old infants try to gain and manipulate another person's attention by doing extreme actions such as screaming and banging. This suggests that infants of this age already know that their body can be an object of perception for the other in interactions. This dyadic relation is triangulated among the self, the other, and the object after joint attention arises between mother and infant (Tomasello, 1995): Infants around nine months of age come to notice the object of visual attention of the mother and to pay attention to the same object. Concerning the meaning of joint attention, Fuchs (2013) points out the following:

> Joint attention transforms objects as well as persons. On the one hand, objects are transformed from ego-bound things for action into ego-distant things for pointing – towards or symbolic interaction. By seeing them "through others' eyes," they become *objects* in the proper sense of the word, namely independent from one's own subjective perspective. On the other hand, in order to show the object to another *person*, the infant has to grasp what this person sees and to take into account her spatial perspective at least implicitly. (Fuchs, 2013, p. 667)

After establishing the capacity of joint attention, infants would gradually become able to understand explicitly the other's visual perspective, and in correspondence with this, they start to imagine their body-as-object viewed from the external perspective. As Schilder (1950, pp. 213–282) considered in his classical work, one's body image is informed and influenced by others in interaction. I am not only looked at by surrounding others, but also look at others' bodies. On the one hand, through looking comparatively at others' bodies, one grasps one's appearance as different from that of others in terms such as height, shape, gender, skin color, and hair style. But on the other hand, I can form my body image as the same kind of person by coupling the appearances of others' bodies and that of mine.

In any case, one's body image is not pictured by oneself alone. What I would like to emphasize here is that one's *body-as-object for others* precedes one's body-as-object for oneself in its developmental origin, and it provides the empirical foundation for one's body image. The image of one's body is actually a product of *social* interactions of looking-at and being-looked-at between the self and others.

Third Ontological Dimension of the Body as the Source of Social Anxiety

Let us continue to discuss the difference between the body-as-object for oneself and that for others. As Ichikawa (1992, pp. 93–95) points out, the experience of tickling is the easiest example with which to illustrate this difference. No matter how ticklish I feel when tickled by others, I am not able to elicit this response by tickling myself. My feeling of being ticklish is made possible only by the other body that is not *mine*. In other words, the ticklish feeling in my body cannot be elicited by the body experienced with a *sense of ownership*. This is not the entire point. Consider the difference between touching oneself (body-as-object for oneself) and being touched by another person (body-as-object for others). In the latter experience, through my tactile perceptions, I feel a variety of intentions that are not precisely predictable before I am touched, such as tickling, patting, slapping, pinching, scratching, rubbing, and so on. The other body that touches my body as an object is experienced with various intentions that are not mine. The other body appears not only as a body lacking my sense of ownership but also as one inhabited by an *agency* other than mine. Thus, it is possible to say that through my body-as-object I directly experience the presence of the *other subjectivity* beyond the limit of my subjectivity (Tanaka, 2018).

Therefore, my bodily experience of being an object is coupled with the emergence of the other subject. Sartre (1943/1956) describes this experience with his notion of the "third ontological dimension of the body." According to Sartre, the body is ontologically constituted of three dimensions. In the first dimension, the body is simply lived and not explicitly known, as described above as the body-as-subject. In the second dimension, both my body and that of others stay within an anonymous region, so to speak. My body appears as an object for others and others' bodies appear to me as objects, but they still lack mutual and personal engagement with each other. In the third dimension, the other body appears to me as the subject for whom my body is an object. He writes, "I exist for myself as a body known by the Other. This is the third ontological dimension of my body" (Sartre, 1943/1956, p. 351).

My body-as-object is an interface through which the other's subjectivity appears to me. However, let us be reminded that Husserl (1950/1960) used to characterize one's experience of the other as "what is not originally accessible" (p. 114) or "a primordially unfulfillable experience" (p. 115). Although I experience the presence of the other's subjectivity with their body, there always will remain certain aspects of it that are not disclosed through social interactions.[1] Simply put, it is impossible for me to perceive my own body in the same manner that the other perceives it. Of course, by exchanging perspectives imaginatively with the other or checking my own appearance in a mirror, one can well know how I am viewed by the other. But such knowledge never shows exactly how the other person looks at me. My body-as-object appearing in the other's perception is not provided to me as such, but akin at best. Along with his concept of the third ontological dimension of the body, Sartre (1943/1956) clearly highlights the problem that arises concerning this point:

> With the appearance of the Other's look I experience the revelation of my being-as-object; that is, of my transcendence as transcended. A me-as-object is revealed to me as an unknowable being, as the flight into an Other which I am with full responsibility. (Sartre, 1943/1956, p. 351)

The point is that my body-as-object perceived by the other is essentially unknowable. The sum of the aspects that is perceived by the other constitutes a "me-as-object" in the other's mind, of which I am not able to know its exact form. In the subsequent paragraph, Sartre (1943/1956) also writes, "my body escapes me on all sides" (p. 352). In relation to the body image, the third ontological dimension of the body is one's body image formed in the other's mind, which is not totally disclosed to oneself.

Here, we find the primary source of social anxiety (in Figure 8.3). One cannot know exactly how one is perceived by others and even less so how one is evaluated by them. In the first moment of social encounter with another, one is suspended in the unknowableness of one's me-as-object and evaluation toward it. Until one receives feedback, one's evaluation remains potentially negative as well as positive. And even though one can receive feedback about oneself from others, this does not change the structural unknowableness of one's body image in the other's mind. This experience

[1] In the context of phenomenology, there may be room for discussion at this point. Unlike Husserl and Sartre, Max Scheler (1948/1954) claimed the possibility of directly perceiving the other's mental states. Gallagher (2008) elaborated his ideas as the direct social perception (DSP) theory, which asserts that others' mental states, such as emotions and intentions of action, are expressive enough to be perceived. The author also defends DSP in considering the most fundamental aspect of social cognition (Tanaka, 2015). However, its claims are defended inasmuch as we consider social situations in which the self and the other engage via bidirectional social interactions. In this chapter, we consider the specific situation in which one's attention is directed mainly to the passive experience of being perceived by the other almost unidirectionally. For this reason, DSP is not the first theoretical choice to pursue our description of the subjective experiences.

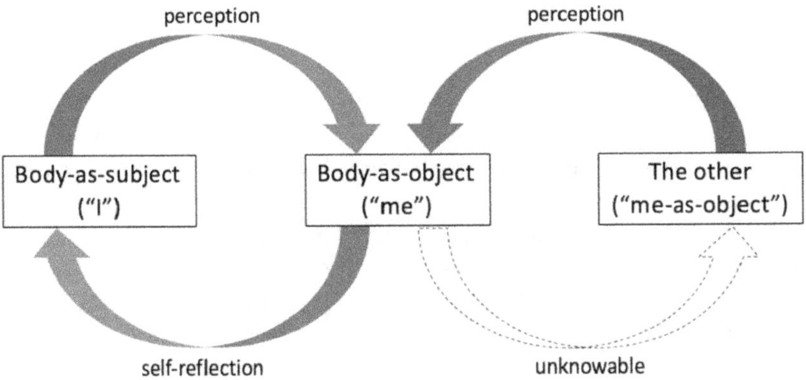

Figure 8.3 The source of social anxiety.

would inevitably cause a basic feeling of tension inside one's body while being exposed to the other's gaze and perception. When the bodily feeling of tension is experienced together with the worries about being evaluated negatively, it generates a feeling of shyness. If the presence of the other becomes overwhelming, the shyness is rather experienced as social anxiety, that is, "more than shyness."

In his well-known work on anxiety, May (1977, pp. 189–193) characterized anxiety as *feelings of uncertainty* in the face of danger. This feature is also observed in the case of social anxiety; one faces uncertainty of the other's mind that may perceive and evaluate her either positively or negatively. The uncertainty of the other's mind that objectifies me-as-object is the source of social anxiety. In this sense, one can say that all of us inevitably experience a slight feeling of social anxiety in the first moment of interpersonal contact. In ordinary cases, however, the initial experience of social anxiety in itself forms a(n) (often unconscious) drive for interaction with the other in anticipation of easing it. If one succeeds in receiving positive feedback, including subtle nonverbal signs such as smiling, one would be released from tension to a certain degree.[2] Now, we need to explicate how one experiences social anxiety in pathological cases.

[2] Note that in this situation we are gradually moving from the unidirectional social situation to the bidirectional one. As one's attentional focus shifts from the passive experience of being perceived to that of actively interacting with the other, there would be more space for DSP. Perceiving nonverbal signs such as smiling means perceiving the other's positive emotional states toward the situation, even though this does not ultimately erase the structural unknowableness of the other's mind.

A Phenomenology of SAD

According to the current DSM-5 (American Psychiatric Association, 2013), "the essential feature of SAD is a marked, or intense, fear or anxiety of social situations in which the individual may be scrutinized by others" (p. 203). The social situations may include those of making conversation in a group, meeting unfamiliar people, dating someone, performing in front of others, and so on. Even though no actual threat exists in these situations, individuals with SAD show psychosomatic symptoms connected with anxiety such as blushing, trembling, sweating, stammering, acting awkwardly, and so on. And these primary symptoms make them even more afraid that they will be evaluated negatively by others. Some individuals may be afraid of making others feel uncomfortable or offended by their symptoms and thus rejected as a result. Social situations almost always provoke anxiety, so individuals with SAD experience anticipatory anxiety and often show a strong tendency to avoid social situations. This symptom causes significant impairment in social or occupational functioning.

From a phenomenological perspective, the first point to be explicated is the relationship between anxiety and fear experienced in SAD. As May (1977, pp. 207–210) emphasizes, the experience of fear is different from that of anxiety. Fear is a reaction to a specific danger normally accompanied with a certain object or a particular situation. For example, one might be afraid of snakes, heights, monsters, ghosts, physical pain, among others. In these cases, fear is clearly directed at a concrete object or situation regardless of whether it is real or not. If one can move away from it, the emotion of fear also disappears or is alleviated. In contrast, although anxiety is also a feeling that arises in the face of danger, it is vague and objectless. For example, one might be afraid of one's own death, but this is an experience of anxiety because one never knows when or how it will happen. Heidegger (1927/1962, p. 295) also emphasizes that "anxiety in the face of death must not be confused with fear in the face of one's demise." Because death is given as the possibility of inexistence of oneself, it is not clearly defined as something as objective as demise. Again, anxiety is a feeling of uncertainty in the face of unspecific danger.

Basically, it is *uncertainty of the other's mind* that lies beneath the experience of social anxiety. To a certain degree, all of us experience this kind of anxiety when encountering someone unfamiliar (but we know how to move beyond that anxiety and engage in subsequent social interactions). However, for patients with SAD, there is a certain trigger within social situations that inflates and exaggerates the uncertainty as danger. Let us consider the relationship between anxiety and fear through the following example. Hofmann and Otto (2008) recount the story of a patient named Barbara, who started to suffer from SAD after being promoted in the company:

> Barbara is a 33-year-old businesswoman who has been living with her husband and two children outside a major metropolitan area. Her husband takes care of the children at home while she works at a large insurance company. She has been extraordinarily successful in her career and recently became the vice president of her company. Shortly after she got promoted, she decided to see a therapist because of her *panic attacks* [emphasis added] that she sometimes gets when she has to give presentations in front of people at work. During the diagnostic interview, Barbara described herself as having been outgoing and popular throughout adolescence and young adulthood, with no serious problems until her third year in college. This is when she began to become extremely tense and nervous when she had to give oral presentations in front of people, especially *large crowds in a formal setting* [emphasis added]. When asked what it was about these situations that make her so nervous, she said that *she was concerned about what the audience would think of her* [emphasis added]. "The audience might sense how nervous I am, and I may not be comprehensible and look foolish." As a result, she spends many hours preparing her speech, writing out explicit scripts for all of her presentations. Curiously, she experiences little or no anxiety in informal social settings, such as parties or large dinner meetings. (Hofmann & Otto, 2008, p. 3)

According to the patient herself, the presence of a large audience is a trigger that causes an intense emotional reaction that is experienced as a panic attack. At a glance, what she experiences seems to be fear because it is directed toward the audience, which is a well-defined object. As a matter of fact, however, she is annoyed by the very uncertainty of "what the audience would think of her" and is especially afraid of their negative evaluation toward her ("I may not be comprehensible and look foolish"). The presence of the audience is a mere trigger, not the actual object that the patient's emotion is directed toward. For patients with SAD, there is something in social situations that makes salient and exaggerates the uncertainty of the other's mind as danger. It is not only confined to others' gazes and facial expressions but also includes patients' own appearances. Their own bodily reactions (blushing, sweating, stammering, etc.) and their bodily features (birthmarks, deformed body parts, body odor, etc.) that they believe to be evaluated negatively by others can also be triggers of the symptom. Therefore, the core feeling experienced by these patients is not fear but anxiety. Even if the patients seem to experience fear, it is a replaced reaction that is triggered by a certain object within the context of social situations.

It is as if the anxiety of death is often replaced by the fear of a certain disease such as cancer.

The second point to be explicated here is the degree of publicness, which seems to affect the symptom of anxiety. The patient quoted above claims that she becomes extremely nervous when faced with large crowds in a formal setting, whereas she experiences little or no anxiety in informal settings. In relation to this point, the DSM-5 newly added the "performance only" subtype of SAD, in which the symptom is restricted to performing *in public* (Heimberg et al., 2014). Generally speaking, the more formal and public the social setting, the more distant and unfamiliar others appear in a given situation. In such a setting, one perceives that each particular person becomes embedded in collectivity. Accordingly, the sum of "persons" starts to appear as "people" in anonymity, whose criteria of evaluation are difficult for one to know explicitly. As the situation becomes more public, it becomes more difficult to be evaluated in a positive manner, especially for those who try to meet expectations at a high level.

There is a related clinical fact that is known in Japanese psychiatry, where research on SAD has a long history with the notion of *Taijin Kyofusho* (literally meaning "phobia of interpersonal relations"). Patients with *Taijin Kyofusho* have a common tendency to suffer from social anxiety the most strongly in ambiguous social settings (Kasahara, 2005, pp. 27–42; Maeda & Nathan, 1999). Although patients do not react with strong anxiety when they are with family members or complete strangers, the anxiety symptom worsens when they are surrounded by acquaintances, typically in schools or workplaces. For these patients, acquaintances appear at a certain public distance, neither far nor close, from where they evaluate the patients in an uncertain manner.

What Sartre (1943/1956) describes as "me-as-object" is essentially unknowable but becomes relatively known with intimate others. One is able to know how the other perceives and evaluates her in the course of close interpersonal interactions. On the contrary, when one is with complete strangers, one's me-as-object remains unknown, but one never really cares about it. Complete strangers are out of the range of shared intersubjectivity, through which they constitute one's me-as-object. Only those who are in the intermediate range, that is, who are neither intimate nor a stranger, can appear as "people" in the public sphere. When one interacts with such people in social situations, the uncertainty of others' perceptions and evaluations toward oneself becomes much more salient than in informal situations. This is why degree of publicness affects the symptom of anxiety.

In addition, what is specific with these patients is that they seem to have internalized the other's perspective that perceives and evaluates them negatively. Remember the patient's claim quoted from above, "The audience might sense how nervous I am, and I may not be comprehensible and look foolish." The uncertainty of the other's mind in social situations involves both possibilities of negative evaluation and positive evaluation. If one can calmly accept both possibilities, one's anxiety would be alleviated in the course of actual interactions with others, even in formal and public social settings. Among patients, the figure of negatively evaluating others is internalized as what Mead (1934, pp. 152–164) terms the "generalized other." According to Mead, "I" conceives of "me" through the perspective of the generalized other, which is constituted through internalizing diverse others' attitudes toward oneself. Within the patients of SAD, the generalized other seems to be biased with a negatively demanding attitude.

Focusing on this point, one can understand anticipatory anxiety in SAD. Because patients are afraid of the generalized other who constitutes their me-as-object in a negative manner, this anxiety can occur even before or without actual encounters with others. For patients, thinking about a social situation would be enough to cause a feeling of social anxiety. In this regard, there is good reason for patients to avoid social situations.

Continuity with Other Disorders

From an embodied perspective, one can locate body dysmorphic disorder (BDD) as a mental illness in close continuity with SAD. Individuals with BDD are "preoccupied with one or more perceived defects or flaws in their physical appearance, which they believe look ugly, unattractive, abnormal, or deformed" (American Psychiatric Association, 2013, p. 243). They are afflicted with the idea that a certain part of their body, such as the nose, ears, hair, or skin, is deformed and ugly. Because the preoccupations are usually difficult to control, they spend an inordinate amount of time checking their body in the mirror and grooming compulsively. Even though the perceived defects appear only slight to others, these patients do not recognize this fact as such because of their significantly low self-esteem (Phillips, 2005, pp. 115–140). A certain number of patients undergo cosmetic surgery to satisfy their desire to change a body part. However, according to a survey by Veale (2000), satisfaction ratings (range, 0–10) after surgery averaged no higher than 3.5 (n = 46). Certainly, the outcomes of cosmetic surgery for these patients are more frequently dissatisfactory than satisfactory. After surgery, they are not only dissatisfied with the result, but even more preoccupied with their perceived defect.

These facts indicate that patients with BDD do not actually suffer from their physical appearance, which they can examine in the mirror. In other words, their preoccupations do not arise from the body-as-object for themselves, but from the *body-as-object reflected in the other's mind*. In fact, most patients try to camouflage their perceived defects with clothes, makeup, hair, a hat, and so on (Phillips, 2005, pp. 84–86). However, remember that this is their third ontological dimension of the body, which is unknowable in its exact configuration. The essential unknowableness of their body image in the other's mind causes the basic feeling of social anxiety, and this anxiety exaggerates the patients' preoccupations with their perceived defects. Because these patients often have a delusion of reference that other people stare at, talk about, and laugh at their body part (Fuchs, 2003), it is appropriate to regard BDD as a severe type of SAD accompanied with a focus on the body image.

This point can be further clarified in terms of the *generalized other*. Patients with BDD are afraid of being perceived and evaluated as ugly or deformed by others, but they have already internalized such evaluating gazes as a part of the generalized other. Although they might be afraid of social situations with others, the actual presence of others does not really affect their symptoms anymore. Because the relationship with others is already internalized in such an extreme manner that generates the delusion of reference, the evaluating gaze is now omnipresent regardless of whether patients are actually exposed to others or not. This is the factor that drives these patients toward compulsive and repetitive behaviors of mirror checking and excessive grooming. They are always monitored by the omnipresent internal gaze. Observing symptoms of BDD after being formed as a mental disorder, it is sorted into a type of obsessive-compulsive disorder as in the DSM-5. However, in describing symptoms of BDD from a genetic phenomenological perspective, it would be more appropriate to understand BDD as a severe type of SAD.

Although olfactory reference syndrome (ORS) is not explicitly classified in the DSM-5, it is appropriate to refer to it along with BDD. Both share structural similarities in their symptoms. According to a review by Feusner, Phillips, and Stein (2010), individuals with ORS are preoccupied with the idea that they emit an unpleasant, foul, or offensive body odor, even though it is not perceived by others. As is the case with BDD, most patients show repetitive behaviors such as smelling themselves and showering excessively. Their preoccupations are often accompanied by delusions of reference that other people would perceive the odor in a negative manner. In the same review, the researchers point out similarities of ORS and BDD in that "the primary symptoms of both disorders involve a belief of a bodily defect which leads to anxious avoidance of relevant (often social) situations" and that both "include preoccupation and repetitive behaviors to check or remediate the perceived problem" (Feusner et al., 2010, p. 595). In addition, there is a curious clinical fact that among patients with severe *Taijin Kyofusho* there are some cases combined with BDD and others with ORS (Yamashita, 1993, pp. 123–143).

Of course, one must acknowledge the difference in modalities in both disorders: BDD has its focus on the visual image of the body, whereas symptoms of ORS appear through olfactory sensations. Although both types of patients are afflicted with the idea that their own body is so extraordinary that it is evaluated negatively by others, it would be easier for patients with BDD to check their own body explicitly and objectively through visual images reflected in a mirror. In contrast, it would be difficult for patients with ORS to check their smell objectively through olfactory sensations. However, beyond the difference in modalities, it is also true that both types of patients suffer from the unknowable feature of one's own body that is perceived and objectified in the other's mind (me-as-object). And in both cases, negatively evaluating others is firmly internalized in an extreme manner, and their symptoms of social anxiety have already culminated in a delusion of reference. In this regard, both disorders can be understood as a severe type of SAD.

Summary and Conclusion

From the very beginning of its development, one's body is thrown into social situations. One begins life as one's body-as-subject but is coupled with others through one's *body-as-object for others*. Consider a newborn baby. She begins life in this world through her body but is held in a caregiver's arms. As we saw already, the body-as-object for others developmentally precedes the body-as-object for oneself. The experience of being looked at by others establishes the visual perspective for one to view one's body from an external perspective. It establishes one's reflexive relation with one's body-as-object for oneself, and thus, the conscious experience of self-reflection through which "I" think of "me" arises. However, the same experience of self-reflection leads one to notice the other's subjectivity through one's body-as-object (Figure 8.3). "I" become conscious of "me" through reflexive bodily experiences, but "I" also notice that me-as-object is reflected in the other's mind.

The image of "me" in the other's mind is unknowable in principle as Sartre (1943/1956) emphasizes. The uncertainty of the other's mind that derives from this unknowableness creates bodily tension and social anxiety in encounters with others in social situations. Although anxiety is alleviated in the course of ordinary social interactions with others, it is rather exaggerated in pathological cases of SAD. Patients lose themselves when their body is perceived by others in social situations. In other words, a patient's "I" cannot continue being "I" when her body is perceived by others for fear of being a negatively constituted image of me-as-object. Because patients have internalized negatively evaluating others as the "generalized other" (Mead, 1934), not only actual social situations but also imagined social situations provoke an anxiety reaction. Patients experience this as anticipatory anxiety and are motivated to avoid social situations in general.

Finally, I would like to emphasize one's body-as-object as the *place of beginning* in the following sense. On the one hand, when my body is perceived as an object, the other begins to appear as the other subject to me. On the other hand, the other subject appears to me accompanied by the unknowable domain. These two facets of otherness that appear through my body-as-object are the *counterpart of myself as a subject*. When I am touched by the other, I immediately become aware of being touched. When I am looked at in the face, sooner or later I become aware of the other's gaze. Note that my awareness derives from my own capacity to touch or look. If I could not feel the other's body when I am touched, or if I could not turn my gaze to the other when I am looked at, I would not be aware of being touched or looked at (consider cases of paralysis or blindness). My passive experiences of being perceived as a body-as-object implicitly inform me that I am a subject capable of perceiving. Furthermore, because my awareness derives from my capability of perceiving, it involves my own perspective, which makes my perception crucially different from that of the other. The other subject could not perceive her body in the same manner as I do. In short, *"I" begin to appear as a subject* in response to the emergence of the other subject. If so, a key to treatment of SAD would be to take patients back to the very moment of interpersonal contact when the subject "I" implicitly appears behind the overwhelming presence of the other.

References

American Psychiatric Association. (1980). *Diagnostic and statistical manual of mental disorders* (3rd ed.). Washington, DC: Author.

American Psychiatric Association. (2013). *Diagnostic and statistical manual of mental disorders* (5th ed.). Washington, DC: Author.

American Psychological Association. (2007). *APA dictionary of psychology*. Washington, DC: Author.

Amsterdam, B. (1972). Mirror self-image reactions before age two. *Developmental Psychobiology*, 5(4), 297–305. doi:10.1002/dev.420050403

Butterworth, G. (1995). Self as an object of consciousness. In P. Rochat (Ed.), *The self in infancy* (pp. 35–51). Amsterdam, Netherlands: Elsevier.

Feusner, J. D., Phillips, K. A., & Stein, D. J. (2010). Olfactory reference syndrome: Issues for DSM-V. *Depression and Anxiety*, 27(6), 592–599. doi:10.1002/da.20688

Fuchs, T. (2003). The phenomenology of shame, guilt, and the body in body dysmorphic disorder and depression. *Journal of Phenomenological Psychology*, 33(2), 223–243. doi:10.1163/15691620260622903

Fuchs, T. (2013). The phenomenology and development of social perspectives. *Phenomenology and the Cognitive Sciences*, 12(4), 655–683. doi:10.1007/s11097-012-9267-x

Gallagher, S. (2005). *How the body shapes the mind*. Oxford, UK: Oxford University Press.

Gallagher, S. (2008). Direct perception in the intersubjective context. *Consciousness and Cognition*, 17(2), 535–543. doi:10.1016/j.concog.2008.03.003

Gallup, G. G. (1977). Self-recognition in primates: A comparative approach to the bidirectional properties of consciousness. *American Psychologist*, 32(5), 329–338. doi:10.1037/0003-066X.32.5.329

Heidegger, M. (1962). *Being and time* (J. Macquarrie & E. Robinson, Trans.). New York, NY: Harper & Row. (Original work published 1927)

Heimberg, R. G., Hofmann, S. G., Liebowits, M. R., Schneier, F. R., Smits, J. A. J., Stein, M. B., … Craske, M. G. (2014). Social anxiety disorder in DSM-5. *Depression and Anxiety*, 31(6), 472–479. doi:10.1002/da.22231

Hofmann, S., & Otto, M. W. (2008). *Cognitive behavioral therapy for social anxiety disorder: Evidence-based and disorder-specific treatment techniques*. New York, NY: Routledge.

Husserl, E. (1960). *Cartesian meditations: An introduction to phenomenology* (D. Cairns, Trans.). Dordrecht, Netherlands: Kluwer Academic. (Original work published 1950)

Husserl, E. (1989). *Ideas pertaining to a pure phenomenology and to a phenomenological philosophy. Second book: Studies in the phenomenology of constitution* (R. Rojcewicz & A. Schuwer, Trans.). Dordrecht, Netherlands: Kluwer Academic. (Original work published 1952)

Ichikawa, H. (1992). *Seishin toshiteno Shintai [The body as spirit]*. Tokyo, Japan: Kodansha.

Ingerslev, L. R. (2013). My body as an object: Self-distance and social experience. *Phenomenology and the Cognitive Sciences*, 12(1), 163–178. doi:10.1007/s11097-011-9228-9

James, W. (1950). *The principles of psychology* (Vol. 1). New York, NY: Dover Publications. (Original work published 1890)

Kasahara, T. (2005). *Taijin Kyofu to Shakou Fuan Shogai [Taijin Kyofu and social anxiety disorder]*. Tokyo, Japan: Kongo Shuppan.

Mach, E. (1959). *The analysis of sensations* (5th ed., C. M. Williams, Trans.). New York, NY: Dover Publications. (Original work published 1906)

Maeda, F., & Nathan, J. H. (1999). Understanding Taijin Kyofusho through its treatment, Morita therapy. *Journal of Psychosomatic Research*, 46(6), 525–530. doi:10.1016/s0022-3999(98)00113-5

May, R. (1977). *The meaning of anxiety* (Rev. ed.). New York, NY: W. W. Norton & Company.

Mead, G. H. (1934). *Mind, self, and society, from the standpoint of a social behaviorist.* Chicago, IL: University of Chicago Press.

Merleau-Ponty, M. (2012). *Phenomenology of perception* (D. A. Landes, Trans.). New York, NY: Routledge. (Original work published 1945)

National Health Service. (2020). *Social anxiety (social phobia).* Retrieved from https://www.nhs.uk/conditions/social-anxiety/

Phillips, K. A. (2005). *The broken mirror: Understanding and treating body dysmorphic disorder* (Rev. ed.). Oxford, UK: Oxford University Press.

Priel, B., & de Schonen, S. (1986). Self-recognition: A study of a population without mirrors. *Journal of Experimental Child Psychology*, 41(2), 237–250. doi:10.1016/0022-0965(86)90038-x

Reddy, V. (2008). *How infants know minds.* Cambridge, MA: Harvard University Press.

Sartre, J.-P. (1956). *Being and nothingness* (H. E. Barnes, Trans.). New York, NY: Philosophical Library. (Original work published 1943)

Scheler, M. (1954). *The nature of sympathy* (P. Heath, Trans.). London, UK: Routledge & Kegan Paul. (Original work published 1948)

Schilder, P. (1950). *The image and appearance of the human body.* New York, NY: International Universities Press.

Tanaka, S. (2013). The notion of embodied knowledge and its range. *Encyclopaideia: Journal of Phenomenology and Education*, 37, 47–66. doi:10.4442/ency_37_13_03

Tanaka, S. (2015). Intercorporeality as a theory of social cognition. *Theory & Psychology*, 25(4), 455–472. doi:10.1177/0959354315583035

Tanaka, S. (2017). *Ikirareta Watashi wo Motomete: Shintai, Ishiki, Tasha [In search of the lived self: Body, consciousness, and the other].* Kyoto, Japan: Kitaoji Shobo.

Tanaka, S. (2018). Bodily basis of the diverse modes of the self. *Human Arenas*, 1(3), 223–230. doi:10.1007/s42087-018-0030-x

Tanaka, S. (2019). Bodily origin of self-reflection and its socially extended aspects. In W. J. Silva-Filho & L. Tateo (Eds.), *Thinking about oneself: The place and value of reflection in philosophy and psychology* (pp. 141–156). Cham, Switzerland: Springer. doi:10.1007/978-3-030-18266-3_9

Tomasello, M. (1995). Joint attention as social cognition. In C. Moore & P. J. Dunham (Eds.), *Joint attention: Its origins and role in development* (pp. 103–130). New York, NY: Psychology Press.

Veale, D. (2000). Outcome of cosmetic surgery and 'DIY' surgery in patients with body dysmorphic disorder. *Psychiatric Bulletin*, 24(6), 218–221. doi:10.1192/pb.24.6.218

Vygotsky, L. S. (1987). Thinking and speech. In R. W. Rieber & A. S. Carton (Eds.), *The collected works of Lev Vygotsky* (Vol. 1) (pp. 101–120). New York, NY: Plenum Press. (Original work published 1934)

Yamashita, I. (1993). *Taijin-Kyofu, or delusional social phobia.* Sapporo, Japan: Hokkaido University Press.

Zahavi, D. (2003). *Husserl's phenomenology.* Stanford, CA: Stanford University Press.

8.1

Commentary on "Body-as-Object in Social Situations: Toward a Phenomenology of Social Anxiety"

Defending Pluralism in Social Anxiety Disorder: Integrating Phenomenological Perspectives

Adrian Spremberg

Shogo Tanaka's engaging chapter defends a phenomenology of social anxiety that aims to go beyond a comprehension of this particular disorder as commonly captured by contemporary classificatory systems, such as the Diagnostic and Statistical Manual of Mental Disorders-5 and the International Classification of Diseases-10. In this short commentary, I wish to emphasize the importance of understanding social anxiety disorder through a *pluralistic* ontological lens, which considers the embeddedness of alterations in bodily experiences not only in their "mineness" but also in their relation to others and to "social bodies." The author has put forward a thought-provoking account of "the body-as-object" in the social realm and achieved an important pluralistic perspective on social anxiety as a disorder arising from "in between" – one's own sense of bodily ownership and agency and the perception of one's "body-as-object" by others. In this commentary, I will "flesh out" some of Tanaka's main arguments and point toward the possibility of further developing his concept of "body-as-object" as key to social anxiety, so as to broaden how a phenomenological account of this particular disorder could be related to other phenomenological dimensions. In order to do this, I suggest, the entire experiential and social (or worldly) dynamics of the patient needs to be considered, so that a more contextualized (or nuanced) approach to social anxiety disorder can be developed.

In order to develop a phenomenology of social anxiety, the author begins his chapter by accentuating the differences between "body-as-subject" and "body-as-object." An important starting point for Tanaka is the idea that the body should not be understood as a purely "naturalized" and physical object but as a body that makes it possible for subjects to perceive and act in the world, in numerous ways. Understanding one's body as intrinsically connected to one's experience of "the mineness of my I" is, very simply put, what enables the experience of being an actual bodily subject. Tanaka's more specific focus in his article is, however, the "body-as-object." For

Tanaka, the embodied subject is usually immersed in a variety of bodily experiences, in which the *objective* aspects of experience are focused on the fact that the body can be perceived by the subject in an array of different manners: It can be felt and touched in different ways; while I am able to experience the "mineness" of my body, it also appears to me as a perception resulting from "multiple modalities of sensation" (Tanaka, 2021, p. 153).

Another crucial point Tanaka makes is that our bodies are *seen* and *perceived* by others, in which case the body appears as an object to those with whom the "I" comes into contact. For Tanaka, the objectivity of my own body is constantly shaped by how others perceive it. This is the case from early on in our development. Before one is able to create a "body-as-object" image of one's own body, one first understands and perceives it via the way in which one socially interacts with others. This is certainly an intriguing argument since it offers the important claim that one's singular sense of selfhood is not to be separated from the "social body": How we interact with others, for example via gestures and behavior, is a crucial part of our own particular sense of selfhood. For Tanaka, it is important to note that one's experience of being a "body-as-object" via contact with others relies on the fact that it is not only the feeling of being *gazed at* by others that generates social anxiety, but the actual physical experience of *feeling someone else's intentions*, for instance via touch. The concept of "body-as-object" that Tanaka brings to the fore is crucial and deserves further exploration, for instance within the realm of phenomenological psychopathology.

Tanaka discusses how the socially anxious subject believes they are "made object" through the gaze of others, and this opens up important issues that a more comprehensive phenomenological perspective could further illuminate. For instance, it seems relevant to explore in more detail the *types* of situation in which anxiety occurs – which situations produce severe anxiety, which produce mild anxiety – and how a subject relates to a particular (social) environment in a specific context. Tanaka argues that patients with social anxiety disorder often feel overly "unfamiliar" in certain surroundings, due to a fear that others might be judging them. It would be interesting to investigate further how different *kinds* of affective and emotional intersubjective alteration might occur in specific cases of social anxiety disorder. For instance, Ratcliffe's (2008) concept of "feelings of being," which comprise a variety of affective background feelings present in psychiatric disturbances, implies a further phenomenological dimension to be explored. It would be fruitful to relate this to Tanaka's notion of "body-as-object" as key to social anxiety disorder.

My criticism of Tanaka's article would be that it seems to miss the opportunity to examine in more detail *why* and *how* specific experiential affective and/or intersubjective modalities such as judgments or evaluations bring about feelings of social anxiety and unease. Tanaka says that the patients are usually so preoccupied with the negative aspects of certain social situations that assessing these situations impartially becomes a hard task. Here would be a good opportunity to further scrutinize the affective intersubjective lived spaces of patients that also play fundamental roles in the manifestation of social anxiety disorder. More concretely, it is crucial to demonstrate how the entire dynamic relationship between "body-as-object" and the other becomes altered in specific situations. For example, a patient may feel comfortable in giving a speech but highly anxious when talking to a stranger on the street. Apart from the feelings of "familiarity" or "unfamiliarity" that the gaze of the other brings, each uncomfortably felt social situation will still be composed in different ways, depending on who is present and on how the patient emotionally attunes to the other(s). Our intersubjective attunement with the world and others is surely embodied, and this is consistent with Tanaka's suggestion of the "body-as-object." The phenomenological primacy he gives to the manifestation of distress in social situations is certainly plausible. I would only add to his perspective the need to investigate the singular dynamics of how SAD appears in each case, depending on the multiple factors involved in this particular group of disorders. I believe that Tanaka's perspective could be further developed by analyzing how other phenomenological dimensions fit into the entirety of the patient's dynamic way of being in the world.

In sum, Tanaka's chapter opens up a useful pluralistic perspective on disorders of social anxiety based on the "body-as-subject" and "body-as-object" distinction. However, as pointed out, I believe the author could complement his phenomenological perspective by more carefully addressing the interrelatedness of other phenomenological dimensions, such as affectivity and intersubjectivity. More comprehensively assessing how the "body-as-object" relates to other phenomenological realms would positively widen and enrich Tanaka's own approach. Given the conceptual and clinical complexities of psychiatric disorders, Tanaka's contribution is a bold step in the right direction, and will hopefully receive proper attention in the growing interdisciplinary field of the philosophy of psychiatry.

References

Ratcliffe, M. (2008). *Feelings of being: Phenomenology, psychiatry and the sense of reality*. Oxford, UK: Oxford University Press.

Tanaka, S. (2021). Body-as-object in social situations: Toward a phenomenology of social anxiety. In C. Tewes & G. Stanghellini (Eds.), *Time and body: Phenomenological and psychopathological approaches* (pp. 150–169). Cambridge, UK: Cambridge University Press.

PART III

Borderline Personality and Eating Disorders

9

Emotion Regulation in a Disordered World

Understanding Borderline Personality Disorder

Matthew Ratcliffe and Anna Bortolan

Introduction

This chapter addresses the phenomenology of "emotion dysregulation," with particular reference to borderline personality disorder (hereafter, BPD). Strong, turbulent emotions, and unstable interpersonal relationships are central to BPD, making it an uncontroversial example of "emotion dysregulation" (see, e.g., Ebner-Priemer et al., 2015; Lieb, Zanarini, Schmahl, Linehan, & Bohus, 2004; Linehan, 1993). Here is how DSM-5 characterizes the condition:

> The essential feature of borderline personality disorder is a pervasive pattern of instability of interpersonal relationships, self-image, and affects, and marked impulsivity that begins by early adulthood and is present in a variety of contexts. (American Psychiatric Association, 2013, p. 663)

Nine more specific symptoms are listed in the DSM-5, at least five of which are required for a BPD diagnosis. They include seeking to avoid real or imagined abandonment, unstable relationships that involve swinging between extremes of positivity and negativity, impulsive behavior, feelings of emptiness, and mood instability.[1]

In what follows, we seek to further illuminate the nature of emotional experience in BPD: Why are emotions (especially those directed at other people) intense and transient, often swinging between extremes in ways that are situationally inappropriate? One might think that the pathological character of emotion dysregulation depends only on features of emotion-processes themselves and how they interfere with evaluation, thinking,

[1] For a wide-ranging survey of recent findings concerning BPD, covering a substantial body of literature, see Leichsenring, Leibing, Kruse, New, and Leweke (2011). For a phenomenological discussion of the kinds of affective experience that are prominent in BPD, such as anger, dysphoria, emptiness, and shame, see, for example, Rossi Monti and D'Agostino (2019).

decision-making, and social behavior. In other words, however the relevant pathology might come about, it is located *within* the person's emotional life. However, we will suggest that emotion dysregulation in BPD should instead be construed as inextricable from a wider ranging phenomenological disturbance. To do so, we will sketch an account of how human emotional experience is ordinarily regulated by the structure of the experiential world. We will further suggest that the dependence is mutual: Emotions act upon a world within which they arise, in ways that maintain, repair, and reshape that world. We add that relations with other people play important roles in regulating both our emotions and the phenomenological backdrop against which they occur.

Putting these points together, it becomes clear how emotional turbulence, of the kind associated with BPD, is *implied* by a certain, distinctive way of being situated in the interpersonal and social world. Those with BPD diagnoses tend to inhabit a world that is lacking in cohesive, practically meaningful structure, where that structure depends on habitually entrenched, integrated, and fairly stable sets of concerns. Moreover, they struggle to relate to other people in ways that are essential to the sustenance of such concerns. So, it would be misleading to conceive of emotion dysregulation as something that arises in isolation from one's wider relationship with the social world. Given the relationships of phenomenological dependence that we will describe, disordered emotion is implied by a disordered world, and a disordered world is implied by a way of experiencing and relating to other people.[2] This conclusion is principally phenomenological; it is concerned with how different aspects of experience interrelate and is thus to be distinguished from a causal explanation of emotion dysregulation. Nevertheless, it complements a range of findings that associate BPD with histories of adverse experiences involving other people, typically dating back to childhood.

It should be noted that the diagnostic category "BPD" is by no means uncontroversial. For instance, Judith Herman (1992/1997, p. 123) expresses the worry that it has pejorative connotations and is sometimes used as "little more than a sophisticated insult." For current purposes, we remain neutral over whether and why the diagnosis and associated terminology should be retained, revised, or discarded. Our aim is instead to illuminate

[2] The account developed here also has implications for how we think of human emotional experience in general: Emotions have a temporal structure and coherence that is obscured by a tendency to think of them as brief episodes that involve being afraid of *p*, happy about *q*, angry with *r*, and so forth. Furthermore, their integrity depends on processes that involve other people in various ways.

a form of emotional experience that is consistent with "BPD as currently conceived of," in order to make points about emotional experience and its regulation that also have wider applicability. If BPD were no longer recognized, this would not compromise the ability to identify and describe the form of experience in question. Furthermore, we do not seek to suggest that the type of emotion dysregulation addressed here is exclusive to those who meet the diagnostic criteria for BPD.[3] Neither do we maintain that *all* cases of BPD are consistent with what we describe, given that the diagnosis admits considerable heterogeneity.[4]

Emotion and World

Our emotional life has an intricate, dynamic structure, which it borrows from the experiential world in which we already *find ourselves* when having specifically directed emotions (see also Ratcliffe, 2019a). Our aims in this section are first to describe, in some detail, the relationship between the two and then to show how it is relevant to the task of understanding emotion dysregulation in BPD.

Emotions – whatever we might take them to be – involve experiencing certain things as salient, insofar as those things possess a certain kind of significance. In other words, the objects of emotion are encountered as *mattering* to us in one or another way. For instance, the fast-approaching, hungry tiger appears immediately threatening. It is not that one first experiences a hungry tiger and then has a separate experience of fear. Instead, the experience of fear consists – in part – in a significance that is experienced as integral to the object of emotion; the tiger *appears* threatening. Experiences of significance are ordinarily not random; they can be appropriate or inappropriate to their objects. One does not and should not experience a glass of water on a table as threatening, or experience joy when approached by the hungry tiger. What one experiences as significant is determined by what we will refer to as one's *concerns* (spanning values and commitments of various kinds, short- and long-term goals, and projects

3 It has been argued that emotion dysregulation plays an important role in other forms of psychopathology, including depression and anxiety (Scheppes, Suri, & Gross, 2015). Although we do not advance any claims concerning the similarities between disordered emotion in BPD and other psychiatric diagnoses, our conclusions may be relevant to the exploration of other pathological alterations of experience.

4 As Rossi Monti and D'Agostino (2019, p. 827) observe, a "wide range of possible combinations of disturbances" are associated with the diagnosis.

that one is invested in to some extent and in some way).[5] We might say that an emotional reaction *makes sense* and is further judged appropriate or inappropriate, in light of whether and how an eliciting entity, event, or situation relates to these concerns.[6] You are afraid of the hungry tiger insofar as it threatens something that you value: your life.

Importantly, experiences of significance and the concerns to which they relate are not atomistic in nature; they have a structure that is both holistic and fairly stable over time. It depends for its integrity on four broad types of factors, which together specify whether and how features of our surroundings are experienced as mattering:

(1) *The body*: Our bodily capacities and dispositions specify what we are able to do, as well as the kinds of bodily performances required. Thus, changes in bodily capacities and dispositions, if accurately reflected in how we experience our surroundings, affect what appears significant and how.

(2) *Projects*: Many of our concerns reflect projects and associated commitments, which depend upon and are often embedded in further projects. Thus, insofar as these projects have a cohesive structure, so do our concerns and our experiences of significance. Long-term projects in which we are heavily invested incorporate goals and aspirations that stretch far into the future. They also encompass numerous subprojects, which relate to one another in ways that are, to varying degrees, coherent.

(3) *Other people*: Sustaining a coherent set of projects and concerns requires certain ways of relating to other people (specific individuals and others in general). What we are able to accomplish is not just a matter of our own abilities; it is also reliant on the abilities and intentions of others. Often, it is *we* who are committed to a project, where that project would be unmanageable or even unintelligible as a solitary pursuit.[7] Our projects and wider concerns also incorporate care *for* others and obligations of various kinds toward them.

[5] Although there are differences in how the notion of "concern" has been conceptualized, it is central to various contemporary theories of emotion. Roberts (1988), for instance, characterizes emotions as "serious concern-based construals." Prinz (2006) also conceives of emotions as forms of perception *representing* certain concerns.

[6] The appropriateness of a given emotion depends not only on how it relates to our concerns but also on whether those concerns are themselves deemed appropriate and coherent according to whichever criteria might be invoked.

[7] An example of unmanageability would be building a space station on one's own. An example of unintelligibility would be becoming the world's greatest footballer without being part of a team.

(4) *Norms, society, and culture*: Although the significance of our surroundings is in some respects idiosyncratic, much of it is shared. Social and cultural norms of various kinds, including artifact functions, norms of performance and etiquette, and moral norms, give the world an enduring, shared structure, which projects and associated concerns presuppose.

These four factors contribute to experiences of significance in ways that are inextricable. For example, suppose one feels a surge of delight when walking into an antiquarian bookshop and seeing a rare philosophy book that one has been seeking for research purposes. Encountering the book in this way is symptomatic of (a) bodily capacities that enable one to read it; (b) commitment to a career as a philosopher and concerns associated with this; (c) interpersonal and social relations that render life as an academic philosopher viable; and (d) shared norms concerning walking into shops, buying things, and so forth. Only with all of this is in place is the book experienced in that particular way. How we experience things emotionally thus reflects a web of concerns, many of which are well established, stable, enduring, and cohesive.[8]

However, experiences of significance are ubiquitous and further distinctions are therefore required in order to capture the more specifically *emotional* phenomenology of BPD. In particular, episodic emotions should be distinguished from what we might call the "emotional background." As one of us (Ratcliffe) writes these words, the glass of water on his desk matters to him in offering the potential to quench his thirst, while his written notes appear immediately relevant to the task of completing this chapter. So, various experiences of significance are integral to how his surroundings are currently encountered. Given this, it might be claimed that, in any such situation, he is *emotional*. However, in addressing

[8] What we have sketched here is largely consistent with Bennett Helm's account of holistic emotional rationality (e.g., Helm, 2001, 2009a, 2009b). Helm maintains that emotions relate to one another in rational ways due to their having a common focus, where the "focus" of an emotion consists in the presupposed values relative to which it is both intelligible and rational. Thus, when something has "import" for us – that is, when we care about something – we are inclined to experience patterns of interconnected emotions. Imagine, for example, that one aspires to be a writer. Positive emotions like pride or excitement will be experienced in circumstances where one is successfully pursuing one's writing-related aims, while negative emotions like shame or sadness will be undergone when failing to do so. However, we further maintain that the foci of emotions are, to a substantial degree, etched into the experiential world. The "rational" structure of emotion is thus parasitic upon the world that we find ourselves in, more so than on concerns that we experience as internal to ourselves. This "presupposed world" is a consistent theme in the phenomenological tradition (see, e.g., Ratcliffe, 2015, Chapter 1).

emotional experience in BPD, we are concerned with something more specific in nature: pronounced, episodic emotions of a kind that can be contrasted with an emotional background. It is these that are described as intense, erratic, polarized, inappropriate, and disruptive.

To distinguish episodic emotions from wider experiences of significance, a contrast can be drawn between experiencing things as mattering in routine, unproblematic ways that reflect our concerns, and experiencing them as pointing to the potential or actual disruption of those concerns. In the context of stable projects, commitments, and concerns, things are experienced as significant in a largely consistent, cohesive way, which reflects – to varying degrees – habitual patterns of activity. We do not need to keep in mind what matters to us, as salient directions and directives are etched into the experienced world, akin to a map (Ratcliffe, 2015, Chapter 2). However, some things do not merely appear significant in light of that structure but, more specifically, in light of their potential or actual impact upon it – their ability to disrupt one's world (in ways that can be positive or negative).

When something has implications for the integrity of one's concerns, intervention may be required to prevent, preserve, repair, revise, or hasten changes in life-structure. This is where episodic emotions come in (or, at least, the kinds of episodic emotions we are concerned with here). They are experiences of things as significant in one or another way, in virtue of their potential or actual impact on holistic patterns of significance, concerns, projects, and commitments (Ratcliffe, 2019a). These experiences also influence how we respond to the events in question; emotions are not just implicated in registering disturbances of one's world but also in negotiating those disturbances.[9]

If something along these lines is right, then our emotional life borrows its structure from patterns of practical significance that are etched into the world we inhabit, like networks of trails through the undergrowth along which we run. In the human case, the appropriateness and proportionality of emotional responses to events are determined not merely by what is happening now but, in addition, by an elaborate set of interrelated concerns. Whether or not those concerns remain viable and how they change over time depends, in part, on our emotional responses to events that impact upon them.

[9] From various perspectives, it has been argued that emotions have a motivational character, inclining us to act in certain ways (e.g., Goldie, 2000; Helm, 2009a; Slaby, 2008).

Disturbances of the habitual world often play out over considerable periods of time. For this reason, many forms of human emotional experience are better thought of as long-term processes than as brief episodes. Grief, for instance, is a form of emotional experience that can persist over time while different emotional episodes are undergone (Goldie, 2012; Ratcliffe, 2017a). Even those who are wary of committing to the view that our emotional repertoire includes unitary, temporally extended processes must at least acknowledge that emotional episodes often fall into temporally organized patterns or sequences. These patterns track, with varying degrees of success, how unfolding events affect our concerns or are likely to affect them. They also influence whether and how we respond to those events, where our responses shape how matters subsequently unfold.

Hence, it is only against the backdrop of an experiential world in which we are *already immersed* that our emotional experiences are intelligible at all and relate to one another in intelligible, structured ways. This position can be accepted without endorsing a more specific account of what emotions *are*. They can play the role ascribed to them regardless of whether we label them as "judgments," "perceptions," "feelings," or something else.[10] The points to note are that (a) a structured emotional life requires a structured experiential world and (b) the sustenance of a structured world in the face of changing events involves responding emotionally to those events in ways that reflect one's concerns. It follows from (a) and (b) that disordered emotions are inextricable from a disordered world. This does not imply any particular causal explanation; disturbances of life-structure will disrupt emotions, while disruptive emotions will undermine life-structure, thus accommodating various different scenarios.

This has implications for how we think of "emotion dysregulation" and for our understanding of BPD. In particular, we would expect the intense, ephemeral, and alternating emotions that mark the disorder to be associated with a habitual world that is lacking in coherence, a world that is not tightly or consistently organized in terms of projects, commitments, and values. Consistent with this, it has been suggested that BPD involves *living in the present*. One's emotional life lacks a

[10] In any case, we think such debates are generally unproductive. A growing number of philosophers, the first author included, maintain that certain emotional feelings are not simply "feelings of the body." Something can be both a bodily feeling and, at the same time, a world-directed intentional experience (e.g., Helm, 2009a; Ratcliffe, 2008; Slaby, 2008). Distinctions between cognition and affect, upon which debates are often premised, are therefore misguided.

meaningful, temporally organized backdrop, against which emotions more usually arise and are judged appropriate or otherwise by oneself and/or others:

> The borderline's behaviors may be sudden and contradictory, since they result from strong, momentary feelings—perceptions that represent isolated, unconnected snapshots of experience. The immediacy of the present exists in isolation, without the benefit of the experience of the past, or the hopefulness of the future. Because historical patterns, consistency, and predictability are unavailable to the borderline, similar mistakes are repeated again and again. (Kreisman & Straus, 2010, p. 44)

Various prominent symptoms of BPD can thus be understood as originating in a certain form of nonlocalized, temporal experience. Emotion, thought, and activity are not organized by the background sense of a meaningfully organized past and future, something that requires a set of enduring and coherently integrated concerns. When the present is all there is, nothing holds back current emotions and, without the anchor of a cohesive life-structure, they oscillate wildly. As Thomas Fuchs (2007, p. 381) writes, "the patients are completely identified with their momentary states of mind, unable to gain a distance from the present situation." Stanghellini and Rosfort (2013, p. 163) similarly emphasize an inability to distance oneself from the "here and now," which includes one's current emotional feelings. Those feelings, they note, do not reflect "values, conventions, and norms" that are more usually integral to the everyday world and constrain emotional experience and behavior.

Such an analysis is consistent with several characteristics of BPD, such as lack of enduring commitments, identity disturbances, feelings of emptiness and superficiality, and frequent changes in jobs, friends, and values (see, e.g., Fuchs, 2007; Kreisman & Straus, 2010; Pazzagli & Rossi Monti, 2000). Even so, several questions remain. Why do the person's concerns (and, with them, the experiential world within which emotions arise) lack structure? Why are emotional responses intense and extreme, rather than merely unstructured? Why does the person not just drift happily through life in an oblivious present, without undergoing the kinds of emotional disturbance associated with investment in fragile, long-term meaning-structures? Why are interpersonal emotions, in particular, so turbulent? Why does the person alternate between the extremes of clinging to and rejecting others? In the remainder of this chapter, we will suggest that the answers to these questions are to be found in a consideration of human emotion regulation and, more specifically, how it utilizes interpersonal and social relations.

Emotion Regulation

Disturbances of the habitual world have differing degrees of severity. In those cases where they are relatively circumscribed, the world retains sufficient structure to provide some sense of the way forward, thus shaping emotion-processes that negotiate disruption. However, when it comes to disturbances that are both profound and wide-ranging, the way forward is not always signposted by what remains intact: Nothing makes sense anymore; there's no way through this; I don't know what to do; I don't know how to feel. How, then, do we steer emotion-processes when concerns that imbue the world with emotion-regulating structure are themselves compromised by emotion-eliciting events? In this section, we will argue that (a) emotion regulation, in these circumstances and also more generally, is inextricable from the interpersonal and the social and (b) other people play indispensable roles in sustaining the habitual world, such that *explicit* regulation of emotion is not usually required.[11] Then, in the final section, we will consider the phenomenology of BPD in light of this.

"Emotion regulation" is a fast-growing field, concerned with a wide range of processes and strategies that influence which emotions arise and when, and how they unfold (Gross, 2014). The term "emotion regulation" can be employed in different ways. Gross (1999, 2001) distinguishes between regulation *by* emotion and regulation *of* emotion, restricting his use of the term to the latter. This still encompasses both conscious and nonconscious strategies, including selection and modification of eliciting situations, direction and redirection of attention, cognitive reappraisal of events, and modulation of emotional responses. Gross (2001, p. 215) draws an overarching distinction between "antecedent-focused" and "response-focused" strategies, the former acting upon emotions before they are fully formed and the latter as they occur. His discussion emphasizes episodic emotions, construed as multifaceted, short-term processes.

Although Gross acknowledges that there are issues to address concerning how other people contribute to emotion regulation, he focuses on the level of the individual. However, others have identified a number of ways in which interpersonal and social processes are involved in emotion regulation. Here, the emphasis is more fruitfully placed on intricate, longer-term patterns or processes than on episodic responses to momentary stimuli. Interpersonal

[11] Of course, emotion-regulation processes are not exclusively phenomenological in nature. Hence, in maintaining that emotional experience depends for its integrity on these processes, we are not suggesting that all aspects of regulation are themselves experienced.

regulation of emotion is especially salient in early attachment, where it is well documented that the emotional behavior of the caregiver elicits emotions from the infant in a structured way (e.g., Hobson, 2002). It has been further suggested that mutual regulation through structured, dyadic interaction is not limited to childhood and continues throughout the human lifespan: "[S]ocial partners continue to serve as external emotion 'regulators' over the life course, through diverse mechanisms" (Diamond & Aspinwall, 2003, p. 145).[12] Indeed, it is arguable that, in many instances, there is no clear boundary to be drawn between self-regulation and regulation by others; the person and her wider environment (including her social environment) are "necessarily entwined in the generation of affect" (Campos, Walle, Dahl, & Main, 2011, p. 27).

The degree of first-person insight into how a given emotion influences and/or is influenced by other people varies. Some studies restrict themselves to deliberate, explicitly motivated manipulation of one party by another (e.g., Reeck, Ames, & Ochsner, 2016). For current purposes, however, we assume a more liberal conception of social emotion regulation, one that is consistent with its ubiquity. As with self-regulation, it need not be construed as explicit in every case. One can regulate others and be regulated by them without being aware of acting or being acted upon in the relevant ways.

Interpersonal emotion regulation might involve a token emotional response being influenced by one-off interaction with another individual. Alternatively, a particular individual might act in a consistent, reliable manner in a certain situation, type of situation, or range of situations. In the case of a close relationship with a partner, there is likely to be an intricate network of variably shared regulatory processes (Ratcliffe, 2019b). Families also serve as frameworks for emotion regulation (Thompson, 2014). The extent to which and manner in which another person or group of people is able to influence one's emotions reflect not just the nature of the relationships in question (e.g., parent, child, spouse, friend) but also their more specific relational qualities (Coan & Maresh, 2014).

So, where one's own regulatory resources fall short, there is often the option of falling back on other people for support. Suppose the world has been disrupted to such a degree that it no longer indicates a route for one's emotions to follow, as might apply following bereavement, breakdown of a long-term relationship, loss of a job, a life-changing accident, or the onset

[12] See also Mikulincer, Shaver, and Pereg (2003) and Varga and Krueger (2013) for the view that early attachment can serve as a model for conceptualizing processes that continue into adulthood and that emotion regulation is interpersonally distributed.

of chronic illness. In such cases, one may still be able to lean on others – to draw on them so as to sustain old paths and forge new ones. For instance, other people can play roles in "coauthoring" coherent, future-oriented narratives that regulate emotional responses and reorganize one's wider engagement with the world (Fuchs, 2007, p. 380).

These considerations might give the impression that the contribution made by others to emotion regulation is limited to intervening periodically, when the world falls short. Indeed, much of the time, emotions are regulated – to a large extent – by the unfolding situations that elicit them. As Kappas (2011, p. 18) notes insightfully, separate regulatory processes are not ordinarily required. Instead, emotions "autoregulate" by self-terminating once one's relationship with an eliciting situation has changed (something that may involve acting upon other people so that they act upon that situation). This is consistent with our proposal that the structure of longer-term emotion-processes or patterns of unfolding emotions is specified, to a large extent, by the practically meaningful structure of an experiential world in which one *already finds oneself* when anticipated or current events elicit emotional responses.

Nevertheless, it would be wrong to assume that interpersonal and social relations only play an indispensable role when we are unable to regulate our own emotions and need others to intervene. And, to understand forms of experience that involve profound and enduring emotion dysregulation, it is important to appreciate why dependence on other people is, in fact, ubiquitous. In addition to relying directly on other people, we draw on a range of other resources to regulate emotions. For instance, Colombetti and Krueger (2015) consider our use of environmental "scaffolding," consisting of a diverse inventory of entities, places, and activities that we rely upon to alter our emotions in predictable ways. They include the likes of clothes, art galleries, cinemas, letters, music, churches, and cafés. It can be added that an impersonal regulator's effectiveness almost always depends implicitly on sets of expectations concerning other people – sometimes particular individuals, groups, or types of people (e.g., partners, friends, teachers, technicians, waiters, musicians, drivers, advisors) and sometimes other people in general (i.e., anyone you might encounter or anticipate encountering during the course of everyday life). For example, you could not have relaxing bicycle rides if you doubted the competence or intentions of all drivers in the vicinity; you would not feel at ease in a favorite set of clothes if you expected everyone to laugh at you for wearing them; you would not feel pleasantly immersed in a film if you experienced the rest of the cinema audience as threatening. Even the regulatory effects of drinking a cup of coffee can depend, in part, on being able to sit in a café and interact with or just *be with* other people in a certain way. In fact, almost everything that we anticipate from the surrounding environment depends in one or another way on what we expect from other people. By implication, so does our ability to utilize environmental resources as regulators on those occasions where our emotions do not self-regulate.

The role of other people further extends to those seemingly straightforward cases where the practically meaningful world does the regulatory work, where additional emotion-regulation processes are not needed. The structure and stability of that world rest on our being able to anticipate, experience, and relate to other people in certain ways rather than others. Many of the concerns that are habitually engrained into our surroundings only *make sense* relative to one or more interpersonal relationships. Things have the experienced significance they do and relate to one another in the ways they do relative to *our* having this project, this set of goals, these commitments. Even where concerns are *mine* rather than *ours*, they often continue to implicate other people: I need you in order to do this; this matters to me in the way it does because I care about your well-being; this is significant to me because I am trying to do that for you; I disapprove of this because I know how you feel about it; and so forth.

Hence, the sustenance of one's concerns and the manner in which situations are experienced as relating to those concerns are both inseparable from relations with particular people. As Thompson (1994, p. 42) remarks, "because attachment figures, friends, parents, spouses, offspring, and significant others constitute invaluable interpersonal resources for coping with emotion, expectations concerning their accessibility, helpfulness, and sensitivity can significantly enhance – or undermine – the capacity to manage emotional arousal." In addition, we are reliant on more general expectations concerning the motivations, capabilities, and likely actions of other people. Almost every project and situation we engage in depends in one or another way on what we expect others to do. We would not have a meaningfully structured, temporally enduring experiential world at all without certain general expectations: Others won't try to mow us down as we cross the road; they won't give us false information when we ask for directions; they won't hurt us for no reason as we pass by them on the street.[13]

[13] All of this is to be construed dynamically. Gross (2014, p. 5) remarks that "emotional responses often lead to changes in the environment that alter the probability of subsequent instances of that and other emotions." Consistent with this, interpersonal interactions shape emotions, which shape the manner in which one's surroundings appear significant. This can modify interpersonal interactions, which regulate emotions, and so forth.

For the most part, what we anticipate from other people involves what is sometimes referred to as a form of *trust*: a nonlocalized, unreflective set of expectations concerning how interactions with others are likely to proceed (Ratcliffe, 2017b). Granted, we do not anticipate all people in this way at all times. Nevertheless, where there is distrust or even the explicit prospect of one or another type of harm, this is the exception rather than the norm, something that disrupts a more generally confident or trusting way of engaging with the social world. But consider what world-experience would be like if this style of anticipation were eroded or even wholly absent, if others offered no prospect of the kinds of relations that might sustain or repair one's world or guide one's response to disruption. All projects, commitments, and concerns, insofar as their stability presupposes a dependable world, would be transient, unstable, or unsustainable.

Fonagy, Luyten, and Allison (2015) propose that BPD centrally involves a lack of interpersonal trust, originating in adverse childhood experience. This, they suggest, interferes with an ability to "mentalize," namely "the capacity of one individual to understand the actions of another in terms of the thoughts, feelings, wishes, and desires (mental states) of that person" (2015, p. 586; see also Fonagy & Allison, 2014). They add that mentalization is integral to a capacity to acquire generalizable cultural knowledge from others and that loss of trust therefore leads to "epistemic petrification" (a predicament involving inflexibility and failure to respond to new information provided by the social environment). What we propose here is consistent with that view. However, our emphasis is different. It is not just a matter of being unable to relate to others in ways that facilitate knowledge of the cultural world. What is also lacking (to varying degrees) is the experience of *having* a cohesively structured, temporally extended world, something that operates as a phenomenological backdrop for any attempt to engage with others or access information. Sustenance of a world depends largely on emotion-processes that detect and navigate disturbances of habitual patterns. The role of trusting relations with others is not exhausted by "mentalizing."[14] These relations also involve anticipating and interacting with people in ways that (a) build and sustain the experiential world that regulates emotion-processes and (b) regulate emotion-processes that sustain, repair, and reshape the world. The common theme, however, is that being able to access something essential from other people requires

[14] This is acknowledged by Fonagy and Target (2007), who address the roles played by early attachment relations in constituting a sense of both "internal" and "external" reality, as well as the distinction between them.

being able to anticipate, experience, and relate to them in a certain kind of "trusting" way, where "trust" consists in a nonlocalized, unreflective, habitual style of anticipation (Ratcliffe, 2017b).

Disordered Emotions and Disordered Worlds

We suggest that the kind of emotional instability associated with BPD can be understood in terms of the regulatory roles played by a structured experiential world and relations with other people. Consider the following possibilities:

(1) Emotional processes are fragile. They may involve navigating a terrain where there is no clear route, where patterns of salience and significance that one's practical reasoning previously took for granted are gone. Such processes might be derailed in any number of ways. They would then have the potential to ripple through one's world in a disorganized manner and further erode its structure, eliciting other emotions that themselves prove disruptive. Sequences of unpleasant life events therefore have the potential to induce further upheaval, in the form of disordered emotional responses to them.

(2) Emotional responses lack phenomenological context from the outset. A coherent, cohesive world, structured by temporally extended projects, commitments, and concerns, was never fully formed. Here, there would be no sense of where emotions are going, what they point toward, what is disrupted, and what remains intact. As emotional experiences would not be embedded in the context of a life, there would be nothing to insulate them, nothing to regulate them.

We suggest that the phenomenology associated with BPD involves some combination of (1) and (2), where lack of regulatory context gives rise to emotions that themselves lack structure and have the potential to further erode the experiential world in which they originate. More specifically, we consider these dynamics to underlie the lack of depth and increased strength, polarization and instability that characterize affective experience in BPD. This is consistent with the view that those with BPD diagnoses do not experience their emotions as situated within a larger, meaningful, temporal context. As Fuchs (2007, p. 381) suggests, emotional experience in BPD has a kind of shallowness: "[T]heir transitory present has no depth."

Pugmire (2005) construes emotional depth as, in part, a matter of the extent to which the object of an emotion impacts upon one's concerns. It therefore requires those concerns to have a certain degree of integration, such that some events affect the structure of one's life more so than others. We suggest that this kind of "depth" is something that can be experienced. This is not to suggest that an emotional response to an event somehow contains a full and immediate appreciation of its implications for one's life. Nevertheless, it can include at least some sense of its import – the extent to which one's life will be affected. This is exemplified by the experience of something "sinking in," where its impact is progressively recognized over time and/or there is an expectation that there will be such an impact. In such cases, there is a feeling, however indeterminate, of where something is leading. One's current emotional experience indicates a path that may not yet be clearly laid out, but which is nevertheless experienced (Ratcliffe, 2019a). This is only possible where an emotional experience occurs within a structured experiential world, of a kind that is inextricable from a structured life. And this is where the shallowness of emotion in BPD comes in: The emotions do not point to anything beyond a current situation. Thus, emotional experiences are not just unusually pronounced and situationally inappropriate; they also have a qualitatively different structure due to their not being anchored to a stable and organized set of concerns.

In BPD, such decontextualized emotions can also be exceptionally strong, where "strength" is construed as a lack of hesitation or perceived ambiguity. More usually, the import of an emotion is circumscribed to varying degrees. Its object has specific implications for aspects of one's life, for parts of a larger whole. Consistent with this, and as outlined above, integral to an emotional experience is some awareness of how it fits into that life. To put it in propositional terms, the experience can include something like "I have lost or might lose P, but the larger framework of concerns relative to which P is important to me remains intact." This puts things in perspective, in ways that shape responses to ensuing events. It can also lend an air of ambiguity to one's interpretations of events and a degree of hesitation to one's responses. A perceived insult may be at odds with one's long-term and anticipated future relationship with a given individual: Perhaps she didn't mean it that way and, in any case, there is more at stake. If this is right, we would expect a "shallow" emotional life, one that lacks context, to be associated with a sense of certainty. The significance of a situation is exhausted by what it currently has to offer and, given a lack of mitigating context, the person is wholly committed to and invested in a current emotional response.

In addition to strength – construed as level of conviction or lack of ambiguity – emotions in BPD are marked by high levels of polarization and instability. Emotional experience has an intensity and felt urgency, something that is consistent with sudden, impulsive reactions to situations. The oscillation between extremes, or "black and white thinking," is often seen as a central feature of BPD, and it is something that concerns not only cognitive but also affective processes (see, e.g., Fuchs, 2007; Kreisman & Straus, 2010). As those with BPD diagnoses tend to shift abruptly between idealization and devaluation of other people – as well as experiencing similarly drastic changes in their view of themselves – they also oscillate frequently between extreme emotions. Indeed, it has been shown that affective experience in BPD not only changes unusually often but also that the difference in valence between the relevant affects is more pronounced (e.g., Ebner-Priemer et al., 2007; Nica & Links, 2009).

What do the shallowness, strength, polarization, and instability of emotion in BPD originate in? And how can these features be integrated into a phenomenological account of the disorder? Fuchs (2007), and also Bortolan (2020), place the emphasis on narrative. Ordinarily, a coherent autobiographical narrative gives one's life a meaningful, long-term structure.[15] In addition, linguistic and narrative expression can impact on the phenomenology of affective states in ways that enable the subject to experience them as less overwhelming and more manageable Bortolan (2019, 2020). These dynamics are impoverished or absent in BPD and so emotions lack their more usual stabilizing context. However, it is arguable that narratives are only part of the story. The regulatory structure that ordinarily shapes which emotions arise and when, and how those emotions relate to other emotions, consists – to a large extent – in the practically significant world that operates as a backdrop to specifically focused experiences, thoughts, and activities. While this world requires a certain degree of coherence in order to be "narratable," it is not itself a narrative, in even the most permissive sense of the term "narrative." Nevertheless, the roles played by narrative can be understood in relation to it. For instance, an explicit narrative might assist in making sense of and negotiating disruptions of world, imposing new forms of coherence, and integrating

[15] Interest in the nature and role of narratives in BPD is connected to the investigation of disturbances of identity that mark the disorder. Various psychological and philosophical accounts share the view that engaging in certain forms of narrative activity is key to the constitution of a distinct dimension of selfhood, and it has been argued on this basis that BPD involves disruptions of "narrative identity" (Adler, Chin, Kolisetty, & Oltmanns, 2012) or, in Fuchs' terms, a "fragmentation" of the narrative self (2007, p. 381).

other people into regulatory processes. Hence, although narrative (however it is conceived of) plausibly plays a range of regulatory roles, what also needs to be acknowledged is the inhabiting of a world that lends itself to narration.

We further suggest that emotional experience in BPD is inextricable from a way of anticipating, experiencing, and relating to other people. Others play important roles in the development, sustenance, and revision of a significant world. As we have emphasized, the constitution and ongoing development of an organized set of concerns, around which one's affective life is structured, is interpersonally shaped in various ways. Where there is emotional upheaval, others can and often do provide some form of support. Where habitual patterns break down and it is not clear what comes next, they can serve as guides, like Virgil leading Dante through the Inferno. And this is where narratives can have an important part to play too. Others whom we trust can assist in the development of autobiographical narratives and other stories that play regulative roles (e.g., Fuchs, 2007, p. 380). Disruptions of a life are also usually mitigated by the continuing applicability of generic social norms and established practices that do not depend on idiosyncratic life-structures. Hence, regulatory processes that are integral to longer-term emotional responses can be and often are interpersonally and socially distributed.

Where the experienced world lacks structure and temporal coherence – resulting, as previously shown, in affective experiences that lack depth and ambiguity – this also implies something about relations with other people. Sustaining coherent projects, commitments, and concerns depends on being able to relate to at least some people in certain ways. These, we have suggested, depend on a form of nonlocalized confidence or *trust*, a set of prereflective expectations concerning the conduct of others. Without this, one could not engage in or anticipate engaging in those types of interactions that offer the potential to build, maintain, restore, and rebuild a habitual world. An unstructured world implies a kind of estrangement from other people in general, and vice versa. It should therefore come as no surprise that reports of loneliness, unbridgeable isolation, being cut off in one or another way from everyone are ubiquitous in BPD.[16]

[16] Kreisman and Straus (2010, p. 79) relate the prevalence of loss of life-structure to forms of social change, noting that we live in a world that places ever-more conflicting demands on a person, where things are more transient and uncertain. They suggest that society as a whole "lacks constancy and reliability" and that BPD is a "pathological" response to such stresses. They further refer to a loss of "historical continuity" and suggest that "devaluation of the past breaks the perceptual link to the future, which becomes a vast unknown, a source of dread as much as hope, a vast quicksand, from which it becomes incredibly difficult to extricate oneself" (2010, pp. 84–85). Fuchs (2007, p. 379) similarly speculates that the increasing prevalence of BPD may be attributable, in part, to "the development of a mainly externally driven, fragmented character in post-modern society."

The suggestion that BPD involves a combination of decontextualized emotion and lack of trust in others is consistent with numerous first-person reports. For example, *The BPD Journals: A Year in the Life*, by Topher Edwards (2015), consists of a series of unaltered entries from an online journal that chronicles his experiences. At various points, the entries convey a lack of life-structure – a fragmented past and no sense of what the future holds:

> Without any idea of where I want to be in five years, it's hard to start doing things to get out of this grave I have been digging for myself. (Edwards, 2015, p. 38)
>
> There are no certainties. I have no plans, no goals, just fears. The past is a good tool for predicting the future, and it looks like I am screwed. (p. 54)
>
> If I cannot fill my past, how the hell do I fill the future? (p. 52)

In conjunction with this, he describes a pervasive sense of social isolation and distrust: "I am afraid to trust anybody anymore. And they should be afraid too. Look at what I have done. Look at the path of destruction behind me" (Edwards, 2015, p. 64). The experience of lack of trust in others, as well as in oneself, is also conveyed by the following report:

> I don't like getting too close to people … I get very threatened. I like to keep a distance. I think that if they got up too close and found out what I was like behind the facade … I don't even know what's behind the facade. I know that they'll think I'm not good enough … that I'll never be good enough. (Crowe, 2004, p. 331)

Here, and elsewhere, estrangement from others is inseparable from how one finds oneself in the world more generally and thus from how one experiences and regulates emotion.

The approach we have sketched can also account for the polarization and instability of emotion in BPD. Why, one might ask, are emotions not only strong but also intense in this way? Furthermore, why do interpersonal emotions not merely lack context but also alternate wildly between the extremes of positive and negative? Lack of trust, and an associated sense of others as hostile, would dispose one toward strong, negative interpersonal emotions, of the kinds associated with BPD. At the same time, though, the need to self-regulate, to preserve what is left of one's world, might remain. And, we have argued, effective self-regulation during times of upheaval requires the assistance of others. Hence, what we suggest is that the person clings to others, desperately seeking out and hanging onto potential regulators. The stakes are high and so emotional responses, including fear of abandonment, are likely to be strong. Yet, with an unstable world and a tendency to experience others as hostile and untrustworthy, interpersonal emotions will also be inconsistent; there is fluctuation between strong but shallow attachments and feelings of anger, betrayal, and distrust.[17] This is consistent with the following characterization of aloneness in BPD, offered by Pazzagli and Rossi Monti (2000):

> The ideal goal of the borderline personality is bonding, but a bonding that has never been achieved, and that has never produced internalization of that fundamental security that guarantees an autonomous life. When faced with an available object, the demand and hope for internalization flares up every time. But it is never achieved, also because it is difficult to internalize a primary object that has been harshly criticized for its failings. (p. 224)

The relevant dynamic is also clearly highlighted by first-person reports:

> In my head are thoughts of: *I am so lonely – won't someone be my friend? Stay away! Come closer. I don't trust you. Why don't you help me? No one cares. I might as well kill myself. I have obligations, I can't kill myself.* (Gunderson & Hoffman, 2016, p. 167)

The resources required to contextualize and regulate negative, other-directed emotions are lacking, a point that applies equally to self-directed emotions. Without regulatory support, they are strong, intense, unambiguous, seemingly inescapable, and yet transient:[18]

> My goals, future, and entire life were all based off of the exact present moment to me, which changed daily. To me, if I wasn't unrealistically achieving major accomplishments (like finishing an entire class in one day with an A), I was useless, meaningless, and not appropriate to the world. (Gunderson & Hoffman, 2016, p. 57)

> Every strong feeling was not only absolute, but eternal. It didn't matter if a person close to me had occupied the pedestal ten minutes ago and been the object of my abundant love. When the emotions changed, it was as if that love had never existed and the hatred I felt today would be the way I felt forever. (Reiland, 2004, p. 89)

A fragile world of this kind could come about in different ways. As noted earlier, the stability of our concerns depends on a range of factors. Thus,

[17] In this chapter, we have focused on how a certain way of finding oneself in the world, involving a pervasive lack of trust, influences the structure of *specifically directed* emotional experiences. However, it should be added that the distrust itself amounts to a form of affective experience. We suggest that this is central to a nonlocalized "dysphoria" that some authors take as key to the phenomenology of BPD (see, e.g., Pazzagli & Rossi Monti, 2000; Rossi Monti & D'Agostino, 2019; Stanghellini & Rosfort, 2013).

[18] Lack of trust can also account for a wider intolerance of ambiguity. Without trust, one cannot live with uncertainty, which takes on the form of threat or menace. One cannot just let things be for a while; the uncertainty has to be resolved. This is consistent with the inflexibility remarked upon by Fonagy et al. (2015).

disruption in one or more of these areas could conceivably result in a world that lacks some degree of structure. This might then leave one vulnerable to the influence of other factors, leading to a process of unravelling or to a process that prevents a stable world from forming in the first place. An emphasis on the extent to which we are reliant on other people to self-regulate is consistent with the well-established correlation between BPD and childhood adversity. Fonagy et al. (2015, pp. 589–590) suggest that "trust may be undermined or destroyed by social adversity, especially attachment trauma" and note that BPD patients are "four times more likely than normal controls to have suffered early trauma," often consisting of emotional neglect or abuse.[19] Others have similarly found a strong correlation between BPD and childhood adversity. For example, Zanarini et al. (1997) conducted a study of 358 subjects who met the criteria for BPD. They report that histories of neglect and/or abuse were "ubiquitous" among these patients, with 91 percent reporting some form of abuse and 92 percent neglect, rates that are far higher than in comparison subjects.[20]

An integral part of experiences of neglect and abuse may be the lack of predictability in caregivers' emotional responses, a factor which can make it particularly difficult to experience the interpersonal world as one in which interactions follow reliable patterns. This dynamic is pointed toward in the following passage, where the author describes her relationship with her father:

> Often his explosive violence had been irrational and triggered by the slightest provocation: a facial expression he found disrespectful, tears he didn't want to see, any expression of emotion he didn't have patience for. And the rules changed all the time. Something that could bring him to smile or laugh one day could provoke him to angrily pull off his belt a few days or hours later. (Reiland, 2004, p. 84)

Regardless of how BPD might be caused in any given case, we have suggested that the type of emotion dysregulation associated with the diagnosis is better

[19] A connection can also be established between the widespread character of these experiences in the history of borderline patients and the centrality of the emotion of shame in BPD (cf. Bortolan, 2017; Crowe, 2004).

[20] Many other studies report correlations between forms of childhood adversity and subsequent diagnosis of BPD. For discussion of the correlations between childhood abuse and neglect and subsequent diagnoses of personality disorders, see, for example, Johnson, Cohen, Brown, Smailes, and Bernstein (1999). Given the likely relationship between BPD and childhood adversity, Herman, Perry, and Van der Kolk (1989, p. 494) propose that we conceive of BPD as a "complicated posttraumatic syndrome," with "direct implications for the treatment of posttraumatic syndromes." Others have proposed an additional role for genetic factors. For example, Chanen and Kaess (2012, p. 46) suggest that "individuals with a 'sensitive' genotype are at greater risk of BPD in the presence of a predisposing environment. Furthermore, the genes that influence BPD features also increase the likelihood of being exposed to certain adverse life events."

conceived of in interpersonal than intrapersonal terms. It involves relating to people in ways that hamper, to varying degrees and perhaps in different ways, the ability to assemble and maintain a stable, significant world of the kind that emotion regulation more usually presupposes. In some instances, it could be that such a world is not fully formed in the first place. In others, there may be damage to a world that was, to some extent, previously established. Sometimes, the causes may be largely interpersonal in nature. In other cases, intrapersonal causes may play a more pronounced role. And, depending on which applies, it could be that aberrant emotions are largely responsible for destabilizing the world or, alternatively, that the world is disrupted in such a way that the formation of coherent emotion patterns is impeded. If what we have said is broadly right, then it is misleading to think of BPD in terms of an individual "personality," given that it involves deprivation or breakdown of regulatory processes that are interpersonal in structure. Recognition of (a) the extent to which emotion dysregulation might be symptomatic of a disordered world rather than vice versa and (b) the essential roles played by other people in sustaining such a world, therefore has the potential to shape how we conceive of and respond to BPD, including where we place the emphasis when referring to "disorder."

Acknowledgment

We are grateful to Gemma Copsey, Christian Tewes, and an anonymous reviewer for helpful comments and suggestions.

References

Adler, J. M., Chin, E. D., Kolisetty, A. P., & Oltmanns, T. F. (2012). The distinguishing characteristics of narrative identity in adults with features of borderline personality disorder: An empirical investigation. *Journal of Personality Disorders*, 26(4), 498–512. doi:10.1521/pedi.2012.26.4.498

American Psychiatric Association. (2013). *Diagnostic and statistical manual of mental disorders* (5th ed.). Arlington, VA: American Psychiatric Association.

Bortolan, A. (2017). Affectivity and moral experience: An extended phenomenological account. *Phenomenology and the Cognitive Sciences*, 16(3), 471–490. doi:10.1007/s11097-016-9468-9

Bortolan, A. (2019). Phenomenological psychopathology and autobiography. In G. Stanghellini, M. R. Broome, A. V. Fernandez, P. Fusar-Poli, A. Raballo, & R. Rosfort (Eds.), *The Oxford handbook of phenomenological psychopathology* (pp. 1053–1064). Oxford, UK: Oxford University Press.

Bortolan, A. (2020). Narratively shaped emotions: The case of borderline personality disorder. *The Journal of Medicine and Philosophy: A Forum for Bioethics and Philosophy of Medicine*, 45(2), 212–230. doi.org/10.1093/jmp/jhz037

Campos, J. J., Walle, E. A., Dahl, A., & Main, A. (2011). Reconceptualizing emotion regulation. *Emotion Review*, 3(1), 26–35. doi:10.1177/1754073910380975

Chanen, A. M., & Kaess, M. (2012). Developmental pathways to borderline personality disorder. *Current Psychiatry Reports*, 14(1), 45–53. doi:10.1007/s11920-011-0242-y

Coan, J. A., & Maresh, E. L. (2014). Social baseline theory and the social regulation of emotion. In J. J. Gross (Ed.), *Handbook of emotion regulation* (pp. 221–236). New York, NY: The Guilford Press.

Colombetti, G., & Krueger, J. (2015). Scaffoldings of the affective mind. *Philosophical Psychology*, 28(8), 1157–1176. doi:10.1080/09515089.2014.976334

Crowe, M. (2004). Never good enough – Part 1: Shame or borderline personality disorder? *Journal of Psychiatric and Mental Health Nursing*, 11(3), 327–334. doi:10.1111/j.1365-2850.2004.00732.x

Diamond, L. M., & Aspinwall, L. G. (2003). Emotion regulation across the life span: An integrative perspective emphasizing self-regulation, positive affect, and dyadic processes. *Motivation and Emotion*, 27(2), 125–156. doi:10.1023/A:1024521920068

Ebner-Priemer, U. W., Houben, M., Santangelo, P., Kleindienst, N., Tuerlinckx, F., Oravecz, Z., … Kuppens, P. (2015). Unraveling affective dysregulation in borderline personality disorder: A theoretical model and empirical evidence. *Journal of Abnormal Psychology*, 124(1), 186–198. doi:10.1037/abn0000021

Ebner-Priemer, U. W., Kuo, J., Kleindienst, N., Welch, S. S., Reisch, T., Reinhard, I., … Bohus, M. (2007). State affective instability in borderline personality disorder assessed by ambulatory monitoring. *Psychological Medicine*, 37, 961–970. doi:10.1016/j.psychres.2006.04.014

Edwards, T. (2015). *The BPD journals: A year in the life*. San Francisco, CA: Blurb.

Fonagy, P., & Allison, E. (2014). The role of mentalizing and epistemic trust in the therapeutic relationship. *Psychotherapy*, 51(3), 372–380. doi:10.1037/a0036505

Fonagy, P., Luyten, P., & Allison, E. (2015). Epistemic petrification and the restoration of epistemic trust: A new conceptualization of borderline personality disorder and its psychosocial treatment. *Journal of Personality Disorders*, 29(5), 575–609. doi:10.1521/pedi.2015.29.5.575

Fonagy, P., & Target, M. (2007). Playing with reality: IV. A theory of external reality rooted in intersubjectivity. *International Journal of Psychoanalysis*, 88, 917–937. doi:10.1516/4774-6173-241T-72

Fuchs, T. (2007). Fragmented selves: Temporality and identity in borderline personality disorder. *Psychopathology*, 40(6), 379–387. doi:10.1159/000106.468

Goldie, P. (2000). *The emotions: A philosophical exploration*. Oxford, UK: Oxford University Press.

Goldie, P. (2012). *The mess inside: Narrative, emotion, and the mind*. Oxford, UK: Oxford University Press.

Gross, J. J. (1999). Emotion regulation: Past, present, future. *Cognition & Emotion*, 13(5), 551–573. doi:10.1080/026999399379186

Gross, J. J. (2001). Emotion regulation in adulthood: Timing is everything. *Current Directions in Psychological Science*, 10(6), 214–219. doi:10.1111%2F1467-8721.00152

Gross, J. J. (2014). Emotion regulation: Conceptual and empirical foundations. In J. J. Gross (Ed.), *Handbook of emotion regulation* (pp. 3–20). New York, NY: The Guilford Press.

Gunderson, J. G., & Hoffman, P. D. (2016). *Beyond borderline: True stories of recovery from borderline personality disorder.* Oakland, CA: New Harbinger Publications.

Helm, B. W. (2001). *Emotional reason: Deliberation, motivation, and the nature of value.* Cambridge, UK: Cambridge University Press.

Helm, B. W. (2009a). Emotions as evaluative feelings. *Emotion Review*, 1(3), 248–255. doi:10.1177/1754073909103593

Helm, B. W. (2009b). Love, identification, and the emotions. *American Philosophical Quarterly*, 46(1), 39–59.

Herman, J. (1992/1997). *Trauma and recovery.* New York, NY: Basic Books.

Herman, J. L., Perry, J. C., & Van der Kolk, B. A. (1989). Childhood trauma in borderline personality disorder. *The American Journal of Psychiatry*, 146(4), 490–495. doi:10.1176/ajp.146.4.490

Hobson, P. (2002). *The cradle of thought.* London, UK: Pan Macmillan.

Johnson, J. G., Cohen, P., Brown, J., Smailes, E. M., & Bernstein, D. P. (1999). Childhood maltreatment increases risk for personality disorders during early adulthood. *Archives of General Psychiatry*, 56(7), 600–606. doi:10.1001/archpsyc.56.7.600

Kappas, A. (2011). Emotion and regulation are one! *Emotion Review*, 3(1), 17–25. doi:10.1177/1754073910380971

Kreisman, J. J., & Straus, H. (2010). *I hate you – don't leave me: Understanding the borderline personality.* New York, NY: Perigree.

Leichsenring, F., Leibing, E., Kruse, J., New, A. S., & Leweke, F. (2011). Borderline personality disorder. *The Lancet*, 377(9759), 74–84. doi:10.1016/S0140-6736(10)61422-5

Lieb, K., Zanarini, M. C., Schmahl, C., Linehan, M. M., & Bohus, M. (2004). Borderline personality disorder. *The Lancet*, 364(9432), 453–461. doi:10.1016/S0140-6736(04)16770-6

Linehan, M. M. (1993). *Cognitive-behavioral treatment of borderline personality disorder.* New York, NY: The Guilford Press.

Mikulincer, M., Shaver, P. R., & Pereg, D. (2003). Attachment theory and affect regulation: The dynamics, development, and cognitive consequences of attachment-related strategies. *Motivation and Emotion*, 27(2), 77–102. doi:10.1023/A:1024515519160

Nica, E. I., & Links, P. S. (2009). Affective instability in borderline personality disorder: Experience sampling findings. *Current Psychiatry Reports*, 11(1), 74–81. doi:10.1007/s11920-009-0012-2

Pazzagli, A., & Rossi Monti, M. (2000). Dysphoria and aloneness in borderline personality disorder. *Psychopathology*, 33(4), 220–226. doi:10.1159/000029147

Prinz, J. J. (2006). Is emotion a form of perception? *Canadian Journal of Philosophy*, 36(5), 137–160. doi:10.1353/cjp.2007.0035

Pugmire, D. (2005). *Sound sentiments: Integrity in the emotions.* Oxford, UK: Oxford University Press.

Ratcliffe, M. (2008). *Feelings of being: Phenomenology, psychiatry and the sense of reality*. Oxford, UK: Oxford University Press.

Ratcliffe, M. (2015). *Experiences of depression: A study in phenomenology*. Oxford, UK: Oxford University Press.

Ratcliffe, M. (2017a). Grief and the unity of emotion. *Midwest Studies in Philosophy*, 41(1), 154–174. doi:10.1111/misp.12071

Ratcliffe, M. (2017b). *Real hallucinations: Psychiatric illness, intentionality, and the interpersonal world*. Cambridge, MA: Massachusetts Institute of Technology Press.

Ratcliffe, M. (2019a). Emotional intentionality. *Royal Institute of Philosophy Supplements*, 85, 251–269. doi:10.1017/S1358246118000784

Ratcliffe, M. (2019b). Grief and phantom limbs: A phenomenological comparison. In T. Burns, T. Szanto, A. Salice, M. Doyon, & A. A. Dumont (Eds.), *The new yearbook for phenomenology and phenomenological philosophy. Vol. XVII* (pp. 77–96). London, UK: Routledge.

Reeck, C., Ames, D. R., & Ochsner, K. N. (2016). The social regulation of emotion: An integrative, cross-disciplinary model. *Trends in Cognitive Sciences*, 20(1), 47–63. doi:10.1016/j.tics.2015.09.003

Reiland, R. (2004). *Get me out of here. My recovery from borderline personality disorder*. Center City, MN: Hazelden.

Roberts, R. C. (1988). What an emotion is: A sketch. *The Philosophical Review*, 97(2), 183–209. doi:10.2307/2185261

Rossi Monti, M., & D'Agostino, A. (2019). Dysphoria in borderline persons. In G. Stanghellini, M. R. Broome, A. V. Fernandez, P. Fusar-Poli, A. Raballo, & R. Rosfort (Eds.), *The Oxford handbook of phenomenological psychopathology* (pp. 827–838). Oxford, UK: Oxford University Press.

Scheppes, G., Suri, G., & Gross, J. J. (2015). Emotion regulation and psychopathology. *Annual Review of Clinical Psychology*, 11, 379–405. doi:10.1146/annurev-clinpsy-032814-112739

Slaby, J. (2008). Affective intentionality and the feeling body. *Phenomenology and the Cognitive Sciences*, 7(4), 429–444. doi:10.1007/s11097-007-9083-x

Stanghellini, G., & Rosfort, R. (2013). Borderline depression: A desperate vitality. *Journal of Consciousness Studies*, 20(7–8), 153–177. Retrieved from www.ingentaconnect.com/content/imp/jcs/2013/00000020/F0020007/art00008

Thompson, R. A. (1994). Emotion regulation: A theme in search of definition. *Monographs of the Society for Research in Child Development*, 59(2–3), 25–52. doi:10.2307/1166137

Thompson, R. A. (2014). Socialization of emotion and emotion regulation in the family. In J. J. Gross (Ed.), *Handbook of emotion regulation* (pp. 173–186). New York, NY: The Guilford Press.

Varga, S., & Krueger, J. (2013). Background emotions, proximity and distributed emotion regulation. *Review of Philosophy & Psychology*, 4(2), 271–292. doi:10.1007/s13164-013-0134-7

Zanarini, M. C., Williams, A. A., Lewis, R. E., Reich, R. B., Vera, S. C., Marino, M. F., … & Frankenburg, F. R. (1997). Reported pathological childhood experiences associated with the development of borderline personality disorder. *American Journal of Psychiatry*, 154, 1101–1106. doi:10.1176/ajp.154.8.1101

9.1

Commentary on "Emotion Regulation in a Disordered World: Understanding Borderline Personality Disorder"

On the Scope of Interpersonal Explanation: Destructivity and Emptiness as Responses to Felt Dependency

Philipp Schmidt

Processes of emotional dysregulation, in their most severe forms, include not only intense, volatile, and uncontrollable emotions but are often associated with serious disturbances in how persons relate to others, the world, and themselves. The syndrome of phenomena that manifest these disturbances, including strong emotions, aberrant feelings of emptiness, unstable interpersonal relationships, and shifting identities, are often considered in terms of a *personality* disorder: borderline personality disorder (BPD). In their rich and insightful chapter, Ratcliffe and Bortolan challenge this influential background assumption, an assumption that affects the way persons with BPD are often seen and treated. They argue that BPD and the different manifestations of dysregulated processes involved should not be understood as emanations of a corrupt nucleus of personality. Instead, they emphasize, emotional turmoil such as BPD should be seen in terms of processes that are *interpersonal* in nature.

To show that disturbances in emotional experience are conditioned by structures that involve others, Ratcliffe and Bortolan address the phenomenology of emotion dysregulation. In their discussion of the latter, two general lines of explanation can be identified.

The first concerns the *experience of the world* and the way it provides the infrastructure for emotional experience. Linking world and emotion by alluding to the notion of "significance," they describe how our experience of the world is always pervaded by concerns, care for others, projects; in short, by things that matter to us. Distinguishing a person's emotional background from their episodic emotions, they describe the latter as the specific experience of significance that arises when something potentially or actually influences what matters to us. Emotions, on that view, evoke certain responses to processes and events of life that affect our concerns, and thus grow out of the experience of significance that constitutes our world experience. A disordered world in which our projects are under threat thus generates strong emotions. It is at that point that the crucial role of others for emotion-processes comes into play: "[T]he sustenance of one's concerns and the manner in which situations are experienced as relating to those concerns are both inseparable from one's relations with particular people" (Ratcliffe & Bortolan, 2021, p. 188). Pursuing our goals in our habitual world, we usually rely on other people to act in accordance with our expectations of them: "[O]thers won't try to mow us down as we cross the road; they won't give us false information when we ask for directions" (p. 188). Relating to others thus involves a certain form of "trust" (p. 189) which allows us to pursue our affairs. If, however, interpersonal relationships are structured in a way that basic trust is eroded, then this has implications for the way we experience significance and the world – with potentially and often severe repercussions for the way emotional experiences are organized.

The second line of explanation concerns *emotion regulation and the role of others* therein. As Ratcliffe and Bortolan emphasize, others are not only relevant to the pursuit of our own projects and the experience of significance involved but also to our emotion regulation, for instance, when our world has been shattered and the things that matter to us are in jeopardy. The crucial insight Ratcliffe and Bortolan offer in this regard is that emotion regulation is not exhausted by activities performed by the individual in isolation from others. On the contrary, "there is no clear boundary to be drawn between self-regulation and regulation by others" (Ratcliffe & Bortolan, 2021, p. 186). Our self-regulation is thus to a great extent socially distributed. Others provide support in times of hardship, for instance, by helping to understand situations and developing scaffolding narratives or simply by being there. Moreover, others are also involved in the utilization of environmental regulatory resources. Ratcliffe and Bortolan mention activities such as going to an art gallery, the cinema, or the café. All these situations are social situations that include certain expectations of how others will behave and react to oneself. Whether related regulatory processes are successful thus depends heavily on others and whether the expectations we have of them are met. Importantly, this experience of others is precisely what is impaired in conditions labeled as BPD – severely and in various ways. Accordingly, regulatory processes that ought to stabilize emotions and secure the integrity of projects are not available to persons so affected.

Although Ratcliffe and Bortolan put emphasis on *inter*personal aspects of the emotional disturbances associated with BPD, they also acknowledge *intra*personal factors which, as they suggest, may sometimes even precede disorders of the social sphere. Hence, their aim is by no means to shift the focus of explanation away from the individual completely. Their approach is compatible with a framework that accepts different directions of causal explanation. But it does raise one obvious question: How far can an interpersonal explanation of the various phenomena of borderline experience take us? Let me evaluate the two lines of explanation offered by Ratcliffe and Bortolan in the light of this question by discussing two issues that prima facie seem to elude an interpersonal explanation and are pertinent to our understanding of BPD. In doing so, my aim is not to suggest a weakness in their account. After all, Ratcliffe and Bortolan do not claim to give an exhaustive account of BPD but only seek to demonstrate – successfully in my view – how crucial interpersonal structures are to the development, maintenance, and regulation of emotional processes. Rather, my aim here is to explore whether the scope of their explanation may actually be wider than Ratcliffe and Bortolan have proposed.

The first issue refers to the experience of the world and others. As Ratcliffe and Bortolan show, ruptures in the way we perceive the world and others do not only manifest themselves in corresponding turbulent emotions but also trigger emotional processes that have further destabilizing effects. Often such ruptures can be traced back to hostile or disappointing others, or life events that threaten the integrity of the individual's concerns. However, while persons with BPD often live in environments that are complicated and even malicious, this need not be the case. Moreover, even when persons with BPD have had troubling experiences that unsettle their trust, they often encounter situations that would allow them to stabilize their world, including the presence of benevolent others, if they let them. Yet persons with BPD often let these possibilities pass and seem to steer toward escalation where this is unnecessary. In these cases, it is the person with BPD rather than their environment that seems to be the epicenter of unsettling processes, including forms of self-destructive behavior that undermine the integrity of their own concerns (Sadikaj, Moskowitz, Russell, Zuroff, & Paris, 2013). Why do persons with BPD sabotage possibilities of stabilization? It might be the case that turbulent emotions can be explained as a result of an unstable world or troublesome interpersonal relationships, but can interpersonal aspects also explain why persons with BPD *themselves* often obstruct the development of a stable world and solid relationships with others?

The second issue concerns the chronic feelings of emptiness prevalent in BPD (Elsner, Broadbear, & Rao, 2018). Ratcliffe and Bortolan explain turbulent emotions by focusing on experiences of significance. Strong emotions are specific kinds of experience of significance that emerge when other people or life events endanger the integrity of a person's concerns and projects. Feelings of emptiness, however, do not seem to be direct responses to endangered concerns or projects. They are experiences of a completely different kind, characterized by a painful *absence* of significance. Whatever concerns or projects are remembered by persons affected in this way are experienced without evoking a feeling of significance. They feel bereft of meaning. It is therefore questionable whether the emotional quality of emptiness can be directly explained by threats to the integrity of a person's concerns and projects. It is easy to see how emotional disturbance may grow out of a threat to projects that have significance to the individual, but if their projects are already experienced as *in*significant, then they can hardly be threatened by others and the interpersonal factor seems to be vanishingly small.

How can one explain these two aspects of BPD experience – destructivity and emptiness? May the two lines of explanation offered by Ratcliffe and Bortolan play a role even though not immediately evident? I want to propose that this is indeed the case.

Interpersonal dependency is an important feature of BPD (Bornstein, Becker-Matero, Winarick, & Reichman, 2010), and Ratcliffe and Bortolan provide an account of why this is the case. However, to see the full explanatory potential of their account, I suggest, one needs to acknowledge that interpersonal dependency is also an *aspect of experience*, that is, that it is not a mere fact underlying the phenomenology but is itself experienced. Once considered as *felt* dependency, we may begin to understand destructivity and emptiness as ways of relating to others.

In healthy individuals, dependence is experienced not solely as a limitation but in the form of others being a resource available to oneself, the utilization of which gives rise to a sense of control and autonomy. In persons with BPD, however, when others are not available in this way, it leads not only to a lack of control in the form of missing regulatory capacities but also to a *sense* of such lack, manifest as *felt dependency*, that is, feelings of exposedness and vulnerability. Once established, these feelings pervade even in situations when the world offers stability or where others show benevolence. Instead of taking these offers as resources, persons with BPD focus on the aspect of dependence implied in the need to rely on a stable world and benevolent others. They are unable to build on such stability because they are irritated by feeling dependent on the stability others provide.

My suggestion is that both destructivity and emptiness can be understood as dysregulated responses to feelings of dependency. *Emptiness* allows the individual to reduce felt dependency by decreasing factual dependence:

If projects cease to appear as significant, then others lose the power to endanger these very projects; likewise, if emotions are numbed down to emptiness, others no longer seem necessary for the regulation of emotional turbulence. *Destructivity* can therefore be explained in at least two ways. First, it may generate experiences of significance by creating turbulence in the world and interpersonal relationships, thereby reintroducing the world and others as things that matter. Second, it may give rise to a surrogate sense of control: When a person suffers from the dependence on others, destroying the stability and harmony that both are reliant on other people might give her the compensatory feeling that she is not completely exposed to them. Feeling the power to destroy might be the only way for persons affected to reassure themselves that they can contribute to or even determine the shared constitution of the world, that is, that they can coauthor their own and other people's experience of significance. Destructivity may induce the compensatory feeling that one can reverse the direction of dependence.

To conclude, both destructivity and feelings of emptiness can be conceived in terms of ways of *relating to the other* and *self-regulation*, as ways of responding to a felt dependency on others. Hence, the account of interpersonal dependence offered by Ratcliffe and Bortolan provides an important basis for the explanation of several phenomena of borderline experience. Crucially, understanding interpersonal dependence not only as an explanatory principle but also as an aspect of experience will add further evidence to the thesis Ratcliffe and Bortolan promote: that BPD is essentially an interpersonal disorder.

References

Bornstein, R. F., Becker-Matero, N., Winarick, D. J., & Reichman, A. L. (2010). Interpersonal dependency in borderline personality disorder: Clinical context and empirical evidence. *Journal of Personality Disorders*, 24, 109–127. doi:10.1521/pedi.2010.24.1.109

Elsner, D., Broadbear, J. H., & Rao, S. (2018). What is the clinical significance of chronic emptiness in borderline personality disorder? *Australasian Psychiatry*, 26(1), 88–91. doi:10.1177/1039856217734674

Ratcliffe, M., & Bortolan, A. (2021). Emotion regulation in a disordered world: Understanding borderline personality disorder. In C. Tewes & G. Stanghellini (Eds.), *Time and body: Phenomenological and psychopathological approaches* (pp. 177–200). Cambridge, UK: Cambridge University Press.

Sadikaj, G., Moskowitz, D. S., Russell, J. J., Zuroff, D. C., & Paris, J. (2013). Quarrelsome behavior in borderline personality disorder: Influence of behavioral and affective reactivity to perceptions of others. *Journal of Abnormal Psychology*, 122(1), 195–207. doi:10.1037/a0030871

10

Nobody? Disturbed Self-Experience in Borderline Personality Disorder and Four Kinds of Instabilities

Philipp Schmidt

Borderline personality disorder (BPD) is a complex psychological condition that severely affects many different aspects of the life of persons suffering from it. Its broad impact is reflected in the *Diagnostic and Statistical Manual of Mental Disorders* (DSM) criteria of diagnosis, which applies if five out of the nine following symptoms are present: unstable personal relationships, identity disturbances, impulsivity, self-mutilation, affective instability due to reactivity of mood, chronic feelings of emptiness, intense anger or difficulties in controlling anger, peculiar behavior to avoid abandonment, and paranoid ideation. Such a variety of symptoms implies heterogeneity in the manifestation of BPD across individuals. Yet in all cases, BPD appears to consist in "a pervasive pattern of instability of interpersonal relationships, self-image, and affects, and marked impulsivity" (American Psychiatric Association, 2013, p. 663), as the DSM's definition suggests. While there is general acknowledgment of the BPD instability pattern in the clinical literature, two related questions have remained unanswered. Both concern its clinical picture: (1) *How does the BPD instability pattern emerge and persist over time?* (2) *How do phenomena associated with the different kinds of instabilities relate to each other?*

Not only do researchers diverge significantly in their understanding of the development of BPD, the causal factors that are taken to underlie the BPD instability pattern are as multifarious as trauma in young age, emotional, sexual or physical abuse, parental neglect or invalidation in the home environment, neurophysiology (lack of oxytocin), and organic brain disease or trauma (Cameron, Calderwood, & McMurphy, 2018; Keinänen, Johnson, Richards, & Courtney, 2012). Moreover, while correlations between instability in identity, affect, and interpersonal relationships have been described by numerous empirical studies, it is still an open question how exactly these symptoms interrelate. Should they be conceived in *atomistic* terms, that is, is the instability pattern and its related phenomena held together by different causes? Or is a *holistic* view more accurate, according to which there is an intrinsic connection between the different forms of instability and related phenomena?

This paper aims to gather evidence for a holistic account of the BPD instability pattern by examining the experiences associated with BPD instability in the spheres of identity, affect, and interpersonal relationships and describing their phenomenological structure. Descriptions of the phenomenological structures involved may not only help us understand what it is like to suffer from BPD but can also help explain how different phenomenological aspects of BPD connect and mutually imply one another (Sass, 2014; Schmidt, 2018, 2020). Showing that different forms of instability are experientially interconnected not only lends support to the holistic view; it also helps solve the mystery of how heterogeneous factors can induce a similar instability pattern. For, on the holistic view, different factors may cause different aspects of the pattern to emerge, which due to their experiential interconnections then trigger the full instability pattern – independently of whether the primary disturbance lies in instability in identity, affect, or interpersonal relationships.[1] Accordingly, conceiving of instability in BPD in holistic terms, that is, considering the pattern as a Gestalt-like complex of structurally intertwined experiential phenomena instead of taking it as a cluster of atomistic symptoms, is also of significance for the understanding of the etiology of BPD.

My analysis of the experiences involved in the different kinds of instabilities is guided by the tradition of phenomenological psychopathology, which focuses on investigating the phenomenological structure of various key dimensions of experience, such as temporality, embodiment, intersubjectivity, self-awareness, agency, affectivity or narrativity, and their modification in psychopathology (e.g., Fuchs, 2007, 2010, 2013; Fuchs & Pallagrosi, 2018; Ratcliffe, 2005, 2008, 2017; Sass, 2014; Stanghellini & Mancini, 2018; Stanghellini & Rosfort, 2010, 2013a, 2013b). As Gallagher (2013) and Gallagher and Daly (2018) emphasize, selfhood is constituted by these various dimensions, and change in any one of them may not only affect the other dimensions but may also radically alter one's self-experience more globally, that is, modify what it is like for the person to be in the world. Put differently, pathological alterations in experiential dimensions

1 With the full BPD instability pattern, I only refer to the four kinds of instabilities that I describe in this paper. To answer whether all BPD-related symptoms can be understood in light of the four kinds of instabilities will require a more encompassing analysis. For instance, in this paper, I will not address paranoid ideation – a possible symptom of BPD – or delusional paranoia – manifest in rather severe cases of BPD. Further research is needed to elucidate the relationship between paranoid ideation or delusional paranoia and the four kinds of instabilities.

are associated with disturbed forms of self-experience. Thus, self-experience is the experiential locus where changes in different experiential dimensions interact and become effective.

It is against this theoretical background that I propose an investigation of the phenomenological structure of self-experience associated with instability in identity, affect, and interpersonal relationships. By focusing on self-experience, I do not want to imply that BPD should be understood merely in intrapersonal terms (I agree with Ratcliffe and Bortolan (2021) on this). What I want to propose, rather, is that by considering self-experience in BPD, we may best understand how different salient BPD phenomena – for example, unstable affect, feelings of loneliness, or distortions in the intentional structure of experience – interact and are connected to each other. Similarly, I do not want to suggest that BPD is primarily a self-disorder, nor for that matter that self-disorder is *the* core feature of BPD, as sometimes has been considered (Meares, Gerull, Stevenson, & Korner, 2011). Instead, I want to say that all pathological experiences involved in BPD amount to changes in self-experience.

At the same time, my focus on self-experience is not merely methodological either. Because BPD seems to be a condition in which self-experience becomes itself a focal point in the experience of suffering. This may be prereflectively present in the form of a lack of self-feeling or low self-esteem, but it is also manifested on a reflective level in the form of self-related thoughts. This is exemplified by a remark from Topher Edwards, BPD sufferer and author of an online diary who, after having written reports for a year, including numerous expressions of anger, sadness, and grief related to the loss of or rejection by others, describes BPD as a "life-long battle – a war raging *between me and myself* [emphasis added]" (2017, p. 159). Problems in life and with others directly translate into issues with oneself. Another post by Edwards is equally revealing: "Misery follows me everywhere. Bad luck clings to me, and everyone I get close to seems to end up wanting nothing to do with me. It's obvious that the common denominator is ME. As in 'it is ME that fucks everything up'" (2017, p. 154). Self-experience, therefore, is not only an indicator of how changes in different experiential dimensions interact in BPD, it is itself an important aspect in the phenomenology of BPD experience and so deserves special attention.

First, I describe how the three kinds of instabilities associated with BPD, instability in identity, affect, and interpersonal relationships, present aspects of disturbed self-experience. Guided by the approach of phenomenological psychopathology, I emphasize that these aspects of disturbed self-experience are experientially interconnected and interwoven. Second, I discuss how the experience of the body features in these aspects of disturbed self-experience and suggest that BPD also involves a fourth kind of instability: a significant instability in embodiment. Finally, I conclude that analyzing the experiential interconnections between BPD-related phenomena and the bodily dimension of disturbed self-experience not only helps in describing and understanding BPD experience but also allows significant insights into how the clinical picture of BPD emerges and persists over time.

The Many Faces of Living as No One: Fragmentation and the Instability of Identity

The most obvious disturbance of self-experience in BPD is the diminishment of the sense of identity. It is a complex disturbance that manifests itself in various ways. From an external perspective, it is not only noticeable in "inconsistency," understood in terms of an "objective incoherence in thought, feeling, and behaviour," but can also be recognized in the "lack of commitment" to, for example, jobs or values. It is equally expressed in the phenomenon of "role absorption," that is, the tendency of persons with BPD to "define themselves in terms of a single role or cause" (Wilkinson-Ryan & Westen, 2000, p. 528). It has also been shown that persons with BPD often demonstrate the tendency to construct different partial identities in which self-attributes with positive and negative valence are organized separately (Vater, Schröder-Abé, Weißgerber, Roepke, & Schütz, 2015). Accordingly, identity disturbance in BPD is more complex than a mere absence of a sense of identity. It concerns the whole process of identity development, which in BPD is often characterized by a "diffuse-avoidant identity style" (Jørgensen, 2009). This includes, apart from a shifting sense of identity, a lack of self-awareness, a tendency to avoid new experiences about oneself or to reject feedback from others on aspects of one's identity. Rather than seeking and integrating information about themselves, persons with such an identity style are driven by their impulses, not only in their decision-making and actions but also in their self-perception (and experience of others).

From a phenomenological point of view, it has been suggested that BPD self-disorder can be understood in terms of a lack of narrative identity (Fuchs, 2007). On this view, persons with BPD suffer from the absence of an integrating and unifying life story that would provide a stable sense of identity. The severe shifts in the person's sense of identity that ensue involve a set of peculiar self-experiences. Among the most important are the following.

First, lack of an integrative narrative implies a form of "self-fragmentation" (Fuchs, 2007, p. 381). Different moments in life feature different ways of conceiving of oneself and different feelings of who one is. Most importantly, though, fragmentation does not mean that the structure of narrative identity vanishes altogether. Rather, the process of understanding oneself in terms of a narrative is severely destabilized, in that narratives may quickly change and are prone to be influenced by current situations. This manifests itself in experience as "painful incoherence" (Meares et al., 2011), adding to the high tension from which persons with BPD suffer.

Second, destabilization is also connected with a distortion of the temporal horizon and a strong focus on the present. As Fuchs highlights, "the patients are completely identified with their momentary state of mind, unable to gain a distance from the present situation" (2007, p. 381). This phenomenon of "instantaneity" (Muscelli & Stanghellini, 2014) or "immediacy" (Lo Monte & Englebert, 2018) implies severe disturbances in reflective processes. Lived experiences determine, in a direct and unreflective way, who a person takes herself to be. Past experiences – of one's own life story, including relationships to others – are barely considered, and when they are picked out selectively or reinterpreted in light of the current situation. This, of course, is not to say that persons with BPD wholly lack a perspective on past or future. Rather, their pasts and futures appear blurred and vague. Take, for instance, the temporal experience involved in sitting in front of a hearth with an old friend, sharing memories, and discussing long-term goals, and compare this with the temporal experience involved in seeing a dog drowning and deciding whether to jump into the ice-cold sea to rescue it. In the latter scenario, of course, past and future do not vanish from the experiential field completely, but they do appear in an empty and indeterminate way, they do not matter in the present moment. The situation is experienced as being one that *makes* who one is: a hazardous life-saver, a coward, or a person of reason? The temporal style prevalent in BPD experience is comparable to the latter kind of temporal experience: as if persons with BPD were constantly experiencing life-changing and identity-forming events. Although the unstable life of persons with BPD does involve an abundance of such kinds of events, clearly not every situation in life has such a momentous character. Nevertheless, the temporal structure of BPD experience with its gravitation toward the present suggests just this. Accordingly, persons with BPD are constantly focused on the life-changing aspects of situations, often where others do not see them (indeed, they sometimes *create* situations that engender such life-changing events). As a result, gravitation toward the present comes with a self-experience that involves a strongly felt vulnerability and exposure to life and to others, a constant threat of losing oneself due to a constant and accelerated process of identity development.

Third, gravitation toward the present and the constant experience of being at the edge of life-change constitute a peculiarly ahistorical mode of being (Fuchs, 2007; Stanghellini & Rosfort, 2013a), corresponding to the lack of an integrative narrative. Prima facie, this seems paradoxical, given that one would think that change implies development. Yet, because of the constant and repeating "life-changes" intrinsic to identity instability, change as such becomes in effect the permanent character of BPD. Recurring change, therefore, constitutes what could be called "stable instability" (Edwards, 2017). However, paradoxically, the very permanence and repetition of changes undermine their character as "change." Losing a loved one after a sudden end of a partnership, for instance, when occurring several times, simply confirms the pattern of instability, rather than allowing any development. This creates a precarious condition in which the most drastic event or escalation of a situation cannot generate progress in the individual's personal history. "There is no continuity over time and across situations, no concept of self-development that could be projected into the future, but only an endless repetition of the same affective states" (Fuchs, 2007, p. 382). Borderline personality disorder instability is therefore no mere *lack* of stability. It is rather a way in which stability is experientially organized and incapacitated, impeding the emergence of a stable and enduring sense of self. The only stability that is left is that of the pattern of instability. This translates into a self-experience of being stuck in a process that is unstoppable.

Fourth, the ahistorical mode of being comes at an additional price. Often persons with BPD not only feel unable to build a stable narrative identity, to gain control over their lives, or to initiate (let alone experience) development, they also suffer from a concomitant lack of self-feeling. In his diary, Edwards puts this in drastic terms: "I feel, for the most part, that I am only just existing. I am part of a continuum but no more, potentially less" (2015, p. 49) or, "That's me … an entity. Invisible to most, simply empty and abstract" (2015, p. 14). The literature is replete with similar examples. The "contradiction between feeling nonexistent and being alive" is "overwhelming," says Emma, a young woman with BPD (Black, Murray, & Thornicroft, 2014, p. 80). Other reports involve descriptions of feeling "deadened" (Singer, 1987, p. 133) or of "rotting away" (Edwards, 2016, p. 27). The ahistorical mode of being thus comes at the price of a feeling of being no one. Persons with BPD are aware that they are alive and yet they feel somehow nonexistent, as if they are leading a *life of no one*. Such self-nihilism sometimes amounts to a feeling of being "not human" (Singer, 1987, p. 133) – a topos manifest in many first-person reports from persons with BPD.

Fifth, and last, lack of self-feeling, the *life as no one*, also alters the way in which any sense of identity that might accrue to a person with BPD is experienced, namely, as a mask-like, fake identity. Jørgensen speaks of the creation of a "false self," which occurs in "an attempt to organize and stabilize the self" (2006, p. 635). A remark by Edwards exemplifies the complexity as well as the tragedy of this condition:

> Sometimes, now more than ever, I feel like a ghost masquerading as a human being.... [T]rying to fool people into thinking it is alive. This play is getting towards the end, when the curtains close and the ghost is thrown back into non-existence.... The ghost should have seen that it can only act for so long until people catch on. (Edwards, 2015, p. 45)

This quotation not only highlights the huge role that others play in temporally stabilizing a certain sense of identity in persons with BPD, it also indicates how any sense of identity incorporated in the encounter with others is experienced as inauthentic, as play. The basic emptiness that smoulders on the grounds of BPD self-experience seems to undermine any sense of identity that might arise. Any indication of meaning and identity is experienced with a taste of suspicion, a feeling of fraudulence. Self-fragmentation and "fragmented selves" (Fuchs, 2007) imply a plurality of identities that all fail to provide a sense of self the person would feel at one with. Accordingly, not only do shifts in identity create painful incoherence corresponding to their respective incompatibility, they each produce a general and abiding feeling of noncoincidence with oneself, creating negative self-related emotions such as inauthenticity, guilt, and fraudulence.

To conclude, unstable identity in the form of a lack of narrative identity encompasses a set of painful self-experiences such as incoherence, impossibility of self-development, vagueness, confusion, and powerlessness.

No Control: Affective Instability and Self-Experience

Self-experience in the context of identity disturbance is associated with a number of disturbing feelings. Affective disorder in BPD, however, goes further than just a person being confronted with discomforting feelings. It involves an affective instability that is structural in nature and has the following main aspects.

First and foremost, affective instability in BPD includes a lack of regulatory capacities: *emotion dysregulation* (Nica & Links, 2009). Both instability and dysregulation are inextricable from each other. On the one hand, it is easy to see that without being able to control and regulate one's own emotions, a person's feelings and emotions develop according to their own dynamics, determined by the situation and conditions out of which they arose. On the other hand, unstable and quickly shifting affects also present major challenges for a person in terms of regulation – and are likely to trigger dysregulative processes. For instance, when in a good mood, a person may have a certain regulatory attitude that is characterized by letting their feelings flow. If then their mood has "dropped like a rock" (Edwards, 2016, p. 31), it may take some time to modify the regulatory attitude from a laissez faire style toward a more monitoring and controlling attitude that gets a grip on the flood of emotion. The sudden flood of feelings makes it very hard for persons with BPD to adopt the right regulatory attitude to stabilize their emotions (Carpenter & Trull, 2013).

A second, related aspect of this is the great *intensity* of emotions in BPD. Difficulties in regulating emotions, obviously, may increase the likelihood that particular emotions become excessively intense, something that is common in cases of BPD. Intensive emotions are much harder to regulate and may in turn trigger further dysregulative processes. The intensity and related dysregulation may also explain the marked irritability of persons with BPD. Lacking the ability to cope with intensive emotions makes even the *possibility* of a negative emotion much more dramatic: Any potentially negative aspect of a situation that could engender negative emotions constitutes its own threat and already represents, for the person with BPD, a destabilizing of the situation. This may also feed into the strong intolerance of ambiguity that is typical of persons with BPD.

A third central aspect of the affective disorder in BPD is the *lack of affective self-knowledge*. Persons with BPD often not only report great confusion about why their mood changes so quickly and why they feel so strongly about things, they also demonstrate difficulties in identifying, labeling, or understanding their emotions (New et al., 2012). Edwards expresses this often-seen alexithymia in BPD: "I hate when I am asked what is wrong and I cannot find the words to articulate the unbearable pain I feel inside" (2016, p. 35). Not being able to describe or understand one's own emotions hinders their regulation. Because if it is unclear what kind of experience one is undergoing, that is, what the situation is and how one feels about it, it is difficult to adjust one's thoughts and feelings accordingly, for example, by focusing on other aspects of the situation or changing relevant beliefs about it. It seems an almost impossible task to find out what to do if it is unclear from the outset what exactly is happening. Moreover, not being able to control one's own emotions tends to make it hard to understand and identify those emotions. It is precisely when regulating feelings that we understand them for what they are. In being able to control and stabilize emerging negative impulses, we gain an understanding of what we are feeling and why we are feeling it. Thus, understanding and regulating emotions are interwoven processes, such that the lack of one hinders the other.

A fourth aspect of the affective disorder is its peculiar *temporality*, a cycle between phases of dysphoria, characterized by high bodily tension and emptiness, and episodes of anger (Rossi Monti & D'Agostino, 2014; Stanghellini & Rosfort, 2013a). This cycle can be explained in terms of a dynamic of uncontrollable, intense, and uncertain feelings and emotions. Explanations tend to focus on two different "movements" in this cycle.

The first explanation focuses on the move from overwhelming anger and intense but barely understood emotions toward emptiness and numbness. Often, persons with BPD feel that there is no remedy to kill the emotional pain other than to numb themselves, for example, via substance abuse and/or by adopting a detached attitude toward everyone and everything that appears to be a cause of the pain. The latter includes playing down the significance of situations, commitments, values, or other persons, but also distancing oneself from one's own desires, ideas, or plans. Put differently, one common dysregulative coping strategy employed by persons with BPD is to "pull the plug" and to no longer care about anything. It is precisely in states of severe anger, grief, or perceived humiliation[2] that feeling numb may provide some relief. In this vein, one can also view uncontrollable, incomprehensible, and overwhelming emotions as having a trauma-like character that induces an involuntary reflex of numbing, akin to posttraumatic stress disorder. It is true that many persons suffering from BPD have undergone severe childhood trauma and their affective style might have its origins in such experiences. But here my point is that the intensity of uncontrollable emotions can be considered to have *its own* traumatizing effect, regardless of whether the occasion (such as sexual or physical abuse) is generally considered severe enough to cause trauma. Numbing, in this sense, might be an ongoing involuntary, dysregulative response to recurring strong emotions.

The second explanation focuses on the move from dysphoria toward anger. Bearing in mind that regulatory practices can be habitualized and become part of emotional experience (Varga & Krueger, 2013), it is easy to see how numbness may transform from a short-term relief to a general condition that is itself experienced as painful. This is because being numb

[2] The important role of shame and humiliation in the experience of BPD, particularly in anger, has recently been highlighted (e.g., Peters & Geiger, 2016).

implies loss of meaning, which over the course of time often translates into a chronic feeling of emptiness, a craving for meaning and self-feeling. Such a feeling involves a high level of tension that can in turn lead to emotional outbursts, because the void of emptiness is often best suppressed by strong emotions that allow one to forget feelings of meaninglessness. As Stanghellini and Mancini put it, "anger is a way of feeling alive and of affirming one's right to exist as the unique person that one is" (2018, p. 11).

Both dysphoria and anger can thus be seen as two sides of the same coin. Emptiness and tension in dysphoria provide the experiential ground out of which a tendency for emotional outbursts grows. Strong feelings and emotions, however, induce a tendency toward numbing and detachment, resulting in states of dysphoria. The person with BPD is caught up in a vicious circle, fluctuating between the experience of meaning and strong (ultimately negative) emotions on the one hand, and the painful experience of loss or absence of meaning on the other. "I feel the repetition getting to me. The upswings and downswings repeating over and over; an endless loop of misery and brief happiness that seems to never end" (Edwards, 2016, p. 9). One further repercussion of this recurring cycle is a growing distrust toward the brief happy episodes, as a further statement by Edwards shows: "Inevitably, I fall back to feeling like shit, leaving me worse off than before. It leads me to wonder if on those rare occasions I am truly happy, or if it is something else" (Edwards, 2016, p. 31). Stanghellini and Rosfort (2013a) accurately call this condition a "desperate vitality."

All four aspects of the BPD affective disorder imply a group of interrelated disturbed self-experiences. Persons with BPD experience their feelings in a particularly passive way. Of course, passivity may be intrinsic to the experience of feeling. However, in healthy individuals, regulation provides some sense of agency in affective experience, despite its generally passive structure. Lacking regulatory possibilities, by contrast, leads to a condition in which one's own affect becomes a threat, a force one has to succumb to. Given the lack of affective self-knowledge, affective processes also induce significant confusion about oneself, since feelings and emotions help make up who we are as persons (Rosfort & Stanghellini, 2009; Stanghellini & Rosfort, 2010, 2013b). Identifying and understanding one's own emotions is vital for the development of a self-concept that includes knowledge about what kind of situation *p* makes one feel in a way *q* and why. Having such knowledge, a person who feels *q* in *p* may "feel herself." For instance, being sad and disappointed by a friend, she may feel great pain, but *knowing* that the kind of behavior her friend was showing is hurtful to her can help her calm down and either accept the given situation or change it.

In such case, despite being the "victim" of the behavior of the other and passively undergoing a strong emotion, she experiences herself responding to the world. *This is me. I don't like it when people do these kinds of things.* Lacking a sufficient understanding of her own feelings, by contrast, would hinder her from feeling herself as the concrete person she is and from gaining knowledge about herself; it would undermine, moreover, her understanding of what the given situation is all about, aggravating her self-confusion. Not understanding what exactly one feels, whether the diffuse pain one is feeling is anger, sadness, disappointment, or anxiety, impedes a more detailed understanding of who one is and who one wants to be. It significantly compromises any sense of identity.

The disruption of the latter in BPD can be further understood in terms of a general modification of the structure of what Ratcliffe (2005, 2008) calls "existential feelings." According to Ratcliffe, existential feelings are "ways of finding oneself in the world that determine the space of experiential possibilities" (2005, p. 61). Existential feelings disclose what we take to be possible. Changes in what we experience as possible are thus manifest on the affective level. In anger, for instance, what we experience is the possibility that we will be attacked and will have to defend ourselves, that we might hurt others or that someone will ask us why we are angry. Accordingly, anger puts us in a certain place in the world and constitutes a certain perspective on the world. Yet, despite undergoing strong feelings that shape how we experience the world, we are usually aware of the fact that we can control, at least to some degree, how we feel. Possibilities of regulation qua experienced possibilities are implemented in existential feelings, though such possibilities may vary in different existential feelings. In anger, for instance, what may seem a possible way to self-regulate might be different to what may seem a possible way to moderate in the case of strong feelings of guilt or sadness. In healthy individuals with well-developed regulation skills, existential feelings will include several experienced possibilities of regulation, some bound to specific existential feelings, others of a more general kind, creating a general sense of control and rendering the current affective state as *one* possible perspective on the world.

In persons with BPD, by contrast, general regulation skills are wanting and what is possible, therefore, is experienced in a significantly modified way. First, experienced possibilities of regulation are mostly exhausted by those intrinsic to the particular emotions: For instance, anger strives toward the release of tension mostly in the form of an aggressive act, while sadness culminates in crying. Second, lack of general regulation skills gives rise to a sense of the impossibility of changing existential feelings. Almost all regulatory possibilities consist in acting out the emotion. For instance, hastily quitting a friendship based on an experience of disappointment may moderate one's anger, but it is a regulation that remains within the boundaries of anger. It hardly changes the existential feeling, and when it does, it ceases to be experienced as a viable form of regulation. This can manifest itself in regret and confusion about one's own behavior as part of the grief about the loss of the friend, which strives toward quite different forms of pain regulations. Third, the general lack of possible transcendence of a given existential feeling also changes the phenomenological character of "finding oneself in the world" characteristic of existential feeling. Instead of being "thrown" into the world as the concrete person that one is, feeling "called" for action and self-determination, as one might characterize existential feeling in a Heideggerian fashion, a person with BPD tends to feel forced into certain responses to the world. Put differently, how a person with BPD takes herself to be and how she *is* tends to be determined by events in the world and the emotions that correspond to them.

Such affective overidentification (Fuchs, 2007; Schmidt, 2020) due to the absolutizing of existential feelings can be described as the structural ground of the ruptures in the individual's sense of identity. Since persons with BPD are absolutely drawn into their strong emotions at a given time, their experience of possibility is completely shaped by the concomitant existential feeling, and so is their sense of identity. Where an affective reaction is intense, all attention gravitates toward the present strong feelings, which weakens the givenness of narrative elements. Memory is blurred and vague, inhibited, which undermines the sense of any narrative identity. Possibilities of regulating general affects are lacking, and so all experiences of possible change are determined by the present affect. The latter dictates how a person with BPD could potentially respond to a given situation and as such defines how the person perceives herself. Ruptures in the sense of identity are therefore concomitant with the often BPD-related shifts in moods and related emotions.

Being Alone with Others: I-Thou and the Instability of the Borderline

Let me now turn to the instability of interpersonal relationships in BPD. Much has been said in the literature on BPD about the recurring and traumatic shifts in relationships with other people, and much needs to be said to grasp the phenomenon in its entirety and clinical relevance. A great deal of the work on intersubjectivity in BPD has focused on the immense role of the significant other, usually the primary caregiver, in shaping a person's ability to identify, label, and regulate feelings and emotions. Borderline personality disorder-related deficits in affective processing have thus often been understood in terms of an aftereffect of interpersonal trauma in early childhood, in which the caregiver has failed to provide a protective environment or to help the infant cope with emotional distress. In a similar vein, Ratcliffe and Bortolan (2021) make a convincing case for the great importance of stable interpersonal relationships for *ongoing* regulative processes. On their view, emotion regulation presupposes a structured world shared with others, and harm done to any of the aspects of the latter may translate into severe impairments in regulative processes.

I am in strong agreement with a line of thinking that emphasizes the major role played by interpersonal issues in the structure of affective experience. Nonetheless, for reasons of balance, and to give a more detailed picture of the structural intertwinement of instability in identity, affectivity, and interpersonal relationships, I wish to emphasize in this section some structural implications of disturbed affectivity for interpersonal relationships. Put differently, my aim is to elucidate the relationship between affect and other by illuminating the opposite direction of explanation that may run from affect to the interpersonal. Shifts in mood are likely to engender interpersonal problems. Not only because emotion regulation is generally interpersonally distributed (Varga & Krueger, 2013), but also because negative emotions may lead to a negative style of communication and behavior that increases the probability of conflicts with others. The potential for interpersonal conflict in BPD, however, seems to run deeper than this general connection between one's own mood and disturbed harmony with others. This raises the following questions: In what sense does the affective disorder in BPD present a social impairment? How does the structure of affective processing in BPD imply a specific style of experiencing and relating to the other?

In fact, it appears as though persons with BPD not only suffer from shifting relationships but also from a peculiar manner of perceiving and attending to others. One major feature of the latter is the increased focus on others' emotional experience. Such attentional gravity toward the other's affect is associated with heightened sensitivity to shifts in the other's mood (Frick et al., 2012) and shows the great importance of the other's affect for persons with BPD. In terms of regulative processes, this can be understood in at least two ways.

First, the other's affect is often perceived as a threat. Given that affect regulation is generally interpersonally distributed, other people's emotions present major challenges for persons with BPD, who lack precisely the corresponding regulation skills and are therefore quickly overwhelmed. Moreover, despite being able to detect changes in other persons' moods, they have difficulties in recognizing and understanding these emotions (Harari, Shamay-Tsoory, Ravid, & Levkovitz, 2010). This is related to a heightened tendency for emotional contagion (Niedtfeld, 2017), which sometimes makes it hard for persons with BPD to differentiate between their own emotions and others' affects (Luyten, 1985, p. 49). Other persons' emotions may therefore quickly develop into one's own emotional crisis.

Second, persons with BPD are often accused of showing an extraordinary proneness to manipulating others. This is a controversial issue and it is unclear whether such a – quite negative – label is appropriate (Potter, 2009, Chapter 6). However, it is fair to say that persons with BPD do indeed often show a heightened interest in influencing the affect of the other, be it by provocative behavior, subtle nudging or withdrawal. Often, such behavior plays an epistemic role: Reactions are tested to find out how strong a relationship is and how much one matters to the other person (Stanghellini, 2014). Moreover, producing emotions in the other also makes said emotions much easier to understand and to control. Such control can also be understood as a way to cope with and compensate for a lack in one's own emotional self-control. If one's own intense feelings and emotions have such an overwhelming character that they render one passive, producing intense emotions in others can allow an experience of activity, of having a say in how things run, and mostly of relief. Influencing others can thus be understood as a form of self-regulation in that it provides a sense of agency, an indirect way of coping with a lack of self-feeling and control.

However, the three symptoms described earlier – (a) lack of self-feeling, (b) defenselessness against one's own and the other's affect, *and* (c) the surrogate-like sense of agency in influencing the other's affect – all seem to blur the I-Thou boundary. Let me explain:

(a) Emptiness involves a severe flattening of experience such that the appearance of the other in social encounters seems to lose its usual salient character. The empty self suffers from feelings of being no one and equally fails to regard the other as another self. Interpersonal encounters are experienced as events no different from any other experiential event in a quasi-anonymous stream of consciousness.

(b) In phases of more intense emotions, persons with BPD might develop a weak sense of self, for instance in anger, and they might feel the significance of the other who falls short in demonstrating the recognition the person with BPD expects (Stanghellini & Mancini, 2018). Nevertheless, in such phases the quality of passivity in affective experience becomes dominant to the degree that the person with BPD may feel consumed by feelings of otherness and alienation, which makes it hard for them to distinguish between the emotions of others and their own affect.

Moreover, the flood of emotion undermines any consciousness able to distinguish between "I am feeling *p*" and "You seem to be feeling *q*." This is not to say that the person with BPD develops the belief that the other is feeling the same way; rather it seems that only one affect is experientially manifest, so that the other's emotions become part of one's own affect. For instance, the sadness of a partner translates directly into acute fear of loss on one's own part, or the partner's sadness is perceived as overwhelming. Instead of perceiving sadness "there" and fear of loss "here," the latter becomes ubiquitous and swallows up the sadness so that the sadness becomes a mere aspect of the fear of loss. Others' feelings and one's own feelings merge together in a diffuse and potentially threatening affect. Hypersensitivity toward the other's affect and emotional contagion imply a direct tie to the affective life of the other, leading to an affective space that lacks any relief: *Either* all intentional focus is on the affect of the other *or* all intentional focus is on one's own affective process. To illustrate the former, consider the example of walking home and suddenly seeing a man on a bicycle being hit by a car. Such a situation normally induces strong empathy and a focus on how the man is feeling, and what could possibly be done to help him. For persons with BPD, the other's affect may have a somewhat similar intentional gravity. Yet consider analogously being the victim in this traffic accident, lying injured on the street. You might still be aware that people around you have their own feelings, but they are not really present to you. Your affective concern is with your pain and your situation. I wish to propose that a person with BPD, if not focused on the other's affect, will experience her strong feelings and emotions in a somewhat similar way. When totally absorbed with one's own intense affects, there is simply no attentional space to consider the emotions of the other. These are present in an unclear, unrecognized, and abstract way, but not in a felt manner. Put differently, persons with BPD have difficulties in being aware of their own affect vis-à-vis the feelings and emotions of the other. Intentionally, one or the other fully determines the experience of affect, impeding any real emotional encounter and exchange between self and other. Whether one's own or the other's affect becomes the center of affective gravity will of course hinge on a number of factors. Given the threatening character of the affects of others and the lack of regulatory skill in persons with BPD, however, it is most likely that affective intentionality sooner or later centers around their own emotions (feelings of passivity, exposure, and vulnerability, etc.) rather than those of others.

(c) Finally, the I-Thou boundary is also blurred as the BPD person attempts to influence the other's affect as a form of maladaptive self-regulation. They do so because producing emotions in the other through their own actions while witnessing the effects of their behavior may provide some sense of control and agency. However, at the same time, it clearly undermines the other's sovereignty. Successful control or even domination of the other, therefore, is always at risk of dissolving the character of the other *as* other. The other may become an object-like entity that can be pushed around arbitrarily. But such behavior comes at a price for the BPD person: By dominating the other, the other also loses her potential for providing recognition. Hence, even though influencing the other may provide some sense of self, it constitutes a self that is unable to interact with the other in a way that would imply a real encounter between two autonomous persons.

All three modes of affective processing thus imply a certain style or structure of relating to the other. Problematically, however, they each imply an interpersonal style in which the I-Thou boundary is significantly blurred. As a result, establishing a relationship with others in which persons with BPD feel truly connected with the other is – so long as they remain in one of said modes – difficult. Nevertheless, connectedness does not only seem to be an important factor in recovery from BPD (Kverme, Natvik, Veseth, & Moltu, 2019), it is also something persons with BPD desperately crave, manifesting itself in painful feelings of loneliness (Pazzagli & Rossi Monti, 2000). As with any individual, persons with BPD often find themselves in situations in which they are alone and rejected. However, as my descriptions of the ways in which persons with BPD typically relate to others indicate, feeling alone need not always be the result of actual abandonment. It seems rather to represent a component implicit in BPD-related affective and interpersonal styles. Loneliness is also a phenomenon of *structure*.

Nobody and No Body? A Fourth Kind of Instability in BPD

Thus far, I have addressed three kinds of instabilities: instability in identity, affect, and interpersonal relationships. I have described how these involve disturbed self-experiences and how the three kinds of instabilities are interconnected, placing emphasis on the changes in relating to oneself and others that are implied in the BPD affective disorder. In this final section, I turn to the bodily dimension of the experiences involved in the BPD pattern. Much needs to be said about the role of embodiment in BPD, and it is surprising how this aspect has received little attention in the clinical literature. Here, my focus lies on the bodily experience involved in the three kinds of instabilities discussed so far. Accordingly, I suggest treating the issue of bodily experience in BPD not in isolation from instability in identity, affect, and the interpersonal, but as an inextricable aspect of all three. The following examples are meant to illustrate such intertwinement, underscoring that BPD is also characterized by a fourth kind of instability: *instability in embodiment.*

(1) The first example refers to chronic feelings of emptiness, which are far from being an absence of feeling. States of dysphoria involve feelings of numbness and meaninglessness, which are no mere negative phenomena but rather involve an abundance of what has been called "mental pain" (Fertuck, Karan, & Stanley, 2016). In contrast to a headache or the pain of a broken arm, mental pain is not attached to any specific body part. Yet it would be a mistake to conceive of it as a nonbodily experience. Dysphoria involves high bodily tension in diffuse form, determining the whole experiential field. Moreover, the lack of self-feeling implied in numbness and emptiness is itself felt bodily. Zandersen and Parnas describe a young woman with BPD who suffers from a "feeling of not being at one with her body" and who conceives of her body as a mere "'tool,' which is there in order for her 'to walk from A to B'" (2019, p. 111). Correspondingly, she "feels as a 'fluent existence,' as a 'fluent blob' in the air," implying that she feels her self "as being outside of her body" (2019, p. 112), though "'there is *nothing* inside of me, nothing like a *soul* or anything'" (2019, p. 111). The lack of self-feeling manifests itself as a diminishment of bodily self-experience.[3]

[3] It should be noted that Zandersen and Parnas (2019) argue that the patient, the young woman diagnosed with BPD, also meets the criteria for a diagnosis of schizotypal personality disorder (SPD). The aim of their paper is to show that phenomenological descriptions can significantly contribute to the differential diagnosis between conditions like BPD and SPD, and they suggest the phenomenological distinctions between minimal self and narrative self play an important role therein. Perhaps more detailed descriptions of bodily experience may also help to differentiate between BPD and SPD. Here, however, my point is more modest, and I only want to say that feelings of emptiness are manifest as certain forms of bodily experience. Whether bodily experiences involved in feelings of emptiness are to be differentiated in BPD and SPD is an issue for future research and depends on how these conditions are conceptualized.

(2) Such diminishment is also experienced in phases of intense emotions. Although these emotions are felt bodily in the form of high arousal, activation of the nervous system, and related feelings of stress, the incomprehensibility and uncontrollability of these bodily feelings amplify the sense of detachment from one's own body. Although the body is felt in an intense manner, it seems to be an alien force to which one is subjected. Edwards writes: "My body is a cage. Inside, it feels like a feral animal is clawing and screaming for release. Yet I suppress it" (2016, p. 29). Lack of regulation of one's affects is experienced as a lack of control over one's body, turning the latter into something "other" and producing feelings of noncoincidence with oneself. As Stanghellini and Rosfort write, it is "felt as … lying somewhere between self and non-self" (2013b, p. 271). Whether the experience of one or the other dominates may also alternate, without being a question of choice. Sometimes it may feel like the "true" self is being held back to fulfill external expectations, with the result that one feels one is wearing a mask. For instance, the identity of being a responsible and caring partner to the other may be perceived as a mask, while one's own egoistic wishes or reckless impulses may seem to be the true self. Conversely, one might identify with the role of the caring partner and feel ashamed of one's own destructive and bodily impulses.

(3) Embodiment also seems to play a major role in pursuing life goals over the course of time. Feelings of emptiness and bodily tension significantly undermine the feeling that goals set in the past are still worth pursuing. If the body feels strange, aroused, or irritable, it is hard to feel anticipatory joy with regards to the achievement of certain aims, and, correspondingly, the means to achieve these lose their enticing character. Bodily feelings may not give rise to certain narrative identities, but how the body feels significantly constrains the constitution of narrative identity and a felt sense thereof. Another quote by Edwards illustrates this well: "Going to school, working, fighting the urge to give in to my Demons … It all feels wrong. Why, with so much progress made in my life, am I still miserable?" (2016, p. 29). Despite having gained a positive perspective on life, his pain still lingers. Indeed, with an irritated body, it is hard to feel at one with previous life goals and plans. One might remember these, but if the body feels estranged, it becomes impossible to embody remembered goals, plans, and the narrative identity that corresponds to them.

(4) Finally, the style of relating to others also involves significant distortions of embodiment. The strong focus on the emotional life of other people, the hypersensitivity in detecting changes in the other, and the risk of emotional contagion present an extended form of embodiment in which the other seems to be "incorporated." Shifts in the other's feelings almost directly inscribe themselves in the bodily experience of persons with BPD. Such fusion-like connection with the other and their body not only dissolves the "centrality" (Zandersen & Parnas, 2019, p. 111) of one's own body but also imports something into bodily experience that is felt yet is not controllable by direct regulation. The blurriness of the I-Thou boundary also has a bodily dimension: One's own body schema becomes fuzzy, involving unclear limitations and an unstable, shifting center.

As these four examples show, instability in embodiment appears to be a concomitant condition of instability in identity, affect, and the interpersonal. The importance of instability in embodiment also appears to be manifest in another bodily phenomenon of BPD: self-mutilation. While self-mutilation is most certainly a maladaptive strategy for moderating uncontrollable affects or for communicating with others, it can also be understood as a response to the instability in embodiment. Self-mutilation seems to transform blurred and vague mental pain into a clearly localizable pain focused on a specific part of the body. It allows the person who self-mutilates to develop a body schema with clear limits, centered around the concrete hurting body. In this manner, self-mutilation restores – albeit in pathological, dangerous form – a sense of agency that is integral to normal bodily experience.

Conclusion: Holism and Etiology

Borderline personality disorder is a complex disorder that shows itself on various levels of life in distinct ways and unfolds differently for each individual person concerned. Yet there is general agreement that three kinds of instabilities – instability in identity, affect, and interpersonal relationships – constitute the condition from which all persons with BPD suffer. Are these kinds of instabilities and their associated phenomena inextricable from each other? Making a case for a holistic view of the BPD instability pattern, I have argued that they are. To that end, I have described the phenomenological structure of some of the experiences constituting each kind of instability – focusing on involved self-experiences – and examined how they are interconnected. I have found all three kinds of instabilities structurally intertwined and put emphasis on the structural implications of the BPD affective disorder for experiencing oneself and others. Moreover, I have given examples of ways in which bodily experience features in the experience of instability in identity, affect, and the interpersonal. Based on these descriptions, I have suggested that BPD is also characterized by a fourth kind of instability: instability in embodiment. Much remains to be said about the mutual implications of (and relationships between) the different aspects of BPD instability. Additional descriptive work may reveal further aspects of the condition that are experientially inextricable from each other or it may come to light that some aspects of BPD are caused by additional factors not implied in the BPD instability pattern. In any case, it is fair to say that the BPD instability pattern is far from being a mere accidental amalgamation of different forms of instabilities. Rather it appears as a general structural disorder that spreads out over different experiential dimensions.

Such a holistic view of BPD, if correct, has significant repercussions for our understanding of the etiology of BPD. For instance, a biological predisposition for heightened body arousal may engender instability in embodiment and failure to develop adaptive emotion regulation skills, despite a healthy social environment with benevolent caregivers. In this case, if holism about BPD is correct, the individual will most likely develop the complete BPD instability pattern, since instability in embodiment and affect imply structural changes in the experience of oneself and others. In other cases, an organically healthy individual may be born into a hostile or unstable social environment, for instance with abusive caregivers who not only fail to support the child in developing emotion regulation skills but who also evoke strong negative emotions by their erratic and hurtful behavior. In such cases, the BPD instability pattern may spread out, starting from a destabilization in the interpersonal domain. Whatever cause generates one of the four kinds of instabilities, according to the holistic view put forward here, it will likely evoke other forms of instabilities in the individual as well. Accordingly, treatment of BPD should always include therapy of all four kinds of instabilities, because the persistence of any single kind of instability may point to an ongoing tendency toward the complete BPD pattern. Hence, the holism proposed in this chapter is not only apt to explain why quite heterogeneous causal factors can induce a similar instability pattern but it also has potential implications for processes involved in recovery from BPD.

Acknowledgment

I am grateful to Thomas Fuchs and Matthew Ratcliffe for feedback on materials on which this chapter is based. Many thanks to the two anonymous reviewers for helpful comments and to Adrian Wilding for his grammatical and linguistic improvements. Special thanks also to Christian Tewes for his feedback and generous support during the publication process.

References

American Psychiatric Association. (2013). *Diagnostic and statistical manual of mental disorders* (5th ed.). Arlington, VA: Author.

Black, G., Murray, J., & Thornicroft, G. (2014). Understanding the phenomenology of borderline personality disorder from the patient's perspective. *Journal of Mental Health*, 23(2), 78–82. doi:10.3109/09638237.2013.869570

Cameron, A. A., Calderwood, K., & McMurphy, S. (2018). A systematic literature review of the etiology of borderline personality disorder from an ecological systems perspective. *Social Work in Mental Health*, 17(3), 1–17. doi:10.1080/15332985.2018.1555104

Carpenter, R. W., & Trull, T. T. (2013). Components of emotion dysregulation in borderline personality disorder: A review. *Current Psychiatry Reports*, 15(1), 1–8. doi:10.1007/s11920-012-0335-2

Edwards, T. (2015). The BPD journals I: A year in the life. Blurb.

Edwards, T. (2016). The BPD journals II: Remission and relapse. Blurb.

Edwards, T. (2017). The BPD journals III: Stable instability. Blurb.

Fertuck, E. A., Karan, E., & Stanley, B. (2016). The specificity of mental pain in borderline personality disorder compared to depressive disorders and healthy controls. *Borderline Personality Disorder and Emotion Dysregulation*, 3, 1–8. doi:10.1186/s40479-016-0036-2

Frick, C., Lang, S., Kotchoubey, B., Sieswerda, S., Dinu-Biringer, R., Berger, M., … Barnow, S. (2012). Hypersensitivity in borderline personality disorder during mindreading. *PLoS One*, 7(8), 1–8. doi:10.1371/journal.pone.0041650

Fuchs, T. (2007). Fragmented selves: Temporality and identity in borderline personality disorder. *Psychopathology*, 40(6), 379–387. doi:10.1159/000106468

Fuchs, T. (2010). Temporality and psychopathology. *Phenomenology and the Cognitive Sciences*, 12(1), 75–104. doi:10.1007/s11097-010-9189-4

Fuchs, T. (2013). The phenomenology of affectivity. In K. V. M. Fulford, M. Davies, R. G. T. Gipps, G. Graham, J. Z. Sadler, G. Stanghellini, & T. Thornton (Eds.), *The Oxford handbook of philosophy and psychiatry* (pp. 612–631). Oxford, UK: Oxford University Press. doi:10.1093/oxfordhb/9780199579563.013.0038

Fuchs, T., & Pallagrosi, M. (2018). Phenomenology of temporality and dimensional psychopathology. In M. Biondi, M. Pasquini, & A. Picardi (Eds.), *Dimensional psychopathology* (pp. 287–300). Cham, Switzerland: Springer. doi:10.1007/978-3-319-78202-7_10

Gallagher, S. (2013). A pattern theory of self. *Frontiers in Human Neuroscience*, 7, 1–7. doi:10.3389/fnhum.2013.00443
Gallagher, S., & Daly, D. (2018). Dynamical relations in self-pattern. *Frontiers in Psychology*, 9, 1–13. doi:10.3389/fpsyg.2018.00664
Harari, H., Shamay-Tsoory, S. G., Ravid, M., & Levkovitz, Y. (2010). Double dissociation between cognitive and affective empathy in borderline personality disorder. *Psychiatry Research*, 175(3), 277–279. doi:10.1016/j.psychres.2009.03.002
Jørgensen, C. R. (2006). Disturbed sense of identity in borderline personality disorder. *Journal of Personality Disorders*, 20(6), 618–644. doi:10.1521/pedi.2006.20.6.618
Jørgensen, C. R. (2009). Identity style in patients with borderline personality disorder and normal controls. *Journal of Personality Disorders*, 23(2), 101–112. doi:10.1521/pedi.2009.23.2.101
Keinänen, M. T., Johnson, J. G., Richards, E. S., & Courtney, E. A. (2012). A systematic review of the evidence-based psychosocial risk factors for understanding of borderline personality disorder. *Psychoanalytic Psychotherapy*, 26(1), 65–91. doi:10.1080/02668734.2011.652659
Kverme, B., Natvik, E., Veseth, M., & Moltu, C. (2019). Moving towards connectedness – A qualitative study of recovery processes for people with borderline personality disorder. *Frontiers in Psychology*, 10, 1–11. doi:10.3389/fpsyg.2019.00430
Lo Monte, F., & Englebert, J. (2018). Borderline personality disorder and lived time. *L'Évolution Psychiatrique*, 84(4), e37–e45. doi:10.1016/j.evopsy.2018.08.001
Luyten, M. F. (1985). Egolessness and the "borderline" experience. *Naropa Institute Journal of Psychology*, 3, 43–70.
Meares, R., Gerull, F., Stevenson, J., & Korner, A. (2011). Is self-disturbance the core of borderline personality disorder? An outcome study of borderline personality factors. *Australian and New Zealand Journal of Psychiatry*, 45(3), 214–222. doi:10.3109/00048674.2010.551280
Muscelli, C., & Stanghellini, G. (2014). La vulnerabilità ai tempi dell'istantaneità: il presente e la condizione borderline [Vulnerability in the time of instantaneity: The present and the borderline condition]. *Psicoterapia e scienze umane*, 48(2), 254–266. doi:10.3280/PU2014-002003
New, A. S., aan het Rot, M., Ripoll, L. H., Perez-Rodriguez, M. M., Lazarus, S., Zipursky, E., … Siever, L. J. (2012). Empathy and alexithymia in borderline personality disorder: Clinical and laboratory measures. *Journal of Personality Disorder*, 26(5), 660–675. doi:10.1521/pedi.2012.26.5.660
Nica, E. I., & Links, P. S. (2009). Affective instability in borderline personality disorder: Experience sampling findings. *Current Psychiatry Reports*, 11(1), 74–81. doi:10.1007/s11920-009-0012-2
Niedtfeld, I. (2017). Experimental investigation of cognitive and affective empathy in borderline personality disorder: Effects of ambiguity in multimodal social information processing. *Psychiatry Research*, 253, 58–63. doi:10.1016/j.psychres.2017.03.037
Pazzagli, A., & Rossi Monti, M. (2000). Dysphoria and aloneness in borderline personality disorder. *Psychopathology*, 33(4), 220–226. doi:10.1159/000029147

Peters, J. R., & Geiger, P. J. (2016). Borderline personality disorder and self-conscious affect: Too much shame but not enough guilt? *Personality Disorders Theory Research and Treatment*, 7(3), 303–308. doi:10.1037/per0000176

Potter, N. N. (2009). *Mapping the edges and the in-between: A critical analysis of borderline personality disorder*. Oxford, UK: Oxford University Press.

Ratcliffe, M. (2005). The feeling of being. *Journal of Consciousness Studies*, 12(8–10), 43–60. Retrieved from www.ingentaconnect.com/content/imp/jcs/2005/00000012/f0030008/art00003

Ratcliffe, M. (2008). *Feelings of being. Phenomenology, psychiatry and the sense of reality*. Oxford, UK: Oxford University Press.

Ratcliffe, M. (2017). *Real hallucinations: Psychiatric illness, intentionality, and the interpersonal world*. Cambridge, MA: Massachusetts Institute of Technology Press.

Ratcliffe, M., & Bortolan, A. (2021). Emotion regulation in a disordered world: Understanding borderline personality disorder. In C. Tewes & G. Stanghellini (Eds.), *Time and body* (pp. 177–200). Cambridge, UK: Cambridge University Press.

Rosfort, R., & Stanghellini, G. (2009). The person in between moods and affects. *Philosophy, Psychiatry, & Psychology*, 16(3), 251–266. doi:10.1353/ppp.0.0257

Rossi Monti, M., & D'Agostino, A. (2014). Borderline personality disorder from a psychopathological-dynamic perspective. *Journal of Psychopathology*, 20, 451–460.

Sass, L. A. (2014). Explanation and description in phenomenological psychopathology. *Journal of Psychopathology*, 20, 366–376.

Schmidt, P. (2018). The relevance of explanatory first-person approaches (EFPA) for understanding psychopathological phenomena: The role of phenomenology. *Frontiers in Psychology*, 9, 1–16. doi:10.3389/fpsyg.2018.00694

Schmidt, P. (2020). Störungen des Selbst in der Borderline-Persönlichkeit: Der Zusammenhang von Affekt und Identitätserleben [Disorders of the self in the borderline personality: The connection between affect and the experience of identity]. In T. Fuchs & T. Breyer (Eds.), *Selbst und Selbststörungen* [Self and self-disorders] (pp. 165–193). Freiburg, Germany: Karl Alber.

Singer, M. (1987). A phenomenology of the self: A personalization, a subcategory of borderline pathology. *Psychoanalytic Inquiry: A Topical Journal for Mental Health Professionals*, 7(1), 121–137.

Stanghellini, G. (2014). De-stigmatising manipulation: An exercise in second-order empathic understanding. *South African Journal of Psychiatry*, 20(1), 11–14. doi:10.7196/SAJP.510

Stanghellini, G., & Mancini, M. (2018). The life-worlds of persons with borderline personality disorder. In G. Stanghellini, M. R. Broome, A. V. Fernandez, P. Fusar-Poli, A. Raballo, & R. Rosfort (Eds.), *The Oxford handbook of phenomenological psychopathology*. Oxford, UK: Oxford University Press. Advance online publication. doi:10.1093/oxfordhb/9780198803157.013.67

Stanghellini, G., & Rosfort, R. (2010). Affective temperament and personal identity. *Journal of Affective Disorders*, 126(1–2), 317–320. doi:10.1016/j.jad.2010.02.129

Stanghellini, G., & Rosfort, R. (2013a). Borderline depression. A desperate vitality. *Journal of Consciousness Studies*, 20(7–8), 153–177. Retrieved from www.ingentaconnect.com/content/imp/jcs/2013/00000020/F0020007/art00008

Stanghellini, G., & Rosfort, R. (2013b). *Emotions and personhood. Exploring fragility – Making sense of vulnerability*. Oxford, UK: Oxford University Press.

Varga, S., & Krueger, J. (2013). Background emotions, proximity and distributed emotion regulation. *Review of Philosophy & Psychology*, 4(2), 271–292. doi:10.1007/s13164-013-0134-7

Vater, A., Schröder-Abé, M., Weißgerber, S., Roepke, S., & Schütz, A. (2015). Self-concept structure and borderline personality disorder: Evidence for negative compartmentalization. *Journal of Behavior Therapy and Experimental Psychiatry*, 46, 50–58. doi:10.1016/j.jbtep.2014.08.003

Wilkinson-Ryan, T., & Westen, D. (2000). Identity disturbance in borderline personality disorder: An empirical investigation. *American Journal of Psychiatry*, 157(4), 528–541. doi:10.1176/appi.ajp.157.4.528

Zandersen, M., & Parnas, J. (2019). Identity disturbance, feelings of emptiness, and the boundaries of the schizophrenia spectrum. *Schizophrenia Bulletin*, 45(1), 106–113. doi:10.1093/schbul/sbx183

10.1

Commentary on "Nobody? Disturbed Self-Experience in Borderline Personality Disorder and Four Kinds of Instabilities"

Who? Nobody? The Existence of Flesh

Milena Mancini

Schmidt (2021) convincingly describes three kinds of instabilities (in identity, affect, and interpersonal relationship) associated with the borderline personality disorder (BPD) and shows how these phenomena are related with body experience. Schmidt argues that all these types of instabilities are experientially interrelated and demonstrates this by providing examples that show how disturbed self-experience is involved in identity, affect, and intersubjective instability. In the light of these descriptions, he suggests that there is a fourth kind of instability in BPD patients that specifically concerns embodiment. I subscribe to these considerations, yet I would like to draw the reader's attention to an additional dimension of bodily experience in persons with BDP: the *living body* (Stanghellini, 2021).

Body and Identity: A Brief Premise

Henry (1973) uses the term "ipseity" to address a basic or minimal form of self-awareness. Ipseity is the most primitive form of self-awareness, the acquaintance with an experience as *my* experience in the first-personal mode of presentation. It is the implicit, prereflexive, immediate, nonconceptual, nonobjectifying and nonobservational sense of existing as a subject of awareness, prior to, and as a condition of possibility of, all other experiences. Two basic and closely related aspects of minimal self-awareness are self-ownership and self-agency. Self-ownership is the prereflexive sense that I am the one who is undergoing an experience. Self-agency is the prereflexive sense that I am the one who is initiating an action. The immediate awareness that my experiences and actions belong to my own self involves that these are in some sense felt as owned and generated by myself. These are the basic components of the experienced differentiation between self and nonself, myself and the object I perceive, and my representation of that object and the object itself. The fact that it is rooted in one's bodily experience and its situatedness among objects and other people is central to ipseity as the basic form of self-awareness. Being conscious is dwelling in (*être-à*) the world through one's own lived body (Merleau-Ponty, 1962). This primitive experience of myself is rooted in my bodily experience. Therefore, embodiment and ipseity are closely interwoven.

Which Body Are We Talking About?

Which kind of body is at play in the borderline condition? It is acknowledged that persons with BDP suffer from so-called emotional dysregulation. In agreement with Schmidt (2021), I wonder if this emotional instability is somehow related to bodily abnormal phenomena. Persons with BPD experience their own body as the source of a chaotic vitality that does not accommodate to prereflexive intentional structures, as a kaleidoscopic universe of raw and unmediated feelings, leaving little possibility for rational action. Bodily *reactions* take dominance over deliberate bodily action. These persons' chaotic vitality, being devoid of intentional structure and content, desperately seeks an object, mostly a person, at which to direct its surplus of energy, its overwhelming intensity (Stanghellini & Mancini, 2017). This is evident especially when persons with BPD are oppressed by *dysphoria* – a mood state characterized by irritability, restlessness, and disquiet (Stanghellini & Mancini, 2017; Stanghellini & Rosfort, 2013a). In the course of dysphoric states, one experiences a force that takes the representation of oneself to pieces, reducing it to an assemblage of disordered emotions and drives. However, one also experiences in oneself a power that expresses an encouraging vitality, seducingly in touch with invigorating sensations (Stanghellini, 2016). Dysphoria is a mood in which violent spasms take control of the body and destroy the embodied structure that organizes one's intentional engagement with the world. As Schmidt (2021) also states, in acute dysphoric states, one's own body, as the source of vitality and conation, is felt out of voluntary control, lying somewhere between self and nonself – the land of otherness (Stanghellini & Rosfort, 2013b).

Deleuze's concept of "the body without organs" (Deleuze & Guattari, 1988) can help us answer the question, "Which body is at play in borderline existence?" With "body without organs," Deleuze means a mere assemblage of organs rather than an *organism*, that is a system or organization consisting of interdependent parts harmonically working together (Deleuze & Guattari, 1988). Each part of the body without organs, including perceptions, visceral sensations, and movements, lives independently from the others and does not belong to an organized and meaningful structure.

Borderline instability is very close to this incessant switching on and switching off of impulses, needs, desires, or emotions, which at one moment possess a powerful intensity, and shut down a moment later or abruptly change their target. Thus, the borderline body, like Deleuze's body without organs, is an intermittent pulsation of pure instantaneous intensity rather than a continuous flow. What is the fate of this overwhelming intensity in borderline existence? A "desperate vitality" is the borderline person's epitaph (Stanghellini & Rosfort, 2013a, 2013b).

Nobody or No-Body? *Nobodyness*

Schmidt's title (2021) – "Nobody? Disturbed Self-Experience in Borderline Personality Disorder and Four Kinds of Instabilities" – recalls the absence of a defined bodily structure. The term "nobody" is composed of two words: "no" and "body." If we consider both of these acceptations (nobody and no-body), we could capture two basic and typical features of BPD: instability in identity and in body. It might be hypothesized that this body not structured into an organism is perhaps the common root of the main psychopathological dimension of BPD: instability in identity, in emotions, and in interpersonal relationships.

No-body addresses the issue of the borderline person's lack of a definite identity (*no body*). Being no-body means having no form, following the logic of the "un-form," the *aneidos* (Stanghellini, 2018). It means being a pure metamorphic body, which entails being an individual that is continuously changed by intense heat or pressure – exactly like a metamorphic rock. The instability of the body implies the instability of personal identity.

Also, no-body addresses a further element of instability in the borderline world, namely, emotional instability. The borderline person's no-body can be understood as a body that is at the mercy of the emotional and humoral spasm – another typical symptom of BPD. Following the logic of emotions, the borderline body is upset by impulses and sensations that deform its own organization. Like an ignited metamorphic rock, it is too hot to be taken by the borderline person into his hand; it cannot be manipulated, it is impossible to give it a stable and solid form.

In the relationships (with others), *nobody* shows its peculiarities in the fickleness of the borderline person when in front of other person. The borderline person oscillates between different "ways to be in front of others," and this depends on the need for recognition. Need for recognition and fear of abandonment force the borderline person to aspire – constantly and insatiably – to a sort of emotional osmosis with the other. The other is needed as a source of recognition. The absence of the other makes the presence of the self impossible. The other's absence, or incomplete presence, is often the reason for feelings of un-recognition and desperate loss of selfhood. The absent other, or the other who does not donate his entire self, is perceived as an abandoning other and an inauthentic other (Stanghellini & Mancini, 2017).

For the borderline person, the other is a source of recognition, that is of attention, acknowledgment commendation, and acceptance. The other is a hoped-for source of selfhood through recognition. The value of recognition is tightly intertwined with the main dimensions of borderline psychopathology, including emotional instability and the instability of one's feeling of one's own self – in a few words: Recognition is a way to deal with being no-body. Recognition is aimed at in order to achieve a sense of being a person through the feeling of belonging, the reciprocation of sensuous experiences as well as the experience of being forgiven and consoled.

In conclusion, the characteristic way borderline persons experience their own body – their "nobodyness" – seems indeed intertwined with their principal afflictions: kaleidoscopic emotions, fluctuating selfhood and identity, and their need for intense relationships to cope with these.

References

Deleuze, G., & Guattari, F. (1988). *A thousand plateaus: Capitalism and schizophrenia, vol. 2* (B. Massumi, Trans.). London, UK: Athlone.

Merleau-Ponty, M. (1962). *The phenomenology of perception* (C. Smith, Trans.). London, UK: Routledge & Kegan Paul.

Henry, M. (1973). *The Essence of Manifestation*. The Hague: Martinus Nijhoff.

Schmidt, P. (2021). Nobody? Disturbed self-experience in borderline personality disorder. In C. Tewes & G. Stanghellini (Eds.), *Time and body: Phenomenological and psychopathological approaches* (pp. 206–229). Cambridge, UK: Cambridge University Press.

Stanghellini, G. (2016). *Lost in dialogue*. Oxford, UK: Oxford University Press.

Stanghellini, G. (2018). *L'amore che cura* [The love which heals]. Milano, Italy: Feltrinelli.

Stanghellini, G. (2021). The heart of darkness of the living body. In C. Tewes & G. Stanghellini (Eds.), *Time and body: Phenomenological and psychopathological approaches* (pp. 60–75). Cambridge, UK: Cambridge University Press.

Stanghellini, G., & Mancini, M. (2017). *The therapeutic interview in mental health. A value-based and person-centered approach*. Cambridge, UK: Cambridge University Press.

Stanghellini, G., & Rosfort, R. (2013a). Borderline depression: A desperate vitality. *Journal of Consciousness Studies*, 20(7–8), 153–177. Retrieved from www.ingentaconnect.com/content/imp/jcs/2013/00000020/f0020007/art00008

Stanghellini, G., & Rosfort, R. (2013b). *Emotions and personhood: Exploring fragility – Making sense of vulnerability*. Oxford, UK: Oxford University Press.

11

Levels of Embodiment
A Husserlian Analysis of Gender and the Development of Eating Disorders

Lanei M. Rodemeyer

Introduction

Husserl scholars, and those who work with Husserl's phenomenology, are generally familiar with the fact that there are different levels of the constitution of our experiences, such as the level of passive synthesis (PS) as opposed to the intersubjective levels. My argument here is that there are several such levels of experience indicated in Husserl's work and that they are much more systematically in place than might first appear. These levels are evident especially in his middle and late periods, and they can be found either implicitly or explicitly in many of his published and unpublished works. In addition to this, I would like to argue that these levels of constitution can be applied to many different areas beyond phenomenology. In this chapter, I will focus on the area of gender, looking specifically at eating disorders. I will also take into account how temporality is involved in our gendered experiences, whether as a historical meaning or as a condition lived by an individual.

My analyses will proceed as follows: First, I will provide an overview of Husserl's levels of constitution, with a brief explanation of each. Then, I will work through these levels in light of gender, connecting this discussion to the condition of eating disorders. In doing so, I would like to demonstrate how a recognition of the phenomenological levels of experience can assist not only in phenomenological description but also in the psychological diagnosis and therapeutic analysis of eating disorders. My goal is to develop a relatively solid understanding of each level, and to demonstrate how it can be applied to areas beyond phenomenology in a way that is useful.

An Overview of Husserl's Levels of Constitution

The levels, from "highest" to "lowest" (to use Husserl's terms), are roughly as follows: At the highest level, we find intersubjective community, which is the historical, intergenerational stratum of meaning or, alternately, an abstract understanding of numerous, possible subjects (abbreviated as IS-2). Husserl refers to a higher level of intersubjectivity in each of these senses (intergenerational and abstract), indicating a level beyond the one-on-one level of intersubjectivity that will be discussed next.[1] This level addresses the meanings that develop within a culture, that transition from one generation to another, and that surface through analyses of history, society, and language. It also includes statistical groupings of subjects and abstract notions of intersubjectivity. We find Husserl discussing this level in his later work such as *The crisis of European sciences* (Husserl, 1970), the latter half of his *Fifth Cartesian meditation* (Husserl, 1999, Chapter 5), and in many of his manuscripts on intersubjectivity. We will turn to specific citations by Husserl in the next section.

At the next level down, we encounter the interpersonal intersubjective level (abbreviated as IS-1). This level describes our interaction with other subjects through empathy, our intersubjective constitution of the world as objective (also addressed at the higher level of IS-2 in a more abstract way), and how our own bodies gain their objective sense through the perception of others. In other words, it addresses our one-on-one relations with others and our experiences of living in a shared world with specific others. This work is carried out most famously in Husserl's Fifth *Cartesian meditation* (Husserl, 1999, Chapter 5), but it is arguably addressed in more detail in his *Ideas II* (Husserl, 1989).

The next level is the most common understanding of Husserl's phenomenology, and it is also his primary entry into many of his own analyses. This is the level of individual meaning constitution. Although much constitutive activity here is actually passive in addition to active, I will refer to it as the level of active constitution (AC). It is here that we take up consciousness' active meaning constitution and the meaningful contents with which it is engaged. I should point out that what is "active" for Husserl is not necessarily what is more energetically in play, but rather, what is in awareness for consciousness, that toward which my attention is directed. Husserl's analyses at this level describe the structures of consciousness required for meaning constitution, such as noesis and noema,

[1] It is possible that these might be two importantly different aspects of IS-2 for Husserl – or even two different levels. For our purposes here, though, the level of IS-2 addresses that aspect of intersubjectivity that is the more general experience of others beyond the individual others in our lives. It not only includes culture, history, and generations but also our understanding of statistical others or abstract groups of subjects.

and he focuses on the individual subject and their constitution of unified experienced objects. *Ideas I* is the text best known for Husserl's extensive analyses in this area, but he refers to this level throughout his work after this one (Husserl, 1983). We should also note that while Husserl's analyses at this level are often carried out through a solipsistic lens, this level is not an argument for solipsism. Indeed, even though the constitution of objects is always informed by intersubjective meanings, it is often from a solipsistic stance that we can more easily recognize certain structures and relations. Husserl's move to analyze this level solipsistically is a methodological move, one that simplifies his access to noesis and noema (and similar structures), so that he can better describe them.

The next layer down is more nebulous; it is the level of PS. This layer addresses what is "passively" in play, such as associations between similar things, habituations of constitution and decisions, and sedimentations of memories. However – similar to the distinction we made above regarding the notion of "active" – for Husserl, "passive" does not mean static or inactive, but rather, that which is "passive" indicates the synthetic work done by consciousness that *goes unnoticed* while consciousness is engaged in direct (i.e., active) experiences. It is all the work done by consciousness to which we do not pay attention. This includes embodied habits as well as tendencies to constitute certain sets of data in one way rather than another. The level of PS requires analyses not only of the structures of consciousness but also of the contents of consciousness and their interplay with one another. This is because it is usually the contents that become sedimented or habituated, rather than the structures themselves. Thus, analyses at this level often point to the interweaving of structure and content in consciousness and in our experiences. These analyses are most famously published in the collection of Husserl's lectures on the *Analyses concerning passive and active synthesis* (2001) but they can also be found throughout his work, especially beginning in his middle period.

Finally, the lowest level of experience is that of the flow of primordial material, often referred to as the "hyletic flow" (HF). This flow is a layer of rudimentary sensory experience that underlies our acts of perception. It is a streaming of primordial sensory impressions, which Husserl sometimes also refers to as sensory "data" or a primordial flow. While Husserl discusses this HF quite a bit already in *Ideas I* (Husserl, 1983), it is in his lectures on PS and in his later manuscripts that we see much more attention directed toward this area.

Here is a simple outline of Husserl's levels of constitution:

Intersubjective Community (IS-2)
Interpersonal Intersubjectivity (IS-1)
Active Constitution (AC)
Passive Synthesis (PS)
Primordial or Hyletic Flow (HF)

Now, although Husserl often refers to "higher" and "lower" levels, they should not be understood in a hierarchical way. The outline given here is merely a schematic in order to present the levels in a simplified form. We could envision these levels alternatively as concentric circles nested in one another, where the movement is "outward" and "inward" rather than "up" and "down."[2] When we visualize these levels in this way, then the flow of sensory material remains a "core" level of experiencing that grounds the other layers, but the mutual influence of these levels on one another is a little more apparent (see Figure 11.1). Here is a possible way to schematize the levels as concentric circles, including a bit of detail for each level:[3] As mentioned earlier, Husserl might focus on only one of these levels in a specific text or set of analyses. However, in some writings, such as those addressing PS or in his Fifth *Cartesian meditation* (Husserl, 1999, Chapter 5), he passes through several levels. For example, he might begin at the level of active meaning constitution (AC), then move down through the level of PS, and finally arrive at the lowest level of primordial sensory contents (HF). Or, conversely, he might move "upward" into discussions of the different levels of intersubjective experience (IS-1 and IS-2). This can be confusing to the reader, as his passage from one level to the next is often unannounced, and even more problematic, we find the same terms, such as "association" or "affectivity" – even "objectivity" – being applied at each level; however, their meaning changes subtly with each move, according to the shift to a new level in his analyses.[4] This leads not only to confusion, but

[2] The descriptive terms of "outward" and "inward" also have their difficulties, especially when they presume, in the case of embodiment, a strict distinction between the body and what is "outside" the body. Regardless of the terms being employed, I am not arguing that these levels or layers are strictly delineated, as should become clear by the end of this chapter.

[3] This diagram includes an inner "core" of an abstract "Urhyle," which is mentioned often in Husserl's late manuscripts. The Urhyle is best understood as an abstraction of the hyle – a pure flow of sensory data prior to any affective unification – such that it is not clear whether it is distinct from the HF as we are describing it here.

[4] See Rodemeyer (2006) for a discussion of how Husserl treats the terms of "association" and "affectivity" differently for different levels of analysis with relation to inner time-consciousness.

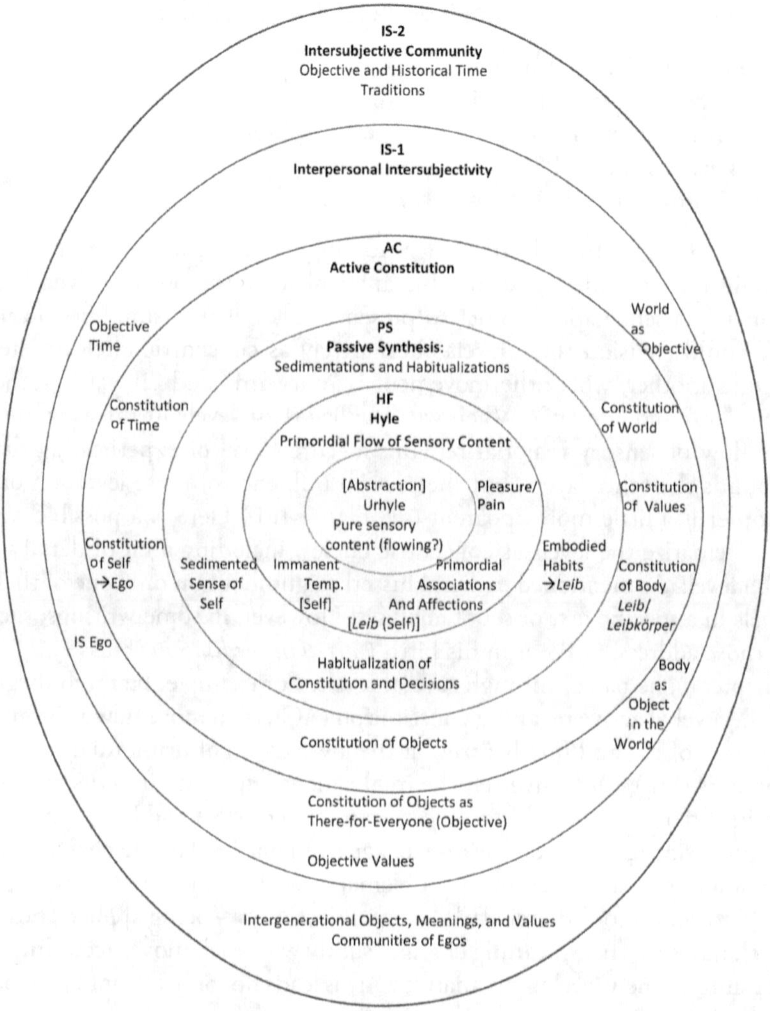

Figure 11.1 Levels of constitution.

it also gives the impression that Husserl is equivocating between multiple definitions of the same term, or that he might be contradicting himself, when in fact, he is not. An understanding of how Husserl moves through these levels in his analyses can hopefully avoid any such misinterpretation.

We turn now to how these phenomenological levels of constitution can be applied to specific phenomena. In the next section, we will work through each level more specifically with regard to Husserl's phenomenological analyses, turning to how each level reveals important yet differentiated aspects of gender and eating disorders.

Application to Gender and Eating Disorders

Intersubjective Community and History (IS-2)

Scholars who focus on Husserl's work in *Ideas I* (Husserl, 1983) or on his Cartesian approach in *Cartesian meditations* (Husserl, 1999) might quickly accuse him of neglecting the importance of social influences upon meaning development, our sense of self, and even our most basic experiences.[5] But Husserl spent excessive amounts of effort analyzing our intersubjective relations – not only at the interpersonal level but also, importantly, at the level of generations, traditions, customs, and history. He also was keenly aware of how the development of ideas through history can affect the way we think about things. We see some of this work explicitly in his *Crisis* (Husserl, 1970). Here, Husserl demonstrates how certain concepts or approaches begin, become developed, and are passed down from generation to generation, where changes and even origins can become lost or covered over in the way that the concepts or approaches are currently employed.

> Thus it could appear that geometry, with its own immediately evident a priori "intuition" and the thinking which operates with it, produces a self-sufficient, absolute truth which, as such—"obviously"—could be applied without further ado. That this obviousness was an illusion … that even the meaning of the application of geometry has complicated sources: this remained hidden for Galileo and the ensuing period. Immediately with Galileo, then, begins the surreptitious substitution of idealized nature for prescientifically intuited nature. (Husserl, 1970, pp. 49–50)

The current work on gender in areas such as feminist, queer theory, and transgender studies points to the historical development of gender, how certain meanings lose or cover over their original meanings, and how gender intersects with multiple other identities in each individual. But

[5] Because I am not an expert in therapeutic approaches, I ask for indulgence in any errors I might make with regard to therapeutic approaches to eating disorders. My goal is not to overturn any approaches already in place: I wish merely to introduce a nuanced perspective that might, first of all, offer a way to gain deeper understandings of the phenomena, and second, present a rubric wherein multiple approaches to an issue can be seen in their relation to each other in such a way that they might be able to work together.

Husserl's analyses already contain the seeds of such insights, when not already laying them out in detail. The fact that he often pointed to this higher level of intersubjectivity, and that he worked through how meanings and approaches are passed down and changed through generations, provides us with a phenomenological approach that can contribute to – and overlap with – contemporary discussions of gender. While Husserl's own statements about gender often fall into traditional, patriarchal claims prevalent during his time, his analyses themselves allow for a more critical approach.[6] From a phenomenological perspective, in other words, we can examine how specific meanings become linked with the notions of the female and male, and with feminine and masculine. Social values determine our understanding of these concepts and even how we experience gendered subjects themselves.

In addition to providing analyses of social meaning structures through generations, Husserl also recognizes the importance of intersubjective discourse in how I experience myself and my embodiment. Here, his work brings a specificity not often offered in contemporary analyses of gender. In *Ideas II* (Husserl, 1989), for example, he demonstrates how my body only truly becomes an objective, *material* body through intersubjective constitution: When I encounter other subjects, I recognize them not only as other subjects like myself but also as other subjects who see me in a way similar to how they constitute objects in the world. Just as our mutual co-constitution gives rise to the objectivity of things in the world (and of the world itself), this co-constitution also folds back onto my own body, and it becomes constituted like other objects in the world. My experience of the world with other subjects brings a new layer to how I experience those objects: They are now experienced as objects there for others and not just there for me. They become objective, material in a new sense. Thus, when we co-constitute the world and its objects as there for everyone, as material, only then can *my body* appear as a material object. In this way – and only through the constitution of other subjects – I am able to constitute my body as an objective thing. As Husserl explains:

> The solipsistic subject could indeed have over against itself an Objective nature, however this subject could *not apprehend itself as a member of nature*, could not apperceive itself as psychophysical subject, as animal, the way this does happen on the intersubjective level of experience. (Husserl, 1989, p. 95)

[6] See, for example, Alia Al-Saji (2010), Janet Donohoe (2010), and Rodemeyer (2018) for approaches that acknowledge Husserl's limitations in his middle and later work on gender while also pointing to how his method can still be applied productively to analyses of gender.

Thus, this higher intersubjective level is essential to how I understand my body, and further, how I experience my body as material and as there for others. Given this, we can now draw a connection between this phenomenological level of intersubjective community and how I experience my embodiment as gendered – and further, how the meanings about gender and my embodiment might play into the development of eating disorders.

Plenty of work has been done to reveal the historical connection between gender, body shape (especially thinness), and beauty. De Beauvoir famously demonstrates that femininity was historically presumed to be natural or essential, when in fact, it is socially constructed:

> But the fact is that [the young girl's] resignation comes not from any predetermined inferiority: on the contrary, it is that which gives rise to all her insufficiencies; that resignation has its source in the adolescent girl's past, in the society around her, and particularly in the future assigned to her. (de Beauvoir, 1989, p. 329)

Since de Beauvoir's work, many other scholars have pointed to the intersections of race, ethnicity, and gender and how these affect our presumptions of (feminine) beauty. And others have connected capitalism, consumerism, and images of female beauty and their effects on how women see themselves. Susan Bordo, in her *Unbearable weight* (2003), for example, draws links between work ethic, asceticism, and self-control on the one hand, and consumerism and lack of self-control on the other.

> Far from paradoxical, the coexistence of anorexia and obesity reveals the instability of the contemporary personality construction, the difficulty of finding homeostasis between the producer and the consumer sides of the self. Bulimia embodies the unstable double bind of consumer capitalism, while anorexia and obesity embody an attempted resolution of that double bind. (Bordo, 2003, p. 201)

The individual who develops an eating disorder is surrounded by attitudes – both in the general "atmosphere" of society and in specific discourses and images – that they take up into themselves.[7] Bordo continues from the citation just given, "Both [anorexia and obesity] are rooted in the same consumer-culture construction of desire as overwhelming and overtaking the self. Given that construction, we can only respond either

[7] In the "Ten Commandments" of a pro-anorexic website, Commandment #1 states: "If you aren't thin, you aren't attractive" (Pro-Ana Lifestyle Forever and Always, 2019a).

with total submission or rigid defense" (Bordo, 2003, p. 201). In other words, I take attitudes about bodies, about specific types of bodies, about beauty and thinness or fatness, and about self-control, and I relate them to my understanding of attractiveness, likability, success, etc., and then they become infused in how I constitute – even feel – my own body. These attitudes become part of how I think, implicit in my decisions, and more importantly, they become integrated into my embodiment as habits, comportment, gestures, and behaviors. Eating disorders, while highly individual, are also a response to – even an enactment of – certain social attitudes that we find at the level of intersubjective community. As Dignon, Beardsmore, Spain, and Kuan (2006) point out, a perspective about anorexia that focuses only on the individual

> fails to theorize socially constructed femininity as a potentially problematic identity. Little account has therefore been taken by psychiatrists of the social context in which anorexia occurs. Feminists however … acknowledge that society conveys contradictory expectations to women, by exhorting them to achieve in the public sphere, while at the same time effectively excluding them from what remains a masculinist culture. (p. 943)

Analyses at this higher intersubjective level can address why certain groups or types of individuals – such as women – may have a higher tendency for developing eating disorders, since it can analyze the discourses that surround women's bodies, expectations of thinness, etc.

In fact, Dignon et al. (2006) quote "Lucy," who recognizes the media as a crucial influence on eating disorders:

> [N]o matter how intelligent you are somehow on some level you do kind of buy that… and… think they they just look so happy and glamorous … you seem to be constantly bombarded by not just images of like slim women but like the whole sort of film industry record industry … it's not something you can escape from… all those images that you're fed, drip fed. (p. 952)

While the authors admit that Lucy rejected the presumption that anorexic people simply buy into media images or are so-called slaves to fashion, they nevertheless include the effect of the media as a common category that can sustain an eating disorder:

> Lucy herself was keen to stress that anorexia amounted to much more than a fashion for slenderness and a slavish adherence to media influence. But even participants like Julie, who felt that media influence was peripheral, were nevertheless aware of the importance of media imagery. (Dignon et al., 2006, p. 952; see also Figure 1, p. 946)

For both Lucy and Julie, then, social discourses were admittedly important in the formation and maintenance of their eating disorders – but they were not the whole story. What Husserl's phenomenology offers is not just the ability to carry out analyses at this level, but rather, an approach to all of the other levels we described earlier as well. Thus, we turn to the next level in Husserl's methodology.

Interpersonal Intersubjectivity (IS-1)

Meanings – of gender and embodiment, for example – are not solely grounded at this higher intersubjective level. Our intersubjective community certainly provides a context and filter that can make eating disorders possible and, in some cases, can even drive forward certain occasions of eating disorders. Nevertheless, we know that there are many people for whom merely this context might not be enough to lead to an eating disorder. Thus, if we were to analyze eating disorders *only* from the perspective of the attitudes of the general community, we would leave many questions unanswered, especially with regard to how different individuals manifest eating disorders in different ways, and how some cases can become much more extreme than others. From a therapeutic perspective as well, it would seem that an analysis of the intersubjective community, of discourses of thinness, might help some individuals, but it would probably not be sufficient to treat the majority of those struggling with eating disorders. As Svenaeus points out,

> the gaze in question does not seem to lead to anorexia for every person exposed to the norms of slenderness in contemporary society—not for most men, … but also not for most women, or even for most young girls exposed to the ideals in question. (Svenaeus, 2013, p. 86)

Simply put, an examination of discourses is not enough to determine the causes and related factors contributing to eating disorders, nor would it be sufficient in developing treatment plans for individuals – even if it remains a root of the disorder.

For this reason, we move to the next level "down," that of the first (lower) level of intersubjectivity: my relations to individual persons and concrete groups of individuals. Husserl's most famous analyses at this level are in his Fifth *Cartesian meditation* (Husserl, 1999, Chapter 5), where he describes my constitution of another person who is standing in front of me. But his analyses in *Ideas II* (Husserl, 1989) are more detailed and complex, taking note of how the way others constitute me can affect how

I view myself. For example, he presents a hypothetical situation where an individual exists alone and constitutes the world as an isolated individual. While purely hypothetical (and practically impossible), he is providing a limit-case of an individual who views the world and has constituted meanings related to that world without a connection to others. Husserl then develops the scenario to describe the encounter of this isolated individual with other subjects. At this point, the individual's meanings and those of the group of subjects conflict with one another, since the individual has had no way to share their meanings with others prior to this moment, and so they hold only a very limited account of the world. Husserl concludes,

> [a]s I communicate to my companions my earlier lived experiences and they become aware of how much these conflict with their world, constituted intersubjectively and continuously exhibited by means of a harmonious exchange of experiences, then I become for them an interesting *pathological* Object, and they call my actuality, so beautifully manifest to me, the hallucination of someone who up to this point in time has been mentally ill. (Husserl, 1989, p. 85)

Husserl, unfortunately, does not develop this hypothetical situation much further than to point out that how we constitute the world is essentially an intersubjective enterprise. However, his description here reveals not only the importance of intersubjectivity to the constitution of objects and the world but also how individuals are constituted by those around them. If an individual sees things qualitatively differently from their fellow subjects, they run the risk of being objectified, even pathologized, by the others. This description runs parallel to those histories wherein women's bodies, raced embodiment, certain sexual orientations, disabled bodies, and transgender embodiment (to name a few) have been objectified and usually pathologized. In this way, then, Husserl's phenomenological descriptions of intersubjectivity provide an entry into discussions of the power dynamics of different groups in their constitution of specific types of embodiment.

When the historical meaning of gender is constituted at the level of interpersonal intersubjectivity, then the values and associated meanings related to gender become applied to me and to others. In this way, cultural associations affect me individually: I might be seen as fat (and therefore, as lazy); as a woman (and therefore, as meek or passive); or as raced (and therefore as criminal or as an impostor). As Bordo shows, many young women with eating disorders seek to overcome presumptions of laziness, meekness, and lack of control.

> For many women ... disidentification with the maternal body, far from symbolizing reduced power, may symbolize ... freedom from a reproductive destiny and a construction of femininity seen as constraining and suffocating. Correspondingly, taking on the accoutrements of the white, male world may be experienced as empowerment by women themselves, and as their chance to embody qualities – detachment, self-containment, self-mastery, control – that are highly valued in our culture. The slender body ... symbolizes such qualities. (Bordo, 2003, p. 209)[8]

When they respond through a focus on thinness, persons with eating disorders such as anorexia have already assumed the meanings that connect power, self-control, and slenderness in their society. They objectify themselves through the eyes of others, intensifying their gendered embodiment and the expectations that go with it. Dignon et al. (2006) cite "Viv" and another patient whose anorexia was a response, at least in part, to instances of bullying and teasing in school:

> Viv explained that: "I got a lot of a lot of ... stick from other kids and bullying and things so that that was bad as well ... at school I'd get called fatty and you know fat-related ... names." Yet another patient was bullied jointly by siblings and school mates: "when I was younger I used to get bullied a lot for being fat ... they used to call me names and everything ... even me own sisters used to pick on me for being fat ... my friends would join in and make fun out of me as well." (pp. 947–948)

Teasing is not the only cause of eating disorders. However, these authors place it under a general "trigger" category of "unhappiness." Individuals develop responses to hurtful intersubjective relations, implicating their own bodies through their control of food.

A therapeutic approach to eating disorders must therefore take into account both levels of intersubjectivity, intersubjective community, and interpersonal intersubjectivity. Thus, it is important to recognize not only the historical interweaving of specific meanings with that of gender but also the interpersonal aspect that affects how an individual takes up those meanings. How the people in a person's life express the discourses relating to their embodiment, as well as how they treat them individually, will have

[8] Commandment #10 of a pro-anorexic website states: "Being thin and not eating are signs of true will power and success" (Pro-Ana Lifestyle Forever and Always, 2019a).

a concrete effect on how they constitute their embodiment for themselves. Dignon et al. (2006) point out that

> The key issue to emerge from all of the interviews was that anorexia was characterized by a strong sense of unhappiness and loss. Something was missing in the life of the anorexic. This may have been the result of definite trauma, such as bullying or abuse, or it may have derived from a more generalized experience of neglect or failure, such as that experienced by some anorexics who felt "passed over" by their parents or age mates. To compensate for this sense of loss the anorexic focused on food as a source of control. (p. 945)

These common causes show the importance of interpersonal relations in the development of eating disorders – even when, as I have been arguing, this disorder can play out at each of the phenomenological levels.

At the interpersonal level, an anorexic person might sometimes respond with a strong desire to be noticed or looked at. As Stanghellini describes, "the Other's look is not only a source of intimidating and shameful 'negation' of their capacity to transcend their facticity or mere objective corporeality, but also a longed-for device through which they can finally define themselves – *an optical self-prosthesis*" (Stanghellini, 2019, p. 71). In all of these cases, the therapist would need to look at both the intersubjective meanings handed down through history regarding a client's gender and embodiment (along with other important markers, such as race and class) and the ways that people in the client's life have constituted them in specific ways.

Active Constitution (AC)

The level of AC is a central point at which intersubjective meanings of embodiment overlap with my own sensory embodiment. As I constitute my embodiment, I may highlight the intersubjective meanings surrounding it, on the one hand, or sensory input, on the other. Or I may find that they integrate with one another, or even that they conflict. I may push certain aspects into the background, remaining relatively unaware of them, while I bring others to the fore. Husserl gives an example wherein a person, in a situation of "impure certainty," may actually decide in favor of a position that is contradicted by other valid positions, because of the strength of his belief.

> Such a certainty is impure insofar as it has the mode of making a decision for an enticement, more specifically, a subjectively secure decision for an enticement, even though opposing enticements are there, and against

> which the ego decides despite their weight; the ego does not accept them, although due to their weight they "demand" being validated. (Husserl, 2001, p. 90)[9]

For Husserl, then, both the belief systems within which we live (which correspond to intersubjective discourses) and the sensory evidence directly experienced are in play when we constitute our current experiences.

My own flow of experiences, retained and recollected, provides a perspective from which I mediate and interpret those meanings with which I come into contact. I cannot access intersubjective meanings from an objective viewpoint: Even if I isolate myself in my own meaning construction, I still engage with intersubjective meanings from the basis of my own history. While recognizing the importance of my cultural context, though, we can see that the development of my own experiences gives me a distinct perspective on the meanings that surround me. From this perspective, my experiences may or may not resonate with the meanings I encounter from my community and other individuals. I may not notice when my experiences are in alignment with social discourses, or when certain meanings oppress me to a point where I have difficulty taking up my experiences as my own; nevertheless, I am called to respond to any overt dissonance. In some cases, my response might be to establish my own world of meaning, attempting to escape the discord. In others, I may accept and adopt intersubjective meanings, sacrificing the validity of my own experiences. Or I may actively revolt against those meanings that exclude my experience. But however I respond, the context of my own experiential history is an essential ground from which I constitute any meaning. My constitution of my own body, therefore, is not just an act of absorbing and living out the intersubjective discourses that surround me (whether from my community or from other individuals), but it is also an engagement from my own perspective.

For this reason, a therapeutic approach to eating disorders must also attend to an individual's history, and to how that person engages with intersubjective meanings from the ground of their own experiences. Svenaeus takes the position, for example, that, "anorexia nervosa is neither a bodily dysfunction, nor a cultural product, only" (2013, p. 81). While we rarely actively constitute our own subjectivity or embodiment – both my sense of self and my body are usually in the background as I engage with the world – the therapeutic situation is one of those moments wherein individuals *are* called to reflect upon and actively constitute themselves.

9 See also Husserl (2001, p. 86): "We lend it validity, believing in it in our subjective certainty; and this inner Yes means a No! for the other testimonies of the opposing enticements."

Thus, therapy is exceptionally poised to reveal those meanings that are employed in an individual's self-constitution of their embodiment. Svenaeus points to a strategy of externalizing the disorder in order to address it:

> A common strategy for dealing with anorexia, … is to view the disorder itself as something alien, externalizing the disorder to make it more manageable (Zimmerman and Dickerson 1994)…. [I]n this image it is not the body, but the anorexia itself, as invading and taking control over the body, that is uncanny. (2013, p. 87)

He further argues that one might constitute the illness as another person, in order to avoid medicalizing the illness to the point of ignoring the experience of it (Svenaeus, 2013, p. 88). Of course, we often resist recognizing or admitting certain meanings about ourselves – this is an important challenge in therapy! But the point here is that the very act of self-constitution in play in the therapeutic situation can already open up a recognition of how a patient interacts with various meanings about their gender and embodiment – and their body itself.[10]

Passive Synthesis (PS)

At the level of PS, we find the synthesis of all meaning that has been constituted through the higher levels, where these meanings are combined according to their similar and associated meanings, becoming part of my consciousness that informs how I deal with new situations by relying on a general impression of the past. In addition to this, PS maintains patterns of behavior, repetitions, habits, and decisions. In this way, experiences that are repeated become part of consciousness so that I no longer need to pay attention to them or reflect upon them. From the definitions of common words and phrases, to decisions that are made regularly, to embodied actions that become habits, I hold general meanings and actions in embodied consciousness as habits and sedimentations of meanings. Embodiment gains depth at this level since here we see how patterns become ingrained, how decisions from the past affect our current engagement with objects, and how actions become part of how we carry and engage our bodies in the world.

[10] In fact, "Patients … [construct] their disorder using the concepts and vocabulary of psychiatry. As well as using psychiatric language, patients also tended to 'clinicalize' their anorexia" (Dignon et al., 2006, p. 954). This indicates yet another level to how individuals take up the intersubjective discourses relating to their situation. However, it is a layer that would complicate the present analysis beyond what can be managed here.

In fact, PS makes it possible for us to maintain habits that we no longer notice and that have become part of who we are. Husserl describes such a situation well:

> There arises some sensuous drive, for example the urge to smoke. I reach for a cigar and light it up, whereas my attention, my Ego-activities … are entirely somewhere else… The Ego always lives in the medium of its "history"; all its earlier lived experiences have sunk down but they have aftereffects in tendencies, sudden ideas, transformations or assimilations of earlier lived experiences, and from such assimilations new formations are merged together, etc. (Husserl, 1989, pp. 349–350)

Husserl is describing embodied habits, habits that I carry out even when I am not paying attention to them. They are part of my history, sedimented into my embodiment, and yet they are connected with what I do now and how I constitute the world and myself.

This level of PS is important in an analysis of eating disorders in two ways. First, the meanings that we have been discussing at the higher levels can become embedded in my consciousness and embodiment in whatever way I have taken them up; they become a part of me. They affect my comportment, how I engage with the world in both my thoughts and actions. The second way that PS provides insight into eating disorders has to do with the patterns of behavior that an individual develops with regard to the disorder itself. Svenaeus cites Halse et al.:

> She started weighing herself regularly – often dozens of times a day – and would stand in front of the bathroom mirror for hours composing long, detailed lists of imagined physical flaws she dreamed of changing. (Halse et al., 2008, 34, as cited in Svenaeus, 2013, p. 87)

> At mealtimes, she'd eat exact things at exactly the same time and there were all these little rituals. She'd get a carrot out of the fridge. She'd peel it. She'd top and tail it, she'd slice it. She'd lay it out in the steamer. She'd cook it for one and a half minutes. She'd get it out and she'd eat. And then she'd go to the fridge and she'd get another carrot out. And she'd top and tail it. And then she'd weigh it before it was cooked and she'd weight it after it was cooked. Then she'd go on to the frozen vegetables. (Halse et al., 2008, 82, as cited in Svenaeus, 2013, p. 87)

Eating disorders do not appear fully formed; rather, they develop through repeated actions, they become ingrained into bodily movement as well as manners of perceiving, thinking, and behaving. A person with an eating disorder might develop revulsion to certain types of food, for example, or establish rituals surrounding meals, exercise, or measuring their size or weight.[11] "Some patients suggested their disorder was as an obsession, and described the complex rituals they engaged in around food" (Dignon et al., 2006, p. 954). Such rituals always begin as momentary actions or reactions, but they are subsequently repeated such that they become part of the individual, embedded in their style of behavior, and they become the means through which they relate to the world and their own embodiment. They become meaningful for themselves. A therapeutic situation must address these rituals and habits along with the belief systems ingrained in the individual with an eating disorder. Once again, we see another layer that is essential to this disorder – one that must be addressed, yet cannot be subsumed under the other levels already indicated.

Hyletic Flow (HF)

Finally, we turn to the lowest level, HF, where we find primordial sensory experience. Here, we have our original flow of sensory content, including not only the traditional "five senses," but also feelings such as nausea, pain, pleasure, and tension. Although the HF is understood by Husserl as simply a flow of pure sensation, he already notices at this level that certain sensory content may be highlighted or primordially associated, and as such, it is set apart from other content.

> But these [immanent data] necessarily have a unity through consciousness, a unity of kinship, as similar to one another or uniform with one another: Several discrete color-data in the visual field are grouped together; they are especially united by virtue of their similarity; [and they are united in] different ways as well. (Husserl, 2001, p. 175)

Sensations of nausea, for example, associate primordially with one another, distinguishing themselves from, say, the color of red, the sound of a ticking clock, or a pain in my toe. Given this, the level of HF can be said to have more than one layer within itself: The pure sensory flowing is the

[11] Under "Tips and Tricks" on a pro-anorexic website, tip #4 states, "Eat in front of a mirror, naked or in underwear if possible.... When you have cravings pinch your fat and look at your problem areas, don't add to them!" And #7 recommends, "Cut a ribbon the size you want your waist to be. Wrap and tie it around your wrist like a bracelet. Every time you look at it you'll be reminded of your goals" (Pro-Ana Lifestyle Forever and Always, 2019b). On another pro-anorexic website, a blogger posted on May 9, 2014, that anorectics should purposefully develop obsessive compulsive disorder behaviors that will occupy them and distract them from their hunger, "You need rules and systems, you might reorganize something 10 times. All of this can take about 3–6 hours of your day. OCD behaviors are addictive so you do not think about food" (My Pro-Ana, 2014) (it should be noted that several subsequent commenters were highly critical of this person's suggestion).

ultimate ground, and the flow of primordially associated sensory contents rises up from that ground. In addition, this primordial level is also the original flow of inner time-consciousness. It is here that sensory contents are originally taken up in temporal relation to one another. Quite a bit is being accomplished at this core level, and each of these aspects would normally deserve their own separate analysis. But for our purposes, when laying out the schematic of these levels as a whole, we merely need to indicate generally what takes place here.[12]

Because this level of the sensory material already contains primordial associations of content, we can argue that this level is also the most fundamental level of embodiment: The sensations arising from the body distinguish themselves from the sensations of other objects, because of their "double sensations." These double sensations are the sensations that come from feeling one's own body externally in touch as well as internally in movement and location (also known as proprioception). The sensory content of embodied constitution therefore originates at this level. In fact, Husserl makes it clear that touch is the sensation that is most fundamental to the constitution of our embodiment: "The Body as such can be constituted originarily only in tactuality and in everything that is localized with the sensations of touch" (Husserl, 1989, p. 158). Thus, it is at this most basic sensory level that our bodies begin to take form for us.

The situation of eating disorders, however, reveals how this primordial level interrelates with the other levels. In some cases, experiences from one level may influence how experiences are constituted at another level, and in others, a certain level might even cover over or overthrow what is experienced at another. As Stanghellini, Castellini, Brogna, Faravelli, and Ricca argue,

> Our results showed that this core psychopathology is related to the dimension of embodiment named "lived-body-for-others," confirming that persons with ED [eating disorders] experience their own body first and foremost as an object being looked at by another, rather than cenesthetically or from a first-person perspective. (2012, p. 155)

The embodiment of a person with an eating disorder will have a phenomenological basis in sensory content, but patterns established through PS, or meanings established at higher levels, can act either to highlight or to cover over aspects of the sensory flow. Hunger might be covered

[12] Husserl carries out many of these analyses in his *Analyses concerning passive and active synthesis*, especially under the heading of "Association," see Husserl (2001, pp. 162–242).

over, for example, while revulsion or desire could leap to the forefront. Or starvation may be employed in order to stay in touch with one's own body. Stanghellini et al. (2012, p. 154) even identify a category of "feeling oneself through starvation," demonstrating a relatively common feature of persons with eating disorders. This need to "feel oneself through starvation" may indicate a fundamental need to stay "in touch" with one's own body. Even though the disorder tends to distance an individual from their own body – through a desire to be "looked at" or through self-objectification – the need to feel one's own body reveals it as an essential component, an essential feeling, that underlies the constitution of the individual. We often find examples where we don't notice our embodiment: Husserl himself, in an earlier citation, describes his urge to smoke not only as a "sensuous drive" but also as a sensuous drive that he does not notice because he is occupied with other things. We also saw much earlier how "impure certainty" can be taken up through a decision that correlates with a person's belief systems, even when there is sensory evidence contrary to that belief. And yet, sensory contents remain at the root of my experiences even as I develop patterns of behavior to avoid or respond to specific sensory experiences. The covered over sensations remain, in other words, but precisely *as covered over*.

Through therapy, a person with an eating disorder can work to recover this foundational sense of embodiment. They might put effort into developing new, opposing patterns of behavior, so that the habit of covering over certain sensations could be counteracted (at least to some extent). A person recovering from an eating disorder, for example, may once again feel hunger pangs (rather than needing starvation to feel their embodiment), or they may overcome the revulsion or desire for certain foods – but in order to do so, they must establish new patterns of behavior to counteract the passive syntheses that covered over their hunger, which required the sensation of starvation, or highlighted their revulsion or desire.

Conclusion

Most therapists who counsel patients with eating disorders, I assume, are already familiar with these several phenomenological levels of constitution (as well as possible others) to some extent. But perhaps outlining these levels as I have done here might offer a rubric from which deeper analyses could be carried out. Some analyses, for example, might focus heavily only on one level. Other analyses could point to the constitution of meaning at one level in its relation to – or influence upon – other levels. We are always experiencing through all of these levels at once, but from a phenomenological perspective, we can examine how the meanings constituted at one level can filter into the others – whether we are following the trajectory "downward"/"inward" (from, say, intersubjective constitution into sensory experience of embodiment) or "upward"/"outward" (from rudimentary sensation into individual and then intersubjective meaning constitution). Thus, we can carry out several types of analyses: First, there are analyses specific to a single level, achieving a deeper understanding of the experience and constitution of meaning that takes place at that level. Second, we can carry out analyses that focus on how a phenomenon might be constituted through multiple levels at once. Finally, we can examine the relations between the levels themselves, looking for breakdowns, lack of fluidity, or domination of one level over the others.

It becomes clear that a straightforward analysis of, say, intersubjective attitudes about beauty and thinness would probably not suffice in treating someone with an eating disorder. As we know, the embodied practices and rituals sedimented in PS – practices that affect not only the physical body but also the thought processes and sensory perception of the individual – are fundamental to the disorder itself. Conversely, addressing only the ritual behavior, the habits, or the embedded patterns of perception and decision-making of an individual – without acknowledging the importance of social context and relations with others – does not address the phenomenon to its fullest extent, either. While the body has its own history – a history sedimented into muscle movement, involuntary reactions to odors and textures, and desires and revulsions – this history is integrated with the meanings found at the higher phenomenological levels. Full analysis must therefore recognize each individual level in some way, as well as how the levels relate to one another.

Thus, we can see the benefits of a phenomenological approach that acknowledges several distinct levels of experience: Recognizing that there are multiple levels of experience, as well as several approaches to those levels, could give a therapist more flexibility as to how to approach a client with an eating disorder.[13] Since each individual has their own embodiment, history, and constitution of intersubjective meaning, how one treats a specific individual might depend upon how that person takes up meaning. One's approach might differ depending on whether, for example, intersubjective

[13] As Bordo points out, "Anorexia nervosa is clearly, as Paul Garfinkel and David Garner have called it, a 'multidimensional disorder,' with familial, perceptual, cognitive, and possibly, biological factors interacting in varying combinations in different individuals to produce a 'final common pathway'" (Bordo, 2003, p. 140).

discourses are given priority in that person's narrative, or contrarily, whether certain sensory experiences have been highlighted, resulting in specific patterns of behavior. From that point, the therapy can then adjust its focus in a variety of ways, depending upon the conversation between therapist and patient. If nothing else, it provides multiple perspectives on an individual case, thus offering different avenues of approach.

A phenomenological approach – and, I would argue, a therapeutic one – is mostly fully carried out when it attends to the different constitutions of meaning at each level, to the movement between these levels, and to the relations of one to another. Each layer relates to the others, influencing them, reacting to them, negotiating with them. They filter into each other without dissipating their distinction entirely. Approaching a phenomenon through a recognition of the levels of its constitution, applying such a nuanced view to conditions such as eating disorders, might increase the chances of a productive therapeutic outcome.

References

Al-Saji, A. (2010). Bodies and sensings. On the uses of Husserlian phenomenology for feminist theory. *Continental Philosophy Review*, 43(1), 13–37. doi:10.1007/s11007-010-9135-8

Bordo, S. (2003). *Unbearable weight: Feminism, western culture, and the body* (10th ed.). Berkeley, CA: University of California Press.

de Beauvoir, S. (1989). *The second sex* (H. M. Parshley, Trans.). New York, NY: Vintage Books.

Dignon, A., Beardsmore, A., Spain, S., & Kuan, A. (2006). 'Why I won't eat.' Patient testimony from 15 anorexics concerning the causes of their disorder. *Journal of Health Psychology*, 11(6), 942–956. doi:10.1177/1359105306069097

Donohoe, J. (2010). The vocation of motherhood. Husserl and feminist ethics. *Continental Philosophy Review*, 43(1), 127–140. doi:10.1007/s11007-010-9129-6

Halse, C., Honey, A., & Boughtwood, D. (2008). *Inside anorexia: The experiences of girls and their families*. London/Philadelphia: Jessica Kingsley.

Husserl, E. (1970). *The crisis of European sciences and transcendental phenomenology: An introduction to phenomenological philosophy* (D. Carr, Trans.). Evanston, IL: Northwestern University Press.

Husserl, E. (1983). *Ideas pertaining to a pure phenomenology and to a phenomenological philosophy. First book: General introduction to a pure phenomenology* (F. Kersten, Trans.). The Hague, Netherlands: Martinus Nijhoff Publishers.

Husserl, E. (1989). *Ideas pertaining to a pure phenomenology and to a phenomenological philosophy. Second book: Studies in the phenomenology of constitution* (R. Rojcewicz & A. Schuwer, Trans.). Dordrecht, Netherlands: Kluwer Academic.

Husserl, E. (1999). *Cartesian meditations: An introduction to phenomenology* (D. Cairns, Trans.). Dordrecht, Netherlands: Kluwer Academic.

Husserl, E. (2001). *Analyses concerning passive and active synthesis: Lectures on transcendental logic* (A. Steinbock, Trans.). Dordrecht, Netherlands: Kluwer Academic.

My Pro-Ana. (2014, May 9). *CuriousYulia* [Forum post]. Retrieved from www.myproana.com/index.php/topic/181525-healthy-pro-ana-lifestyle-forever/

Pro-Ana Lifestyle Forever and Always. (2019a). "*The Lifestyle*" [Blog post]. Retrieved from https://foreverandalwaysproana.wordpress.com/%e2%99%a5the-lifestyle%e2%99%a5/

Pro-Ana Lifestyle Forever and Always. (2019b). "*Tips&Tricks*" [Blog post]. Retrieved from https://foreverandalwaysproana.wordpress.com/%e2%99%a5tipstricks%e2%99%a5/

Rodemeyer, L. (2006). *Intersubjective temporality: It's about time* (Phaenomenologica Vol. 176). Dordrecht, Netherlands: Springer.

Rodemeyer, L. (2018). *Lou Sullivan diaries (1970–1980) and theories of embodiment: Making sense of sensing*. Cham, Switzerland: Springer.

Stanghellini, G. (2019). The optical-coenaesthetic disproportion in feeding and eating disorders. *European Psychiatry*, 58, 70–71. doi:10.1016/j.eurpsy.2019.02.005

Stanghellini, G., Castellini, G., Brogna, P., Faravelli, C., & Ricca, V. (2012). Identity and eating disorders (IDEA): A questionnaire evaluating identity and embodiment in eating disorder patients. *Psychopathology*, 45(3), 147–158. doi:10.1159/000330258

Svenaeus, F. (2013). Anorexia nervosa and the body uncanny: A phenomenological approach. *Philosophy, Psychiatry, and Psychology*, 20(1), 81–91. www.muse.jhu.edu/article/51126

Zimmerman, J. L. & Dickerson, V. C. (1994). Tales of the body thief: Externalising and deconstructing eating problems. In *Constructive therapies* (ed. M. F. Hoyt), 295–318. New York: Guilford.

11.1

Commentary on "Levels of Embodiment: A Husserlian Analysis of Gender and the Development of Eating Disorders"

Agency, Environmental Scaffolding, and the Development of Eating Disorders

Joel Krueger and Lucy Osler

Rodemeyer has made an important contribution to phenomenological work on gender and the development of eating disorders (EDs). Drawing upon Husserl's analysis of "levels of constitution" – the subjective processes by which phenomena are made present as objects of experience – she convincingly argues that these levels not only help us get a better grip on the development and experience of EDs generally, but also refine our methods of diagnosis and treatment. Additionally, Rodemeyer develops a clear account of how these different levels of constitution systematically interrelate. Her chapter, therefore, has important phenomenological, practical, and exegetical significance.

A virtue of Rodemeyer's account is that it develops a pluralist framework that can accommodate individual differences in how EDs develop and acquire their distinctive character. Current discussions sometimes lack this ecumenical sensitivity. Instead, they place excessive emphasis on a specific cause or explanation: for example, biological factors such as irregular hormone function or genetics; psychological factors such as negative body image, poor self-esteem, or an obsessive desire for thinness; or environmental factors such as sexual abuse or family history of disordered eating. As a result, these narrow approaches oversimplify the complexity and multidimensional character of EDs. Additionally, they tend to adopt a third-person perspective that overlooks the lived experience of these disorders. However, with her multilevel Husserlian-inspired analysis, Rodemeyer gives us a powerful conceptual framework that can accommodate these different dimensions while remaining sensitive to their distinct phenomenological features.

In what follows, we discuss two themes that we suggest will help enrich Rodemeyer's analysis while remaining faithful to her pluralist outlook. Specifically, we are concerned with highlighting the (1) agentive and

(2) environmentally scaffolded nature of EDs. The former helps capture how EDs such as anorexia nervosa are very often complex, temporally extended projects: practices, strategies, and deliberately cultivated habits of self-starvation by which individuals gradually objectify their bodies and experiences in order to exert a kind of radical self-control. The latter helps show how these projects are actively driven and supported by environmental factors – pathways of reinforcement like media, online spaces, peers, and family – that embody harmful narratives of femininity (McBride & Kwee, 2019) and organize gender-based atmospheres persistently nudging (predominantly) girls and women toward practices of disordered eating (Piran & Cormier, 2005). None of what we say below is incompatible with Rodemeyer's account. Indeed, most of what we say is already implicit in her analysis. Focusing on these two themes simply brings to light additional descriptive resources potentially downplayed in Rodemeyer's Husserlian approach – in particular, its emphasis on the "passivity" of meaning-constitution in EDs.

We begin by focusing on the connection between agency and EDs. As Rodemeyer notes, much of Husserl's analysis focuses on the passive character of meaning-constitution. To be clear, "passive" here does not mean static or inactive. Rather, as Rodemeyer tells us, Husserl is concerned with "the synthetic work done by consciousness that *goes unnoticed* while consciousness is engaged in direct (i.e., active) experience" (2021, p. 236). This work occurs "passively" in the background insofar as it gives consciousness the structure, stability, and salience we take for granted as we interact with the things and spaces of our lifeworld. So, while this notion of passivity is not equivalent to inactivity, it nevertheless picks out organizational dynamics at the heart of experience over which subjects have little or no control.

Certainly, this notion of passivity can be descriptively useful in the context of EDs. For example, as Rodemeyer demonstrates, it can provide insight into how individuals gradually develop and refine unthinking habits – revulsion to certain types of food; rituals surrounding meals, exercise, or measuring weight – that shape styles of bodily comportment distinctive of EDs (2021, p. 242). However, focusing excessively on passivity in the context of EDs risks depicting these disorders in overly static terms.

For example, Stanghellini, Castellini, Brogna, Faravelli, and Ricca (2012) argue that a profound disturbance of embodiment – disproportionately experiencing one's body as an object subject to the evaluative gaze of others – is *the* core feature of EDs, the causal origin of symptoms such as a tendency to overvalue body shape and weight, an obsessive desire for thinness, and abnormal patterns of eating. Disturbances of embodiment may well be an important part of the experience of EDs for some. But this emphasis on passivity (i.e., the individual caught in the grip of an anomalous world-organizing experience she did not start and cannot control) loses sight of the dynamically *malleable* character of EDs: the way these experiences develop over time as interrelated dimensions of control, self-preservation, bodily distrust, obsession, and vulnerability assume prominence throughout the pathology's evolution. So, focusing excessively on one putative root cause of EDs "does not make sense from the patient's perspective, in her world, but only in the objective and objectifying world of the psychiatrist" (Legrand, 2013, p. 186).

What drops out of the picture on such accounts is the first-person reports of, for instance, anorectics who describe the first stages of anorexia nervosa not simply as a disorder they found themselves with but as a project they actively took up. Consider Hornbacher's (1998) description of her own experience of anorexia nervosa:

> Anorexia was my Big Idea, my bid for independence, identity, freedom … You don't just get it, the way you get a cold; you take it into your head, consider it as an idea first, play with the behaviours awhile, see if they take root. (p. 69)

Part of capturing the progression of anorexia nervosa, then, involves recognizing how the disorder can start as an active project pursued by the anorectic that eventually – and tragically – reverses, leaving the anorectic subject to the disorder itself. Rodemeyer's framework, with its delineation of the various levels of constitution, allows us to make sense of such a progression by accounting for how the disorder manifests and sediments at different levels of constitution at different times.

To further clarify this point and highlight the key role that agency plays in this temporal development, consider a distinction Rodemeyer briefly mentions at the end of her discussion: hunger versus starvation. The former is a sensation we're all familiar with. It indicates a need to eat. For most, it's also a moderately unpleasant sensation that we look to eliminate as quickly as possible. However, as Rodemeyer observes, even at the lowest of Husserl's levels of constitution – *hyletic flow*, or the primordial stream of sensory content, as well as feelings like nausea, pain, pleasure, and tension – this sensation is never given neutrally, independent of associations or connections with other sensations and levels of constitution that shape its meaning and felt character. Rather, the "embodiment of a person with an eating disorder will have a phenomenological basis in sensory content, but patterns … or meanings established at higher levels, can act either to highlight or to cover over aspects of the sensory flow" (Rodemeyer, 2021, p. 251). So, for someone with an ED, the felt intensity or salience of an occurrent hunger experience might be subdued while revulsion or desire assumes greater prominence.

Importantly, however – and this is the key link with agency – this phenomenological transformation is not simply given. It is something that must be *cultivated*. It occurs when occurrent episodes of hunger are repeatedly taken up into a larger existential project: namely, the ongoing practice of self-starvation. This project of self-starvation is complex and multidimensional. It develops across multiple timescales and takes many forms: different rituals, practices, strategies, and deliberately cultivated values and habits by which individuals gradually objectify their bodies – including episodic sensations like hunger – in order to exert a radical self-control. So, in this way, the felt manifestation of hunger is transformed at multiple timescales and via deliberate agentive interventions. Instead of remaining an unpleasant experience or something to be stoically ignored, it takes on a new salience: a felt reward or affirmation that one has successfully committed to, and maintained, the ongoing project of self-starvation.

Of course, our agency – as well as the projects that flow from it – is always situated. This takes us to our second theme: the role environmental factors play in driving the temporal development of EDs. In the past few decades, so-called situated approaches to cognition in philosophy of mind and cognitive science have moved away from a neurocentric focus and instead emphasize the ineliminable role physical and social factors in the environment play in shaping cognition. While these approaches are diverse, all agree that cognition cannot be understood without considering the crucial way environmental resources "scaffold" (i.e., actively shape and regulate) the form and function of our cognitive capacities. A recent trend is a focus on the role environmental resources play in scaffolding emotions and affect (Colombetti & Krueger, 2015; Krueger & Szanto, 2016; Stephan, Walter, & Wilutzky, 2014).

For our purposes, the key point is that projects of self-starvation are not accomplished solely via the agency of solitary individuals. They involve carefully curating specific environments designed to scaffold the practices and values that make up these projects. This scaffolding can take many forms: obsessively weighing and scrutinizing one's body in front of the mirror or taking selfies to find flaws; maintaining a diary of desired body-focused improvements; using technologies for hyperdiligent calorie counting; developing complex, excessively intricate eating rituals (supported by various artifacts and technologies) intended to slow down the eating process and minimize consumption; regularly inhabiting online spaces (pro-anorexic websites, blogs, social media, or chat groups; image-blogging platforms like Instagram and Tumblr) for tips, strategies, inspiration, or emotional support. These environments are comprised of technosocial resources designed to synchronically and diachronically regulate how individuals enact their food-related behavior in specific contexts and relate to food-related behavior – and their bodies and bodily experiences – more generally. This scaffolding can be located at different levels of constitution, in accordance with Rodemeyer's framework. For instance, the role of social media falls within the intersubjective layer, whereas ritualistic eating might start at the level of active constitution but, over time, become sedimented as a bodily habit at the level of passive synthesis.

Focusing on the environmentally scaffolded nature of EDs also productively highlights an important tension regarding agency and EDs. As we've noted, the physical and social environments individuals set up to scaffold EDs often reflect deliberate choices and interventions: for example, choosing to participate in certain pro-anorexic online spaces. However, many of these environments – particularly online spaces where billions of people regularly go to connect with others and share emotions and experiences (Osler, 2019) – are set up and regulated by *others* (e.g., technology companies like Google or Facebook), and reflect *their* interests, values, and ends. Moreover, these environments, in turn, may subtly influence values, behavior, and emotions – including those that drive projects of self-starvation – without the individual's full awareness or consent (Krueger & Osler, 2019; Slaby, 2016).

To give just one example: Consider popular "beautifying" filters in Snapchat, an instant-messaging app primarily used by individuals aged between 18 and 24 (roughly 70 percent of users are female). These filters remove "imperfections" (blemishes, wrinkles, discoloration), change or soften skin tone, and manipulate the physical structure of the user's face (slimming cheeks and nose; increasing eye size). Users can, in this way, not only experiment with unrealistic ideals of beauty and thinness (e.g., manipulating their cheekbones or eye size to anatomically impossible configurations) and reinforce insecurities about their own appearance; they can also easily share these images with others and, in so doing, propagate potentially harmful representations of beauty and thinness. So, while these filters are fun to use – and clearly serve Snapchat's interests in driving user engagement – they also feed into much larger networks of technosocial scaffolding that reinforce unhealthy narratives of femininity and, along with a sea of other gendered content in media and online spaces, persistently nudge girls and women[1]

[1] Although rates of EDs are increasing among males (Limbers, Cohen, & Gray, 2018; Mosley, 2009).

toward practices of disordered eating in order to embody these unhealthy narratives. Accordingly, this scaffolded perspective emphasizes that EDs – including the practices and values that sustain them – are disorders of a society, and not simply an individual (Piran & Cormier, 2005).

To conclude, nothing we say here is incompatible with Rodemeyer's rich phenomenological account of EDs and gender. Again, we've simply tried to highlight some additional conceptual resources and themes that will, we hope, supplement her contribution and trigger further consideration of this important topic.

Acknowledgment

Both authors contributed equally to this work.

References

Colombetti, G., & Krueger, J. (2015). Scaffoldings of the affective mind. *Philosophical Psychology*, 28(8), 1157–1176. doi:10.1080/09515089.2014.976334

Hornbacher, M. (1998). *Wasted: Coming back from an addiction to starvation*. London, UK: Flamingo.

Krueger, J., & Osler, L. (2019). Engineering affect: Emotion regulation and the techno-social niche. *Philosophical Topics*, 47(2), 1–53.

Krueger, J., & Szanto, T. (2016). Extended emotions. *Philosophy Compass*, 11(12), 863–878. doi:10.1111/phc3.12390

Legrand, D. (2013). Inter-subjectively meaningful symptoms in anorexia. In R. T. Jensen & D. Moran (Eds.), *The phenomenology of embodied subjectivity* (pp. 185–201). Basel, Switzerland: Springer.

Limbers, C. A., Cohen, L. A., & Gray, B. A. (2018). Eating disorders in adolescent and young adult males: Prevalence, diagnosis, and treatment strategies. *Adolescent Health, Medicine and Therapeutics*, 9, 111–116. doi:10.2147//AHMT.S147480

McBride, H. L., & Kwee, J. L. (2019). Understanding disordered eating and (dis)embodiment through a feminist lens. In H. L. McBride, & J. L. Kwee (Eds.), *Embodiment and eating disorders* (pp. 17–34). Abingdon-on-Thames, UK: Routledge.

Mosley, P. E. (2009). Bigorexia: Bodybuilding and muscle dysmorphia. *European Eating Disorders Review: The Journal of the Eating Disorders Association*, 17(3), 191–198. doi:10.1002/erv.897

Osler, L. (2019). Feeling togetherness online: A phenomenological sketch of online communal experiences. *Phenomenology and the Cognitive Sciences*. Advance online publication. doi:10.1007/s11097-019-09627-4

Piran, N., & Cormier, H. C. (2005). The social construction of women and disordered eating patterns. *Journal of Counseling Psychology*, 52(4), 549–558. doi:10.1037/0022-0167.52.4.549

Rodemeyer, L. M. (2021). Levels of embodiment: A Husserlian analysis of gender and the development of eating disorders. In C. Tewes & G. Stanghellini (Eds.), *Time and body: Phenomenological and psychopathological approaches* (pp. 234–255). Cambridge, UK: Cambridge University Press.

Slaby, J. (2016). Mind invasion: Situated affectivity and the corporate life hack. *Frontiers in Psychology*, 7, 1–13. doi:10.3389/fpsyg.2016.00266

Stanghellini, G., Castellini, G., Brogna, P., Faravelli, C., & Ricca, V. (2012). Identity and eating disorders (IDEA): A questionnaire evaluating identity and embodiment in eating disorder patients. *Psychopathology*, 45(3), 147–158. doi:10.1159/000330258

Stephan, A., Walter, S., & Wilutzky, W. (2014). Emotions beyond brain and body. *Philosophical Psychology*, 27(1), 65–81. doi:10.1080/09515089.2013.828376

12

Phenomenology of Corporeality (and Spatiality) in Anorexia Nervosa with a Reference to the Problem of Its Temporality

Otto Doerr-Zegers and Héctor Pelegrina-Cetran

Introduction

There are few psychiatric pathologies in which disturbances of corporeality are so evident and dramatic as in anorexia nervosa. Two phenomena related to the topic have been mentioned in the earliest descriptions of the illness (Gull, 1873 as cited in Thomae, 1961; Lasègue, 1873). One is the obsessive search for an extreme thinness, and the other, the paradoxical physical hyperactivity accompanying the process of systematic slimming down. In the 1960s, along with an increased incidence of this illness, a third phenomenon was described in the relation of the patient to his or her body, that is, the distortion of the body image: Identified patients would look at themselves in the mirror and find themselves fat (Gallwitz, 1965). This distortion could reach the extreme that patients would see others, particularly women, as much thinner than they are.

In this chapter, we will not explore psychodynamic factors potentially involved in the genesis of this illness, or the role of the family therein, as these topics have been the subject of previous investigations (Doerr-Zegers, 1972a, 1972b, 1985, 1988, 1994; Doerr-Zegers, Petrasic & Morales, 1976; Doerr-Zegers & Pelegrina, 2016). The question we want to address presently is that of the relationship of the anorectic patient with her body and with the world. Any question relating to the human body must acknowledge the distinction made by the French philosophers Maurice Merleau-Ponty (1945/1957) and Gabriel Marcel (1955) between the subject-body and the object-body. In Latin languages, there is only one word – *cuerpo* in Spanish, *corp* in French, *corpo* in Italian – for these two bodies, whereas, in German, the subject-body and the object-body have always been distinguished by the words *Leib* and *Körper*. It is interesting that *Leib* is derived from *Leben*, which means "life" or as a verb, "to live," whereas *Körper* is derived from the Latin word *corpus*, which in English is transformed into corpse, a dead body. But already in the etymology of the Latin word *corpus*, there also appears the sense of the cadaveric. The lived subject-body not only means the body I feel but also the body that appears (in front of others) and is expressed, in the sense of Zutt's (1963) "in Erscheinung stehender Leib" (the standing and manifesting body). I perceive and act through my lived body, but without reflecting on it. I am always living through it in my life world. Consequently, the lived body means a corporealized being-in-the-world, that is, an embodied subject who feels the stimuli of the world that affect him and corporeally goes to it from his desires. The object-body or soma is something that the subject has as a *possession* without *constituting it* or something proper that can be used as an "instrument" of execution of tasks or converted into an object of extreme actions over it as in anatomy or physiology. This body can also be transformed into the object of visualization of another person or in what betrays me in the illness.

Thomas Fuchs (2003) has presented phenomenological analyses of what occurs with this polarity subject-body/object-body in two human phenomena; shame and guilt, and their respective relationship with dysmorphophobia and depression. Shame is intimately related with the glance of another person, and appears in situations in which one is surprised or unmasked. From the phenomenological point of view, an alienation and "objectualization" of the lived body occurs, which in a way loses its insertion in the world and is found – in the moment of shame – transformed into a mere object of the glance of another person. Unlike shame, guilt would not be linked to the immediate presence of the other person. Instead of being exposed and paralyzed by the glance of another person, the guilty subject feels abandoned by the other. The person who feels guilt is thrown toward his own body and separated from the others. And as shame burns, guilt weighs.

Dysmorphophobia is a distortion of shame, and melancholia is the distortion of guilt. Shame occurs in a precise interpersonal context and the person recovers their self-esteem when they escape from the shameful situation, whereas in dysmorphophobia, a part of the body is objectified and remains the center of attention in the glance of any other person and in any circumstance. In melancholia, an "objectualization" and/or stiffening of all the lived body occurs, which is experienced by the patient as decay, anxiety, pain, vital symptoms, etc., and which in a way catch the lived body and push it toward its mere condition of object-body. This same phenomenon was described by one of us (Doerr-Zegers, 1980) as the process of cadaverization or "chrematization" in severe depressions. In a body transformed into an object, time is detained, as Viktor von Gebsattel (1954) and Erwin Straus (1960) described, and the subject is invaded by their past from which little failures arise transformed as unforgivable sins and delusions of guilt.

Psychopathological peculiarities of Anorexia Nervosa

An analysis of the corporeality of anorexia nervosa must be made in the psychopathological structures of this illness. The definition in DSM-V (American Psychiatric Association, 2013, pp. 338–339) is very simple: restriction of the caloric ingestion, which leads to a significant weight loss, fear of getting fat and measures that interfere with weight increase, alteration of the body image, and negation of the seriousness of the patient's condition. Undoubtedly, all this is true, but the psychopathology of this illness is much richer than that. The structures that do not appear in this definition and are indeed fundamental for their understanding are as follows:

(1) *Intellectualization*: The rejection of the body is accompanied by an overvaluation of the intellectual sphere. People with anorexia are the best students, they reason admirably; they show an extraordinary ability to lie, eluding controls and reaching their purpose of continuing weight loss. Their style of communication is merely intellectual, and they refer to their own affectivity as "from outside," something they think, but do not feel and, therefore, do not express (alexithymia). In a study about anorexia and the family carried out by one of us (Doerr-Zegers, 1985), we found this characteristic in 90 percent of the patients studied, and 50 percent showed an overvaluation of the intellectual and cultural sphere. An impressive example of this phenomenon is found in the diary of famous Binswanger's case, Ellen West: "When I try to analyse all that nothing is achieved but a *theory, something purely thought*. I only can *feel* unrest and anxiety" (Binswanger, 1957, p. 78).

(2) *Eagerness for control*: In the same way that anorectic patients tyrannize their physical body from outside, up to the point of not allowing it to satisfy any of its basic appetitive needs, such as nutrition and sexuality, they do this with their environment: they dominate their parents, brothers, caregivers, and therapists. However, these are forms of controlling the world with their reason, and in particular, they seek to control the body even to the point of wanting to make it disappear. These characteristics have been found in all the cases studied by one of us (Doerr-Zegers, 1985). Furthermore, patients with anorexia try to control not only their instincts, needs, and the environment but also the physical space and the symbolic space that they inhabit. They seek to create a private space that protects their body from the community space,

which they experience as an enemy. At the same time, they seek to construct a cognitive, symbolic space, in which they exercise their absolute domination to the point of allowing themselves every type of transgression. Other authors have also drawn attention to the phenomenon of control, as for instance Svenaeus when he wrote: "[T]he body in the anorectic patients becomes an *obstacle* and an *enemy* that needs to be controlled" (Svenaeus, 2013, p. 89). And he had also previously mentioned this controlling tendency by referring to the anorexic person's entire life: "Two striking elements in all narratives of anorexia I have come across are weak self-confidence and an urge to control one's own (and sometimes others') life in a perfectionist way" (Svenaeus, 2013, p. 86).

(3) *The paradoxes of anorexia nervosa*: There are several paradoxes in the existence of patients with anorexia. The Chilean specialist in this field, Rosa Behar (1988), referred to this as "the antithetical in anorexia nervosa." We will describe the main characteristics:

(a) The *first paradox* that is observed in patients with anorexia is the coincidence between an extreme thinness, which can result in cachexia, and marked hyperactivity. This last was already identified in the first descriptions of anorexia and contributed, in the case of Lasègue (1873), to consideration of this syndrome as an independent illness when comparing it with cases of extreme loss of weight consequent to the hardships of the Franco-Prussian war and in which passiveness predominated. Pelegrina (2006a) agrees, emphasizing that that hyperactivity would not be explained only by the eagerness to lose weight, but rather as an expression of an eagerness to construct a personal physical space, of mechanical activities, elaborated from outside of this space, as a sort of island supporting and protecting their bodies. Anorectics aim to manufacture a space where they feel nothing but emptiness and *personal* desolation, *a space of physical structures, with operative, not affective interrelationships.*

(b) The *second paradox* is given between anorectics' tremendous affective dependence on others, particularly on the mother, and their rejection of every other real affective bond. Thus, they generally do not have partners or friends, and in the psychotherapeutic relationship, the rational moment dominates over the affective, configuring the alexithymia that characterizes these patients. In our experience, this incapacity to establish adult affective relationships can lead to a complete solitude when the only being with whom they have been able to emotionally connect themselves, generally their mother, becomes ill or is absent. The above-mentioned case of Binswanger's, Ellen West, expresses this feeling in a way difficult to surpass:

> I feel myself excluded from every form of real life. I am seated inside a glass sphere. I look at the persons through a glass wall and I hear their voices in a muffled way. I aspire to reach them and I cry but they do not hear me. I extend my arms toward them but my hands only collide against the walls of my glass sphere. (Binswanger, 1957, p. 80)

(c) The *third paradox* manifests itself between anorectics' great intellectual maturity and their extreme emotional immaturity, which appears among other forms as a desire to not grow up, to remain preadolescent, and to not be incorporated into the adult world. Although, strictly speaking, anorectics are neither in the adult world nor in the adolescent one. They enter neither into the adult world, because they do not want to accept the challenges that this implies, that is, marriage, maternity, and professional life, nor into the adolescent world, because they consider pubescents and adolescents as intellectually very immature. It seems as if they desire to live in an adult world but with infantile dynamics.

(d) In the *fourth paradox*, patients with anorexia appear to have a need to make their body disappear (a phenomenon Pelegrina (2006b) has described as "ex-corporation of the Ego" or the disembodied subject), to not be physically seen by others in their volume. At the same time, they feel the need to draw attention, to be objectified by the gaze of others. Svenaeus (2013) has pointed to something similar, when he stated that "the different ways of becoming bodily alienated interact in anorexia in establishing an uncanniness of the body that is both conspicuous (to people around the ill person) and hard to escape (for the person herself)" (p. 89). They want to be corporeally absent and at the same time become present in a nonflesh manner, to provoke scandal in others.

(e) The *fifth paradox* can be appreciated in the framework of treatment and rehabilitation. The attitude of the anorectic patient is ambivalent. On the one hand, patients are interested in treatment, regularly attend sessions, smile at the physician, call him their "saviour," express their desire to recover, etc. On the other hand and according to Rosa Behar (1988), the problem is that, insofar as their wellbeing is linked to losing weight, any success of treatment that is expressed as weight gain is going to mean for them, first, uneasiness and unhappiness, and second, a confirmation that their fight for losing weight must continue at any price.

The Relationship between Anorectics and Their Bodies

As we saw in the introduction, the investigator who approaches the problem of the human body in an unprejudiced way appreciates the distinction between the body I have or object-body (my eyes, for example) and the body I am or subject-body (my gaze). The differentiation between these two bodies implies a complex philosophical problem and has many nuances. Gabriel Marcel (1955), one of the philosophers who has inaugurated the phenomenology of corporeality, also saw a certain danger in reducing the multiplicity of aspects that the human body has to this single duality, when he affirmed: "In the measure that I am a lived body I have a body, but at the same time I only have the appearance of this, precisely because I am a lived body" (Marcel, 1978, p. 49). But this is not the only ambiguity we have to deal with. Blankenburg indicates other ambiguities, for example, the fact that

> the object-body belongs, on one side, to the world and as such, can be an object of scientific investigation and, on the other, it belongs to the Ego and as such it is not an object, but the assumption and basis—and, at the same time—organ of that same investigation. (Blankenburg, 1989, pp. 174–175, my translation)

Another ambiguity is given in the framework of the lived body itself, between one that is a consciously experienced body and another that is inadvertently lived – a silent body that is a part of one's state of health. Finally, there exists that ambiguity indicated by Jürg Zutt (1963) between a lived body, which carries and charges us, and that other body referred to in the world, "which appears, moves, and allows voluntary activity." A way of overcoming these ambiguities would be to consider this separation as a dynamic polarity: At one extreme is the subjective experience of the body and of the world and, at the other, the body as object of the gaze of others or of the action of the surgeon over the operating table. I am and I have a body at the same time. Each one is a condition of possibility of the other. Without a functioning brain, subjective life would be impossible and, inversely, without openness to the world, which affords a lived body, the other body – Ortega y Gasset's extra-body (1964) – would be a mere thing. Today, these polar dynamics are precisely the current trans-phenomenological vision of the process of human life with its progressive "autopoietic" emergency of the different levels of organization and actualization of the communicative poles of life. In this new ontological and epistemological paradigm, "nature and nurture (incorporated culture) are in relation one with each other as product and process" (Varela, Thompson, & Rosch, 1991). This new approach deals with enactive dynamics of the "new ontological-methodological paradigm" of the "general theory of systems," to which one of us (Pelegrina) dedicated the second chapter of his *Fundamentos Antropológicos de la Psicopatología* (Anthropological Foundations of Psychopathology) (2006b, pp. 88–147).

Now, what happens with the body of patients with anorexia? As we saw, both in dysmorphophobia and in melancholic depression, there is a sort of "corporealization" or rather becoming a thing of the lived body, in the sense of a predominance of the object-body over the subject-body. In the first case, a part of the object-body (the nose, the eyes, the jaw) is emancipated from the rest and is transformed into the center of the attention of both the patients themselves and others. This transformation in a mere object of glance of others necessarily leads to a separation of the world and to a loss of one's insertion in it. In the second case, and as Doerr-Zegers (1980, 1993) and Fuchs (2003, 2005) have described, the lived body is "objectualized" and absorbed by the object-body up to the point of becoming a thing and eclipsing any relationship with the world until the patient is transformed – in a stupor – into a mere immobile object.

In the anorectic patient, there is no predominance of one body over the other, but a fragmentation of that dynamic polarity, which, in the state of health, constitutes a perfect unity. The anorectic does not live in this unity, but in two opposing and mutually hostile realities. Herself – her lived body – rejects her physical-volumetric body and wants to be only a subjective experience, only a spirit, and then, she treats it like a fetish, like something that can be manipulated at will. We believe that in these patients their own body becomes a "thing" separated from the ego itself. This fully coincides with the observations by Hanna Bowden in the sense that "the anorectic … constantly has this feeling of her body being obvious and object-like, and in being visible it becomes 'too big'" (Bowden, 2012, p. 234). There is also an empirical study carried out by Stanghellini, Castellini, Brogna, Faravelli, and Ricca, in which a questionnaire for evaluating identity and embodiment in eating disorder patients was applied, which demonstrates that anorectic patients experience "one's body first and foremost as an object being looked at by another (rather than coenaesthetically and from a first-person perspective)" (Stanghellini et al., 2012, p. 156). Later, Stanghellini came back to the subject and underlined the object character of the body in anorectics when he manifests:

> These persons feel extraneous from their own body and their bodily feelings are discontinuous over time. This suggests that the Other's look is not only a source of intimidating and shameful "negation" of their capacity to transcend their mere objective corporeality, but also a longed-for device through which they can finally define themselves—an optical self-prosthesis. (Stanghellini, 2019, p. 3)

In a similar way, Dorothée Legrand argues: "The patient [with anorexia] experiences her body's physicality as her belongingness to the realm of objects" (Legrand, 2010, p. 732). On the following page, she completely coincides with our opinion, when she claims: "The objectifying stance over the body has far-reaching consequences in that it disintegrates physical from subjective dimensions of bodily self-consciousness" (Legrand, 2010, p. 733). Hannah Bowden refers to the same phenomenon of both forms of corporality we mentioned before, when she stated:

> The anorectic, in experiencing her body as corporealized also seems to partially lose a sense of identification with her body. The objectified nature of her body prevents her from fully living through it. Instead, she experiences it almost as if it were a separate object. (Bowden, 2012, p. 234)

Patients suffering from anorexia seek a merely ideal existence, without flesh throbbing with desires and affections, an existence without intimate intentions directed to the world, which is not properly a "life world." This anorectic phobia to any corporal manifestation in the exterior space crystallizes in a fear of being a volumetric body, that is, ex-pansive and ex-positional. The body of anorectic patients is their greatest enemy. It is an inappropriate body, a body of another, which is external to its personal dimension. And to this point, the fragmentation is united with the eagerness to control, because when one experiences his/her own body as an alienated one and full of animadversion against its owner, the patient with anorexia needs to establish a continuous and total control over it. Instead of conducting the lived body, in which she exists, from inside toward the world, she tries to control it from the outside.

But it is not just a matter of wanting to be thin or very thin, for the simple reason that persons with anorexia are never satisfied with their weight or with the attained skeletal figure. Pelegrina has adequately expressed this phenomenon in one phrase: "[Patients] do not try to be very thin, but to continuously lose weight, since the immediate presence of the threat of their voluminous bodies ... (only) allows them ... the continuous attempt to diminish the spatial dimension of the threat … reducing volume" (2006a, p. 53, my translation). We think that the anorectic does not attempt to reach a properly ideal weight, but rather seeks a physical body without volume or weight. This disembodied existence of the anorectic can be understood as an enactive dynamic of the field of life, which actualizes both a disembodied subject and a devitalized world, that is, a subject who has only a physical body in a physical world.

Differences and Similarities between the Body in Anorexia and in Other Pathologies

With Respect to the Body in Dysmorphophobia

In dysmorphophobia, it is a part of the body that is extracted from the harmony of the whole, whereas in anorexia it is the totality of the body that is alienated, constituting rather a "morphophobia" (Pelegrina, 2006a, p. 53). Patients who suffer from dysmorphophobia reject the "expressive figure" of that part of the body that would manifest their own being in an unpleasant way under the presumed judgment of others. In anorexia, in contrast, there is no shame for what the figure of her body expresses, but rejection of occupying volume in physical space. In the dysmorphophobic patient, the world is reduced because a part of it is interfering with the fluidity of the consciousness–world relationship. People with anorexia are, on the one hand, obsessed with dominating this object-body, which is marginal to her disembodied subjectivity and, on the other hand, throw themselves into the world using multiple intellectual interests and eagerness to dominate and control the people around them, in particular their mother. In this context, and unlike what happens in dysmorphophobia, it seems interesting to mention the "communicative" character that the anorectic body can reach, as has been expressed by Legrand and Briend:

> It is precisely if they are "listened" to as modes of *addressing* others, that is, as modes of *speaking* with others, and if they are *responded* to as subjective manifestations, rather than being observed in an objectifying manner, that bodily symptoms participate to the communicative dynamic which animates the speech of the subject as well. (Legrand & Briend, 2015, p. 59)

With Respect to the Body in Depression

Differences with respect to the body of depressed people are even greater. In the latter, the lived body, as it is felt and as it is expressed, sinks in the object-body, producing a process of *Verdinglichung* (becoming a thing) or "chrematization" (Doerr-Zegers, 1980, 1993) or objectualization (Fuchs,

2005) which, in extreme cases, such as stupor, completely cuts off any appetitive relationship with the world. From this process of becoming a thing derives the alteration of the *Befindlichkeit* (officially translated as "state of mind") described by Doerr-Zegers, Enríquez, and Jara (1971), Doerr-Zegers (1979, 1980) and by Berner (1983) and that classical "not-being-able-to" (*das Nicht-Können* following Binswanger, 1960), which corresponds more or less to psychomotor inhibition or retardation. In patients with anorexia, the body is simply not felt and there is not only no inhibition, but on the contrary, this condition shows a hyperactive daily life, which can include exercises and jogging. In summary, anorectics treat their bodies as "slaves," as something separate that can be manipulated at their discretion. However, in no case are they – as occurs in depressed patients with stupor – "imprisoned" in their bodies, but rather are threatened by its physical size, which tends to annul their purely thinking being. The anorectic pretends to realize the famous Cartesian formula, "I think, then I exist," which inaugurates – curiously – modernity, and in which the psychopathological form of "anorectic existence" just appears.

With Respect to the Body in Schizophrenia

The phenomenological differences with respect to the body in schizophrenia are more complex. An author who has extensively worked on this theme is Thomas Fuchs (2005). Fuchs postulates that patients with schizophrenia are characterized by having a "disembodied subjectivity." They do not inhabit their body in a natural form, nor do they employ it for the performance of the tasks they have to fulfill in the world. Parnas (2000) and Sass (2001) conclude that much of the schizophrenic symptomatology derives from what they call "self-affection" or "self-referentiality" and from a compensatory hyperreflexivity. Consequently, tacit self-consciousness or self-referentiality, present in each experience of daily life, is much weakened or even lost. This results in the alienation of perception and of action. The fragmentation of the intentional arc in perceiving, feeling, thinking, and acting is also derived from this phenomenon of the "disembodied mind" (Fuchs, 2005). In the case of emotions, healthy people experience them and connect emotionally with the phenomena of their corporal sensations and their resonances. The same is valid for impulses and desires. In schizophrenia, according to Fuchs (2005) and Sass (2001), this intentional arc of emotion and of impulses is fragmented, and somatic sensations are extracted from their motivational context. This leads to a sensation of artificiality and distance, both in the experience of emotion and its visible expression for others. This dissociation is observed in an exaggerated way in the coenaesthetic forms of schizophrenia (Diebold & Doerr-Zegers, 1965, p. 25). A patient of one of us (Otto Doerr-Zegers) who suffered from this illness reported that he had to make sure that his arms and legs were his own, for the sake of which he moved and observed them with attention and frequently put his fingers into his mouth to bite, assuring himself that they belonged to him (Diebold & Doerr-Zegers, 1965, p. 25). With respect to his relationship with the world, he said:

> The world is very much away, without meaning and empty. For example, if I observe a farm, I see with great exactitude the house and the persons, but only as something material. Beyond that, everything is poor, desert and without meaning. (Diebold & Doerr-Zegers, 1965, p. 31)

This clearly implies a "dis-ontologicalization" of the world and of one self, as it has also been postulated by Pelegrina (2017), and which can lead in these patients to a "dis-structuration" of the reality of the world, to a sort of "destruction" of the world and of the meanings that identify the real entities that constitute it.

Nothing of this sort occurs in anorexia nervosa. There is no alteration of the intentionality of perception, or of actions, neither of the ontology of the world, nor of the anorectic's own body, which, although alien, is not cognitively strange to the patient. Patients do not present the self-referentiality mentioned by Parnas (2000) and Sass (2001). The anorectic patient knows that they are the one who perceives and feels or acts with their body. They can manage or mold as they want the world around them, including other persons, and do this with a firm will. Their surrounding world is a synthetic structure, integrated by particular things differentiated from each other and with respect to the anorectic patient as a perceiving and acting being. It is an intelligible, logical world of real character and constituted by entities with their own identities, which are seized rationally with great capacity and ability. But this world that anorectic patients inhabit is a world lacking vitality and meaning, in which they do not feel its structure as affecting their life.

The Question of Temporality in Anorexia Nervosa

We will not refer here to the conscious experience of time in people with anorexia as Stanghellini and Mancini (2019) have recently reported. We rather want to inquire about disturbances in temporality itself, in the sense of the phenomenological investigations made by Thomas Fuchs and Mauro Pallagrosi (2018) about the alteration of temporality in schizophrenia, melancholic depression, and borderline personality. These authors postulate that in schizophrenia, implicit or prereflexive temporality appears as severely disturbed. This perturbation affects the threefold structure of time consciousness (*presentation*, *retention*, and *protention*) and manifests itself as fragmentation of the intentional arc, which leads to the typical schizophrenic symptoms, such as thought disorder, thought insertion, auditory hallucinations, and passivity experiences. In melancholic depression, however, the temporal structure remains intact and, in consequence, there is no fragmentation of the intentional arc. What is altered are the conative–affective dynamics of the implicit temporality in the sense of a retardation or inhibition of the stream of consciousness.

In borderline personality disorder, it is not the implicit temporality that is altered, but the explicit one. One of the essential elements of this temporality is the enduring self-identity. The French philosopher Paul Ricoeur (1990) places the very essence of the human being in the temporal relationship that we have toward ourselves through a narrative identity that implies the process of integration or at least a quest for coherence of the personal past, present, and future. In borderline personality disorder, according to Fuchs and Pallagrosi, one finds marked disturbance of identity: "[T]hey lack the strength to establish and maintain a coherent self-concept. They tend to switch from one present to the next" (Fuchs & Pallagrosi, 2018, p. 296). They also show an inability to contain and regulate overwhelming moods and affects.

What occurs with temporality in anorexia nervosa? The first thing we can establish is that the implicit or prereflexive temporality – this perfect articulation of *retention*, *protention*, and *presentation* – is intact. They not only do not manifest a fragmentation of the intentional arc as in schizophrenia, but, on the contrary, they show an incredible will for achieving their goals in general and in particular, that of losing weight with all means imaginable: from extreme fasting to hyperactivity – that, as we said, drew the attention of one of the authors who first described the disease (Lasègue, 1873) – passing through the use of laxatives, the betrayal of their family, hiding food instead of eating it, and the act of vomiting. The explicit temporality, specifically altered in borderline personality disorder, following Fuchs and Pallagrosi (2018), also does not appear as disturbed in anorexia. Anorectics do not suffer under identity diffusion, as in borderline personality, nor under intense and abrupt changes of mood. One does not observe this failure in the conative–affective element of the implicit temporality as occurs in melancholic depression: Anorectics are, in contrast, too decided and goal-oriented, all the more because their goal can mean their own death.

Nevertheless, facing the severity of this disease and the almost delusional character of the anorectic ideas referring to one's self and to the world, one would have to think that anorectic patients must have an alteration of this fundamental dimension of human existence, which is temporality. If we approach an anorectic patient without prejudice, the first thing that draws our attention is, besides their extreme thinness, their pubertal, immature, and somehow asexualized aspect. All substance has disappeared from their body; there are only lines, angles, and corners. In the early forms – around puberty – this is much evident, but in the late beginning forms, one can also appreciate an involution of their bodies toward the infantile and pre-pubertal. If one adds to this the denial of sexuality, amenorrhea, sterility, the denial of maternity/paternity, one would have to conclude that the temporality fundamentally altered in anorexia nervosa is that of the maturational process, that is, the process of becoming. This is connected on one side with the more biological element of maturation, and on the other – beyond any implicit temporality – with this ideal of being a disembodied spirit as we described before in relation to the phenomenology of corporeality in anorexia nervosa.

The body they have is a thing that occupies a place in Newtonian space, full of other physical things but without vital relations, without desires, or stimuli. This spatial relation of a mere physical type necessarily leads to a lack of lived time in the self-construction of life. The anorectic patient rejects the maturation process of the body they have and of the structure of their living, because their intellectual rationalist existence does not experience temporality as biographic structuration or as procursive actualization of their identity.

In this sense, the enactive process of their existence does not actualize their life as a dynamic satisfying correlation between an organism pretending to incorporate what is desired from the environment and what they feel as an embodied subject. The merely physical things have relationships of position, distance, and volume between them, but lack structuring dynamic relations of one's life, as it occurs in the "open systems" of living beings, that is, in organisms. These build themselves through the behavior *in* and/or *with* the ecological niche, as the two poles characterizing all living systems. The enactive relationships between the living corporeality of the others and the own living corporeality constitutes an "intercorporeality," as Fuchs has postulated (Fuchs, 2013; Fuchs & De Jaegher, 2009) following the "new ecological paradigm," which was in turn inspired by classical authors such as Merleau-Ponty (1945/1957), Von Weizsäcker (1950), Buytendijk (1956), and other modern authors like Francisco Varela et al. (1991). This paradigm was initiated by Whitehead at the first part of the twentieth century in his book *Process and Reality* (1929/1978), manifesting that "in reality there are no things, only processes" and was expressly manifested by Varela, Thompson, and Rosch when they wrote: "[T]he term enactive emphasizes the growing conviction that cognition is not the representation of a pregiven world by a pre-given mind but is rather the enactment of a world and of a mind" (Varela et al., 1991, p. 9). And later, Varela et al. said:

> The key point is that such systems (self-organization with autonomy) do not operate by representation. Instead of *representing* an independent world, they *enact* a world as a domain of distinctions that is inseparable from the structure embodied by the cognitive system. (1991, p. 140)

In anorectic patients, body and world are actualized without vitality, that is, without affectivity or appetites, but also without historical temporality. However, the patient does not lack a narrative identity in the sense of Ricoeur (1990). Their narration is completely narrowed around the theme of losing weight and of reaching the condition of being a disembodied spirit, a spirit without flesh, without any desires. Their thinking as well as her acting turn untiringly and years-long around the same subject, somehow resembling paranoid developments as in the sense of Karl Jaspers (1963).

Conclusions

(1) In anorexia nervosa there is a total division between the subject-body (*der Leib*) and the object-body (*der Körper*), between the lived-body and the body as mere soma. The subject is merely intellectual and disembodied, and the factual body that the subject necessarily has is experienced as a physic-volumetric structure strange to it, something that is useless and obstructs their existence. There is a need to eliminate that object-body (*Körper*). This relationship between both bodies, as we saw, is very different from that in other mentioned pathologies. Different authors have reached similar conclusions (Bowden, 2012; Legrand, 2010; Svenaeus, 2013).

(2) Patients with anorexia treat their body as a thing elaborated from their instrumental reason, as a fetish, which can be molded and given any appearance. Their attempt to control goes beyond the weight and volume of their body; they try to control all their structure and to submit it under their will to design and manufacturing production (Heidegger, 1954). Fredrick Svenaeus (2013) has also emphasized this

aspect in anorexia nervosa. This phenomenon has a clear relationship with characteristics of postmodernity, the era in which this illness appeared (Doerr-Zegers, 2011). Other characteristics of anorexia nervosa, such as hyperactivity and intellectualism, also have a certain correspondence with postmodernity.

(3) Patients with anorexia try to maintain an absolute power over their body and their needs. Thus, they do not respect hunger, or rest, or the appeal of sex. Their fight against hunger is "to the death," and they employ several techniques for overcoming it, as spending all day filling their mouths with minimal quantities of food (fragments of bread, little pieces of apple, etc.) or dreaming at night of banquets. Some patients of one of us (Otto Doerr-Zegers) used to dream in an insistent and paradoxical way that they ate enormous wedding cakes. This fascination for the dominion and the control of everything (body, persons, and world) comes to the extreme of feeling true pleasure when it occurs in transgressor behaviors, such as kleptomania, for example. All things – good and bad – are to be controlled.

(4) Patients with anorexia experience their body as something obscene, as a degrading show of their intimacy in the public space. Every protuberance, every roundness is lived as an exposition over the public scene (*ob-scene*) of their own personal intimacy, as something disgusting. It is an open and ostensible, bold, and interminable war of the ego with its body. And the obscenity is another characteristic of our postmodernity, as Jean Baudrillard (1988) has shown. We have developed this issue in its relationship with anorexia in another paper (Doerr-Zegers & Pelegrina, 2016).

(5) All these characteristics lead patients with anorexia to a deep sense of abandonment and lack of hope, which no one has described better than Ludwig Binswanger (1957), à propos the case of Ellen West. The patients deal with a cosmic solitude, "lacking every fundamental bond to a global comprehensive structure, which contains, supports, welcomes, and gives sense to their existence" (Pelegrina, 2006a, p. 59). Their world has ceased to be a dwelling.

(6) The question of temporality in anorexia nervosa is a complex one because both kinds of temporality (the implicit and the explicit), which are disturbed in a respectively specific way in the different psychopathological syndromes – such as schizophrenia, depression, and borderline personality (Fuchs & Pallagrosi, 2018) – remain intact. What we find altered is the maturation process, which is detained at the adolescent or pubertal stage. Patients with anorexia do not exist in

the procursive (biographic) time of the creative process of human life. Their life is detained in a sort of adolescent or preadolescent world, and within it their only worry turns and keeps turning around their fight against their object body.

References

American Psychiatric Association. (2013). *Diagnostic and statistical manual of mental disorders* (5th ed., pp. 338–339). Washington, DC: Author.

Baudrillard, J. (1988). *El otro por sí mismo* [The other by himself]. Barcelona, Spain: Anagrama.

Behar, R. (1988). Lo antitético en la anorexia nerviosa [The antithetical in anorexia nervosa]. *Revista Chilena de Neuro-Psiquiatría*, 26, 201–204.

Berner, P. (1983). Wiener Forschungskriterien. Endogenomorph-Zyklothyme Achsensyndrome von Berner [Berner's Vienna research criteria. Endogenomorph-cyclothimic axial syndrome]. In P. Berner, E. Gabriel, H. Katschnig, W. Kieffer, K. Koehler, G. Lenz, & C. Simhandl (Eds.), *Diagnosekriterien für Schizophrene und Affektive Psychosen* [Diagnostic criteria for schizophrenic and affective psychoses] (pp. 165–171). Genf, Switzerland: Weltverband für Psychiatrie.

Binswanger, L. (1957). Der Fall Ellen West [The case Ellen West]. In *Schizophrenie* [Schizophrenia]. Pfullingen, Germany: Neske Verlag.

Binswanger, L. (1960). *Melancholie und Manie* [Melancholia and mania]. Pfullingen, Germany: Neske Verlag.

Blankenburg, W. (1989). Phänomenologie der Leiblichkeit als Grundlage für ein Verständnis der Leiberfahrung psychisch Kranker [Phenomenology of corporeality as fundamental for an understanding of body experience of psychic patients]. *Daseinsanalyse*, 6(3), 161–193.

Bowden, H. A. (2012). A phenomenological study of anorexia nervosa. *Philosophy, Psychiatry & Psychology*, 19(3), 227–241. Retrieved from https://muse.jhu.edu/article/489100

Buytendijk, F. J. J. (1956). *Allgemeine Theorie der menschlichen Haltung und Bewegung* [General theory of human posture and movement]. Berlin, Germany: Springer.

Diebold, K., & Doerr-Zegers, O. (1965). Zum Problem schizophrener Begegnungsweisen [About the problem of schizophrenic forms of encounter]. *Jahrbuch für Psychologie, Psychotherapie und Medizinische Anthropologie*, 12(1–3), 23–36.

Doerr-Zegers, O. (1972a). *Beitrag zum anthropologisch-dynamischen Verständnis der Anorexia Nervosa mit besonderer Berücksichtigung der Familienkonstellation* [Contribution to an anthropological-dynamic understanding of anorexia nervosa]. Jahrbuch der Dissertationen der Medizinischen Fakultät. Heidelberg, Germany: Universitätsverlag.

Doerr-Zegers, O. (1972b). Sobre una forma particular de perversión oral en la mujer joven; hiperfagia y vómito secundario [About a particular form of oral perversion in young women; hyperphagia followed by vomiting]. *Revista Chilena de Neuropsiquiatría*, 11(2), 27–41.

Doerr-Zegers, O. (1979). Análisis fenomenológico de la depresividad en la melancolía y en la epilepsia [Phenomenological analysis of depressivity in melancholy and in epilepsy]. *Actas Luso-Españolas de Neurología, Psiquiatría y Ciencias Afines*, 7(2a. Etapa), 291–304.

Doerr-Zegers, O. (1980). Adicción y temporalidad [Addiction and temporality]. *Psicología Médica*, 5(3), 361–397.

Doerr-Zegers, O. (1985). The role of the family in the pathogenesis of anorexia nervosa. In P. Pichot, P. Berner, R. Wolf, & K. Thau (Eds.), *Psychiatry, the state of the art* (pp. 459–465). Amsterdam, Netherlands: Elsevier.

Doerr-Zegers, O. (1988). La familia de las anorécticas nerviosas [The family of the patients with anorexia nervosa]. *Acta Psiquiátrica y Psicológica de América Latina*, 34(1), 33–40.

Doerr-Zegers, O. (1993). Fenomenología de la corporalidad depresiva [Phenomenology of depressive corporeality]. *Salud Mental*, 16(3), 22–30.

Doerr-Zegers, O. (1994). About a particular type of oral perversion in the female: Hyperphagia followed by vomiting. *International Journal of Eating Disorders*, 16(2), 117–132.

Doerr-Zegers, O. (2011). Die Postmoderne und die Frage nach dem Sinne [Postmodernity and the question of the meaning]. In *Das Wort und die Musik* [The word and the music] (pp. 165–178). Würzburg, Germany: Königshausen & Neumann.

Doerr-Zegers, O., Enríquez, G., & Jara, C. (1971). Del análisis clínico-estadístico del síndrome depresivo a una comprensión del fenómeno de la depresividad en su contexto patogénico [From the clinical-statistical analysis of depressive syndrome to an understanding of the phenomenon of depressivity in its pathogenetic context]. *Revista Chilena de Neuropsiquiatría*, 10(1), 17–39.

Doerr-Zegers, O., & Pelegrina, H. (2016). Anorexia nervosa: Historical, clinical, biographic and phenomenological considerations. In G. Stanghellini & M. Aragona (Eds.), *An experiential approach to psychopathology* (pp. 127–147). New York, NY: Springer.

Doerr-Zegers, O., Petrasic, J., & Morales, E. (1976). Familia y biografía en la patogénesis de la anorexia nerviosa [Family and biography in the pathogenesis of anorexia nervosa]. *Revista Chilena de Neuropsiquiatría*, 15(1), 3–26.

Fuchs, T. (2003). The phenomenology of shame, guilt and the body in body dysmorphic disorder and depression. *Journal of Phenomenological Psychology*, 33(2), 223–243. doi:10.1163/15691620260622903

Fuchs, T. (2005). Corporealized and disembodied minds. A phenomenological view of the body in melancholia and schizophrenia. *Philosophy, Psychiatry & Psychology*, 12(2), 95–107. doi:10.1353/ppp.2005.0040

Fuchs, T. (2013). Depression, intercorporeality, and interaffectivity. *Journal of Consciousness Studies*, 20(7–8), 219–238.

Fuchs, T., & De Jaegher, H. (2009). Enactive intersubjectivity: Participatory sense-making and mutual incorporation. *Phenomenology and the Cognitive Sciences*, 8, 465–486. doi:10.1007/s11097-009-9136-4

Fuchs, T., & Pallagrosi, M. (2018). Phenomenology of temporality and dimensional psychopathology. In M. Biondi, M. Pasquini, & A. Picardi (Eds.),

Dimensional psychopathology (pp. 287–300). Cham, Switzerland: Springer. doi:10.1007/978-3-319-78202-7_10

Gallwitz, A. (1965). Versuch einer experimentellen Erfassung des body image bei weiblichen Magersüchtigen [Attempt of an experimental apprehension of body image in female anorectics]. In J.-E. Meyer & H. Feldmann (Eds.), *Anorexia nervosa* (pp. 139–141). Stuttgart, Germany: Georg Thieme.

Heidegger, M. (1954). Die Frage nach der Technik [The question concerning technology]. In *Vorträge und Aufsätze* (pp. 9–40). Pfullingen, Germany: Neske.

Jaspers, K. (1963). Kausale und "verständliche" Zusammenhänge zwischen Schicksal und Psychose bei der Dementia praecox (Schizophrenie) [Causal and "understandable" coherences between fate and psychosis in dementia praecox]. In *Gesammelte Schriften zur Psychopathologie* [Collected writings on psychopathology] (pp. 329–344). Berlin, Germany: Springer.

Lasègue, C. (1873). De l'anorexie hystérique. *Archives of General Internal Medicine*, 21, 385.

Legrand, D. (2010). Subjective and physical dimensions of bodily self-consciousness, and their dis-integration in anorexia nervosa. *Neuropsychologia*, 48(3), 726–737. doi:10.1016/j.neuropsychologia.2009.08.026

Legrand, D., & Briend, F. (2015). Anorexia and bodily intersubjectivity. *European Psychologist*, 20(1), 52–61. doi:10.1027/1016-9040/a000208

Marcel, G. (1955). *Être et avoir* [To be and to have]. Paris, France: Montaigne.

Marcel, G. (1978). Leibliche Begegnung: Notizen aus einem gemeinsamen Gedankengang [Bodily encounter: notes from a shared way of thinking"?]. In A. Kraus (Ed.), *Leib - Geist - Geschichte: Brennpunkte anthropologischer Forschung* [*Lived body - Mind - History: focusing on anthropological research*]. Commemorative Publication for the 60th Anniversary of Hubertus Tellenbach (pp. 47–73). Heidelberg, Germany: Hüthig.

Merleau-Ponty, M. (1957). *Fenomenología de la percepción* [Phenomenology of perception]. Ciudad de México, Mexico: Fondo de Cultura Económica. (Original work published 1945).

Ortega y Gasset, J. (1964). La aparición del otro [The appearance of the other]. In *Obras Completas. Tomo VII* (pp. 124–140). Madrid, Spain: Revista de Occidente.

Parnas, J. (2000). The self and intentionality in the pre-psychotic stages of schizophrenia. In D. Zahavi (Ed.), *Exploring the self: Philosophical and psychopathological perspectives on self-experience* (pp. 115–147). Amsterdam, Netherlands: John Benjamins.

Pelegrina, H. (2006a). *Mundo de vida y psicopatologia: la anorexia nerviosa* [Life world and psychopathology: The anorexia nervosa]. Madrid, Spain: Monografias de Psiquatría.

Pelegrina, H. (2006b). *Fundamentos antropológicos de la psicopatología* [Anthropological foundations of psychopathology]. Madrid, Spain: Ediciones Polifemo.

Pelegrina, H. (2017). *Psicopatología regional. Estructuras dimensionales de la psicopatología. Logopatías y timopatías* [Regional psychopathology. Dimensional structures of psychopathology. Logopathies and Tymopathies]. Buenos Aires, Argentina: Editorial Polemos.

Ricoeur, P. (1990). *Soi-même comme un autre* [Oneself as another]. Paris, France: Seuil.

Sass, L. (2001). Self and world in schizophrenia: Three classic approaches in phenomenological psychiatry. *Philosophy, Psychiatry & Psychology*, 8(4), 251–270. doi:10.1353/ppp.2002.0026

Stanghellini, G. (2019). Embodiment and the other's look in feeding and eating disorders. *World Psychiatry*, 18(3), 364–365. doi:10.1002&wps.20683

Stanghellini, G., Castellini, G., Brogna, P., Faravelli, C., & Ricca, V. (2012). Identity and eating disorders (IDEA): A questionnaire evaluating identity and embodiment in eating disorder patients. *Psychopathology*, 45(3), 147–158. doi:10.1159/000330258

Stanghellini, G., & Mancini, M. (2019). Abnormal time experiences in persons with feeding and eating disorder: A naturalistic explorative study. *Phenomenology and the Cognitive Sciences*, 18(4), 759–773. doi:10.1007/s11097-019-09618-5

Straus, E. (1960). Das Zeiterlebnis in der endogenen Depression und in der psychopathischen Verstimmung [The experience of time in endogenous depression and psychopathic dysthymia]. In *Psychologie der menschlichen Welt. Gesammelte Schriften* [Psychology of the human world. Collected writings] (pp. 126–144). Berlin, Germany: Springer.

Svenaeus, F. (2013). Anorexia nervosa and the body uncanny: A phenomenological approach. *Philosophy, Psychiatry & Psychology*, 20(1), 81–91. doi:10.1353/ppp.2013.0012

Thomae, H. (1961). *Anorexia nervosa*. Bern, Switzerland: Huber-Klett.

Varela, F. J., Thompson, E., & Rosch, E. (1991). *The embodied mind. Cognitive science and human experience*. Cambridge, MA: Massachusetts Institute of Technology Press.

von Gebsattel, V. (1954). Störungen des Werdens und des Zeiterlebens im Rahmen psychiatrischer Erkrankungen [Perturbations of becoming and of experience of time in the framework of psychiatric illnesses]. In *Prolegomena einer anthropologischen Medizin* [Prolegomena of an anthropological medicine] (pp. 128–144). Berlin, Germany: Springer.

Von Weizsäcker, V. (1950). *Der Gestaltkreis. Theorie der Einheit von Wahrnehmen und Bewegen* [The Gestaltkreis. Theory of the unity of perception and movement]. Stuttgart, Germany: Georg Thieme.

Whitehead, A. N. (1978). *Process and reality* (corr. ed.). New York, NY: Free Press. (Original work published 1929)

Zutt, J. (1963). Über den Stand des in Erscheinung stehenden Menschen [About the position of man as a being that manifests himself]. In *Auf dem Wege zu einer Anthropologischen Psychiatrie* [Towards an anthropological psychiatry] (pp. 410–416). Berlin, Germany: Springer. doi:10.1007/978-3-642-85694-5_22

12.1

Commentary on "Phenomenology of Corporeality (and Spatiality) in Anorexia Nervosa with a Reference to the Problem of Its Temporality"

Anorexia Nervosa: Linking the Phenomenology to Cultural and Neuropsychological Aspects of the Disease

Adrian P. Mundt

Otto Doerr-Zegers and Héctor Pelegrina-Cetran (2021) elaborate a phenomenology of corporeality and temporality in anorexia nervosa. With respect to the corporeality, they describe a fragmentation of the polarity between subject-body as a corporealized being in the world and the object-body as a mere thing. In patients with anorexia nervosa, the self develops disgust and rejection of the volumetric-physical body, which is accompanied by intellectualization and rationalization. Instead of living through the own body in the world, patients with anorexia develop an eagerness to control their own bodies, such as a fetish, as from the exterior. This can result in the continuous desire to eliminate the spatial dimension of the own body that is perceived as a threat.

Remarkable are five paradoxes of anorexia nervosa developed here that invite the reader to think about anorexia in an innovative way: the antitheses between cachexia and motor hyperactivity; affective dependence, often on the mother, and incapacity to engage in real affective bonds or intimate relationships; intellectual maturity and emotional immaturity including desires to not grow up; the need to make disappear the own body and to appear with cultural achievements; interest in regular treatment, but uneasiness with weight gain, which is defined as successful outcome of treatment processes.

The authors present differential alterations of the corporeality in anorexia nervosa, body dysmorphic disorder, depression, and schizophrenia that are clinically useful. Regarding the differentiation between anorexia nervosa and body dysmorphic disorders, findings presented here can complement and inform neurobiological psychometric and imaging research developed for this purpose (Vaughn et al., 2019) and psychometric research (Toh, Grace, Rossell, Castle, & Phillipou, 2020). The dysmorphic concern in anorexia nervosa is typically about zones that are linked to weight gain, whereas in body dysmorphic disorders the typical concerns are about facial features, hair, and skin (Toh et al., 2020).

Doerr-Zegers and Pelegrina-Cetran also contrast the temporality in patients with anorexia with those with schizophrenia, depression, and borderline personality disorder. They refer that implicit temporality is disturbed in schizophrenia resulting in a fragmentation of the structure that time consciousness typically has in the form of retention, presentation, and protention. In melancholic depression, the flow of time consciousness is retarded and inhibited. In contrast, for borderline personality disorder, a disturbance of explicit temporality was described consisting of difficulties to form a coherent self-concept and identity. The authors do not find any disturbance of implicit or explicit temporality in anorexia nervosa. This delineation is surprising given that many people with borderline personality disorders go through episodes of anorexia and may be useful for differentiating the two disorders. The authors further describe a lack of living temporality in anorexia nervosa manifesting as a rejection of growth, maturation, and constructive evolution.

It may add to this chapter that the influence of Western culture has widely been recognized in anorexia nervosa (Banks, 1992). In medieval to Victorian times, self-starvation in women had religious value. Food refusal and sexual abstinence were forms of religious asceticism. The rejection of bodily desires was linked to purity and higher forms of spirituality. The historically described religious asceticism may correspond to the intellectualization and ambitiousness for cultural achievements in contemporary manifestations of anorexia described by Doerr-Zegers and Pelegrina-Cetran. An extreme form of dualism was overcome by eliminating the body and becoming pure spirit. The religious type of motivational component may be less frequent nowadays, but still has a role in contemporary forms of anorexia nervosa (Banks, 1992). In contrast, the popular ideal of thinness currently in vogue as dieting may be the main cultural component in most current types of more transitory and adolescent anorexia. The influence of parents, peers, and the media has been described as the key sociocultural components for the internalization of a thin ideal and appearance comparisons that can lead to appearance dissatisfaction (Munro, Randell, & Lawrie, 2017). Recent research has focused less on causing, but on disease maintaining factors, such as carer accommodation, which is a process of assisting or participating of parents or close others in symptomatic behaviors (Fox & Whittlesea, 2017; Salerno et al., 2016).

Self-criticism and perfectionism have been identified as key phenomena in eating disorders (Dahlenburg, Gleaves, & Hutchinson, 2019). The developmental counterpart of perfectionism and its pathological elements are parental criticism and concern over mistakes (Sapuppo, Ruggiero, Caselli, & Sassaroli, 2018). Self-criticism associates with low self-esteem and rumination and may be even harsher in eating disorders compared with depression and perceived as part of the personality (Thew, Gregory, Roberts, & Rimes, 2017). The weight-related worries lead to a long-standing negative self-evaluation. Recent research has proposed to add further cognitive and metacognitive variables (Sapuppo et al., 2018): the need for control, negative beliefs about worry, uncontrollability and danger, and self-esteem. As Doerr-Zegers and Pelegrina-Cetran stated, the need for control can go beyond the eating behavior itself. It can include large parts of the intrapersonal and emotional life as well as the interpersonal world, which can lead to social isolation, especially in the restrictive type of anorexia nervosa (Fairburn, Cooper, & Shafran, 2003). The perception of lack of control has been linked to anxiety. The continuous monitoring of body weight can improve the subjective sense of being in control in a world that is perceived as uncontrollable. Worry is a perseverative preoccupation in patients with anorexia about food, body weight, and aspects of the body. High levels of negative beliefs about worrying can lead to an escalating cycle and increase the sense of uncontrollability (Sapuppo et al., 2018). When worrying is perceived as dangerous, but it is not considered safe to stop worrying, the fear about fatness may increase.

Furthermore, there is a large body of evidence on dysfunctional processing and regulation of emotions in anorexia nervosa (Munro et al., 2017). Those include experiences and beliefs of being inadequate, disgusting, needy, greedy, and shameful. This experience has also been called a "feared self" who will be criticized by others. From a behavioral perspective, starvation and over-activity may be maladaptive coping with this experience of vulnerability and inadequacy (Munro et al., 2017). An impaired reflexive function has been described resulting in closeness of emotional and physical experiences (Skarderud, 2007). Anxiety and depression in anorexia nervosa were associated with higher levels of body image disturbance or dysmorphic concern (Beilharz et al., 2019). Levels of dysmorphic concern also predict relapse in anorexia nervosa (Beilharz et al., 2019).

In conclusion, the phenomenological contributions to the understanding of anorexia nervosa presented here by Doerr-Zegers and Pelegrina-Cetran are original. They can interact with and complement research on cultural, social, psychological, and biological models of anorexia nervosa. Moreover, the contribution has the potential to inform the refinement of psychotherapeutic interventions for the disease.

References

Banks, C. G. (1992). 'Culture' in culture-bound syndromes: The case of anorexia nervosa. *Social Science and Medicine*, 34(8), 867–884. doi:10.1016/0277-9536(92)90256-p

Beilharz, F., Phillipou, A., Castle, D., Jenkins, Z., Cistullo, L., & Rossell, S. (2019). Dysmorphic concern in anorexia nervosa: Implications for recovery. *Psychiatry Research*, 273, 657–661. doi:10.1016/j.psychres.2019.01.102

Dahlenburg, S. C., Gleaves, D. H., & Hutchinson, A. D. (2019). Anorexia nervosa and perfectionism: A meta-analysis. *International Journal of Eating Disorders*, 52(3), 219–229. doi:10.1002/eat.23009

Doerr-Zegers, O., & Pelegrina-Cetran, H. (2021). Phenomenology of corporeality (and spatiality) in anorexia nervosa with a reference to the problem of its temporality. In C. Tewes & G. Stanghellini (Eds.), *Time and body: Phenomenological and psychopathological approaches* (pp. 263–281). Cambridge, UK: Cambridge University Press.

Fairburn, C. G., Cooper, Z., & Shafran, R. (2003). Cognitive behaviour therapy for eating disorders: A "transdiagnostic" theory and treatment. *Behaviour Research and Therapy*, 41(5), 509–528. doi:10.1016/s0005-7967(02)00088-8

Fox, J. R., & Whittlesea, A. (2017). Accommodation of symptoms in anorexia nervosa: A qualitative study. *Clinical Psychology & Psychotherapy*, 24(2), 488–500. doi:10.1002/cpp.2020

Munro, C., Randell, L., & Lawrie, S. M. (2017). An integrative bio-psycho-social theory of anorexia nervosa. *Clinical Psychology & Psychotherapy*, 24(1), 1–21. doi:10.1002/cpp.2047

Salerno, L., Rhind, C., Hibbs, R., Micali, N., Schmidt, U., Gowers, S., … Treasure, J. (2016). An examination of the impact of care giving styles (accommodation and skilful communication and support) on the one year outcome of adolescent anorexia nervosa: Testing the assumptions of the cognitive interpersonal model in anorexia nervosa. *Journal of Affective Disorders*, 191, 230–236. doi:10.1016/j.jad.2015.11.016

Sapuppo, W., Ruggiero, G. M., Caselli, G., & Sassaroli, S. (2018). The body of cognitive and metacognitive variables in eating disorders: Need of control, negative beliefs about worry uncontrollability and danger, perfectionism, self-esteem and worry. *Israel Journal of Psychiatry and Related Sciences*, 55(1), 55–63.

Skarderud, F. (2007). Eating one's words: Part III. Mentalisation-based psychotherapy for anorexia nervosa – An outline for a treatment and training manual. *European Eating Disorders Review*, 15(5), 323–339. doi:10.1002/erv.817

Thew, G. R., Gregory, J. D., Roberts, K., & Rimes, K. A. (2017). The phenomenology of self-critical thinking in people with depression, eating disorders, and in healthy individuals. *Psychology and Psychotherapy*, 90(4), 751–769. doi:10.1111/papt.12137

Toh, W. L., Grace, S. A., Rossell, S. L., Castle, D. J., & Phillipou, A. (2020). Body parts of clinical concern in anorexia nervosa versus body dysmorphic disorder: a cross-diagnostic comparison. *Australas Psychiatry*. 28(2), 134–139. doi:10.1177/1039856219839477

Vaughn, D. A., Kerr, W. T., Moody, T. D., Cheng, G. K., Morfini, F., Zhang, A., … Feusner, J. D. (2019). Differentiating weight-restored anorexia nervosa and body dysmorphic disorder using neuroimaging and psychometric markers. *PLoS One*, 14(5), 1–16. doi:10.1371/journal.pone.0213974

PART IV

Depression, Schizophrenia, and Dementia

13

Intrinsic Temporality in Depression

Classical Phenomenological Psychiatry, Affectivity, and Narrative

Edward A. Lenzo and Shaun Gallagher

Introduction

Studies of depression suggest that in depressed persons abnormal dynamical synchronies exist between the various factors of first-person perspective, bodily/emotional agency, and reflective (narrative-related) agency, as evidenced in both phenomenology and dynamical connections across correlated brain areas (Fingelkurts & Fingelkurts, 2017; Gallagher & Daly, 2018). With reference to these anomalies, there is a long-standing view in phenomenological psychopathology, reinforced by empirical studies, about disruptions of the experience of temporality in depression. Erwin Straus (1947, p. 254), for example, characterizes depression as an alteration in the "basic structure of space and time." Common complaints include those of time slowing down or stopping, the past as distant, the future as empty and hopeless. Fuchs (2013) describes this as a reification of time. More recently, a growing (although still somewhat scattered) consensus around this view links problems with the intrinsic temporality of experience to disorders involving affect, affordances, and narrative aspects of experience, understanding these links in terms of enactive approaches to cognition and dynamical systems theory.

In this chapter, we offer a phenomenologically inspired enactivist interpretation of how disordered temporal experience relates to the structure of intrinsic temporality, which much of phenomenological psychopathology takes as its starting point. Our intention is to make the aforementioned consensus more apparent and to offer some specification to the phenomenological analysis.

Intrinsic Temporality

In most of the phenomenological discussions of disturbances in temporal experience, reference is made to Husserl's analysis of intrinsic temporality ("internal time-consciousness"). We start with a brief primer of Husserl's analysis.

Husserl analyzes intrinsic temporality by making evident the structure of the living present or current moment of experience. The living present is constituted by a threefold temporal synthesis – the recent past, present, and immediate future. The living present thus has a unified structure consisting of three forms of intentionality, each unique, but concretely inseparable from one another: primal impression, retention, and protention.[1] Primal impression is our directedness toward what is now, retention toward the past, and protention toward the open-ended future. As the moment fades away, what was disclosed "runs-off" into the past, with retention appresenting these more and more distant pasts precisely *as past*, and as increasingly removed. Protention points toward the future as a possibility of change, as the present will pass away. This anticipation of change is informed by what is already disclosed through current impression and retention.

To illustrate this intrinsic temporal structure, consider Husserl's favorite example: consciousness of a melody. At a given moment, you are aware of a particular note, for example, B, as the one that currently sounds. However, in order to perceive that note as part of a melody rather than as a singular note in isolation, you must also be aware of the notes that were previously given, for example, G. Furthermore, the past note G cannot currently be given in precisely the same way as the currently sounding note, B, or else they would be given together not as a melody but as a chord. G is thus cointended alongside B, but specifically *as* already past, as prior to B. That is, while your impression is of B, you retain G, as a modification of the previous impression of G, and this is necessary for the constitution of the melody as a temporal object. In the other direction, upon hearing B, following G, you are directed toward the future as a possibility of change. Minimally, protention is the current awareness of the possible future that shapes the current experience. Perhaps the melody will continue or is already complete; perhaps B will linger or will be cut off as quickly as it arose. If you have studied some music, you might be conscious of the possibility of a particular note sounding, for example, you might expect

[1] Retention, primal impression, and protention may be considered forms of operative (*fungierende*) intentionality distinguished from act-intentionality. Specifically, these moments of intrinsic temporality involve an intentional direction toward past, present, and future, respectively, although they are not acts of consciousness in the full sense of having a noetic-noematic structure or of being a kind of object-awareness. Husserl calls protention a "passive intentionality," for example (Husserl, 2001, p. 181), and describes retention as involving a double (transverse and longitudinal) intentionality (*Querintentionalität* and *Längsintentionalität*).

the completion of the G major arpeggio, protentionally directed toward D. If D does not subsequently sound, then the arpeggio may be experienced as incomplete. If the next note is flat, the entire melody – not any isolated note – will be dissonant. Our awareness of the melody as a unified temporal phenomenon depends on the threefold structure formed by impression, retention, and protention.

This structure – "the form of time-consciousness" – belongs to what Husserl calls *primary passivity* and is characterized as "the most universal genetic structure" (Husserl, 2001, p. 184). Other syntheses of primary passivity include those of sensory association and affection, the latter of which we will treat in depth in the third section. According to Husserl, syntheses of primary passivity occur without any contribution of the "ego," and thus are contrasted with the active syntheses that presuppose egoic processes. Syntheses of primary passivity establish the form of consciousness in general; the ego then plays a role in modifying what is thus constituted. This modification first belongs to the sphere of "active synthesis," or genuine activity on the part of the ego. There is also a sphere of "secondary passivity," which consists of sedimentation and habitus, or meanings and motivations that have been built up over time through active synthesis. A key feature of Husserl's analysis is that the temporal structure (or form) of experience is intentional, so it is never without the something that is being experienced (call this intentional content). Form and content are, in this sense, inseparable from one another. Yet, they are abstractly distinguishable, and Husserl distinguishes them for purposes of analysis. For instance, at the formal level, he writes that the form of time-consciousness is

> the most general and most primary synthesis that necessarily connects all particular objects of which we become conscious originally in passivity as being, no matter what their content may be and however else they may be constituted as unitary objects with respect to content. (Husserl, 2001, p. 173)

However, he also acknowledges that "mere form" is "an abstraction" (Husserl, 2001, p. 173). For Husserl, the formal structure of intrinsic temporality is thus independent of any *specific* content of experience, though always only experienced in concrete unity with some content or other; it is the foundational framework in which any content can be experienced at all, or, as he puts it:

> In the ABC's of the constitution of all objectivity given to consciousness and of subjectivity as existing for itself, here is the "A." It consists, as we might say, in a universal, formal framework, in a synthetically constituted form in which all other possible syntheses must participate. (Husserl, 2001, p. 170)

Nevertheless, other syntheses are necessary for the constitution of objectivity and subjectivity, including the primary passive syntheses of association and affection, which are inseparable from the contents of experience. He writes that "these syntheses run their course together with the synthesis constituting the temporal form of all objects, and thus must co-relate to the temporal content, the temporally formed content of the object" (Husserl, 2001, p. 171). The form of intrinsic temporality is thus abstractly distinguishable, but concretely inseparable, from temporal (or, generally, experiential) contents. Put another way, there is no "how" of experience without some "what." We note, in anticipation, that we will offer a more complex notion of content than the one that ties neatly to form in Husserl's analysis – one that involves not only affectivity, but action-related aspects of embodiment and affordance-based conceptions of environmental contexts.

To summarize, regarding form, retention and protention are understood as designating horizonal structures against which the present becomes meaningfully articulated: The present takes on its meaning and position against a background of the past and an open horizon of the future. In this respect, intrinsic temporality constitutes the living present as a synthetic unity and constrains an ordering of experience in terms of temporal positioning. With regard to content, retention and protention take on somewhat more familiar meanings: Retention discloses what has recently passed, and protention discloses what could soon occur. The unification of experiential content – "the constitution of all objectivity given to consciousness and of subjectivity as existing for itself" - depends on more than mere, formal temporality, however. Additional syntheses are required for such achievements.

Husserl's account motivates a three-way distinction between form, content, and the *filling of form*, with the latter depending also on association and affection.[2] Articulating the filling of form as a kind of intermediary between form and content allows us to understand how there can be alterations to lived or experiential temporality without positing a disruption of the most fundamental temporal structure of experience. As we will show, this allows us to interpret reports and characterizations of depressive

[2] Husserl (2001, p. 212) explains the filling of form in this way: "[T]he filling of these forms, which makes the concrete formed unities possible, is subject to the special conditions of concrescence and contrast. Affection accompanies the connections; only insofar as the conditions of materially relevant or figurative homogeneity are fulfilled such that syntheses of coinciding can be formed in being adjoined or at a distance, can the affective framework exist and can the affections propagate, can the current affective force be augmented, etc." The second and third sections shed some light on the significance of this passage.

experience without positing such a fundamental disruption; indeed, the reports themselves do not, it seems to us, require such a posit.[3]

Phenomenological Psychopathology and Intrinsic Temporality

Many of the most influential classic thinkers in phenomenological psychopathology have taken Husserl's intrinsic temporality as a starting point for their analyses. Here, we will summarize the views of Minkowski, Binswanger, Straus, and Jaspers, focusing on their respective characterizations of depressive experience in terms of temporal alterations and distortions. The work of these phenomenological psychiatrists is open to different interpretations, specifically with respect to the kind of phenomenology at stake in their work (see, e.g., Tatossian, 1979). On the one hand, it is possible to read Minkowski, Binswanger, and Straus as embracing a transcendental–philosophical phenomenology that emphasizes form or intentional structure more than affective processes. Both Jaspers and Tatossian read them that way. On the other hand, one can highlight the emphasis on clinical observation and description that is found in their work. We acknowledge this tension, and in our own interpretation, we steer away from the transcendental interpretation, although we find this easier to do, for example, with Straus than with Minkowski.

Minkowski (1970) uses Husserl's analysis to identify problems with intrinsic temporality in depression, which, he argues, is the generative disorder in depression. It is notable that empirical studies confirm that persons with depression have a slowed experience of time flow and that they tend to underestimate time spans (Bschor et al., 2004; Mahlberg, Kienast, Bschor, & Adli, 2008). In comparison with control subjects, depressed patients tend to be preoccupied with past events, and less focused on the present and future events (Wyrick & Wyrick, 1977). These empirical studies are consistent with the interpretation proposed by Minkowski from a clinical–phenomenological perspective.

Consistent – but Minkowski does not address precisely the same aspects of temporality. Experimental studies often emphasize changes in perceived (measurable) duration, whereas Minkowski focuses on

[3] On a strictly transcendental reading of Husserl's analysis, one might argue that primary passive temporal synthesis is a necessary condition for any consciousness whatsoever. As such, a dissolution of this synthesis would result not in altered experience, but in the lack of experience altogether. We don't endorse such a strong position. Instead, our claim is that positing such a dissolution is not warranted by the available evidence.

changes in the intrinsic structure of temporal experience. His focus is on disordered structural or generating aspects. In the case of depression, this is a disorder of experiential temporality rather than the ideo-emotional content; that is, it is more about *how* the subject is experiencing rather than *what* the subject is experiencing. In other words, experience in depression involves modifications to structural aspects of experience and not simply to intentional content or phenomenal aspects. To get some clarity on this, Minkowski references Husserl's analysis of the temporal structure of consciousness. Disruptions or distortions of retentional or protentional aspects can result in temporally distorted experiences. Connected with a slowing of experiential time, there is a reorientation away from the future (protentional) toward present and especially past (retentional) dimensions. Describing Minkowski's view, Cardinalli (2012, p. 30) notes that for patients with depression, "the future is perceived as blocked; their attention is directed to the past and the present feels stagnant." As a result of this deeper disorder of temporality in depression, time "seems to slow down remarkably, even to stop; and this modification of the temporal structure seems to be interposed between the subjacent biological order, on the one hand, and the usual clinical symptoms on the other" (Minkowski, 1970, p. 298). Minkowski suggests, without further specification, that the temporal modification is reflected in a biological disorder.

It is important to note here that, while there is apparently a difference in the *how* of experience, and this undoubtedly involves temporal alterations, this does not necessarily indicate a difference in the fundamental form of intrinsic temporality, that is, a disruption of primary passive temporal synthesis. For Husserl (2001, pp. 170–172), the formal aspect of intrinsic temporality is a necessary feature of any and every consciousness. Importantly, the maintenance of intrinsic temporality as a formal synthesis of past, present, and future modes of intentionality can be witnessed even in a slowing of the experience of time, underestimation of time, or orientation within time: Precisely, these all presuppose time as already constituted. Any phenomenon of duration or temporal orientation, or the positioning of events and objects in time, presupposes a temporality that divides between (in terms of intentional modality) but also unifies concretely the past, present, and future. In depression, redirection away from the future and toward the past presupposes an already constituted future, present, and past, a kind of temporal milieu in which orientation toward any temporal feature becomes intelligible at all. That the form of time-consciousness is here maintained (as evidenced by Husserl's conceptual framework as well as Cardinalli's and Minkowski's description of the phenomena), however, does not mean that depression is incorrectly characterized in terms of temporality: Retention and protention are relevant when we consider not just the form of time-consciousness or the content experienced and ordered in time, but also the ways in which content comes to be experienced in time, that is, when we consider the filling of form. In the third section, we develop the claim that we can best understand depressive experience in terms of primary passive syntheses of affectivity, rather than intrinsic temporality, which, as inseparable from the filling of form necessary for "all objectivity" and "subjectivity as existing for itself," conditions the *how* of our temporal experience.

Ludwig Binswanger also takes the work of Husserl, as well as Heidegger, as the starting point for his "existential analysis," or *Daseinsanalyse* (Bloc, Souza, & Moreira, 2016). Accepting Husserl's analysis of temporality, he characterizes depression and melancholia as a disruption in the normal interplay of protention, primal impression, and retention. The ways in which this interplay can be transformed are understood as two directions of "infiltration," termed "retrospection" and "prospection." As Bloc et al. (2016, p. 295) write of Binswanger's position:

> Melancholic retrospection is characterized by infiltration of retention into protention … it produces a discussion of empty possibilities, protentive acts of a past without any possibilities.… In melancholic prospection the future is seen as lost, impossible.… The melancholic "knows that foreseen loss in the future is already a reality" (Binswanger, 1960/2005, p. 48).

Again we here see a conceptualization of depression in terms of disruptions to processes of retention and protention. Although this is not an inapt description, we must keep in mind the ways in which such disruptions are both conceptually possible and empirically justified. One way of understanding Binswanger's claim is that what is objectively past is experienced in the mode of protention, that is, in the mode of the possible future, or that what is objectively future is experienced in the mode of retention, that is, as already past, dead, "impossible." But again, we see that this presupposes an already constituted intrinsic temporality according to which there is a future in which loss may be foreseen; there is a past, albeit empty. What is described here is not a loss of retention or protention, considered as strictly formal, but rather alterations in temporal associations between past and future, resulting in a change to the way in which temporal contents are experienced. We are again led to an analysis of depressive experience that is not reducible to that of a disruption of the formal structure of time-consciousness, while nevertheless undeniably involving temporal peculiarities; an analysis according to which what is in question is precisely the normal interplay between these temporal modes of intentionality such that the way in which contents are experienced is fundamentally altered.

Erwin Straus' view of depression pinpoints the way in which these disruptions are plausibly instituted. According to Straus, depression involves a "disharmony" within temporal experience. Here, however, the posited disruption is not to primary passive temporal synthesis but rather occurs between "immanent" and "experience-transcending" or "objective" time (Moskalewicz, 2018, p. 68; Moskalewicz provides a table that tracks Straus' expression of this dualism throughout his works). Husserl also refers to "objective time," and by understanding its relationship to intrinsic temporality, we can better situate Straus' position. Husserl writes: "In the flow of time, in the continuous sinking down into the past, a nonflowing, absolutely fixed, identical, objective time becomes constituted. This is the problem" (Husserl, 1991, p. 67). The constitution of objective time depends on the form of intrinsic temporality, as does the constitution of all objectivities, but bridging this gap – the filling of form – is a problem his theory must address. Straus hones in on this gap as the site of the disruption posited as characterizing depressive experience. He theorizes that depressive (as well as schizophrenic) experience involves a loss of the ordinary, healthy connection between one's lived experience of time and the ordinary time that we track by dates, clocks, etc. (Moskalewicz, 2018).

Interestingly, this conception of temporal disruption in psychopathology nicely corresponds to some experiments that attempt to measure temporal discrepancies in persons with depression. For example, Hsu, Lee, Lane, and Missal (2019) conclude that temporal processing is altered in persons who undergo major depressive disorder, and that this alteration is connected to abnormal time experience in such persons. They write:

> Based on questionnaires, depressed patients report often a "slowing down" of subjective time (Blewett, 1992; Ratcliffe, 2012; see review in Droit-Volet, 2013). This desynchronization between the subjective experience of time and physical time seems to be a characteristic of depressive states without being systematically studied and compared with other cognitive functions. (Hsu et al., 2019, p. 10)

Understanding this desynchronization as closely related to Straus' "disharmony," their findings constitute a striking confirmation of Straus' phenomenological analysis and are also consistent with the theses, as interpreted earlier, of Minkowski and Binswanger. Thomas Fuchs also characterizes depression as resulting from a desynchronization between "organism and environment" or "individual and society" and relates desynchronization to "disturbances of time" (Fuchs, 2001). In this respect, we take Fuchs to be in agreement with Straus' account.

We turn finally to the thought of Karl Jaspers, who is sometimes credited with founding the field of phenomenological psychopathology with the publication of his *General Psychopathology* (1913/1997). Jaspers takes up Husserl's early descriptive methodology (as found in his *Logical Investigations* (Husserl, 1900–1901/1970)) but does not endorse Husserl's later development of the transcendental phenomenological approach (see Luft, 2008; Thoma, 2014), which he takes Minkowski, for example, to practice. Jaspers partially characterizes certain psychopathological conditions, including depression, in terms of a loss of the ordinary sense of time; he takes seriously reports from patients of a "loss of time," and of time "going backward" or "standing still" (Jaspers, 1913/1997, p. 84). He writes that "Some psychathenic or depressive patients describe this experience as follows: 'It feels as if it is always the same moment, it is like a timeless void'" (1913/1997, p. 84). While this may seem somewhat consistent with Minkowski, Binswanger, and Straus, Jaspers rejects what he takes to be the formal analysis of intentionality embraced by those thinkers (see Jaspers, 1913/1997, pp. 540–546).

In later editions of *General Psychopathology*, Jaspers distinguishes between descriptive phenomenology that aims at understanding an entire person in the context of their personal world from scientific explanation or causal analysis.[4] Phenomenological understanding is limited, but so is scientific explanation. Specifically, he writes that "The basic disturbance that is theoretically deduced is ill defined and of shifting significance" (Jaspers, 1913/1997, p. 543) and that "An empirical proof of a definite disturbance in becoming cannot be produced" (Jaspers, 1913/1997, p. 544). As Thoma explains:

> In understanding, we come up against the unintelligible time and time again. At these points, Jaspers claims that we must revert to models of explanation based on that which is outside of consciousness. He moreover considers the prospects of explanatory psychology to be limited in a different sense: namely, in determining man as a whole. This whole is, for him, both incomprehensible (*unverstehbar*) and inexplicable. (Thoma, 2014, p. 91)

[4] Elsewhere in *General Psychopathology*, Jaspers establishes that psychological understanding is situated somewhere between existential or philosophical understanding and causal explanation.

The second part of Jaspers' objection – that "empirical proof of a definite disturbance in becoming [of the kinds posited by Minkowski and Straus] cannot be produced" – is interesting for at least two reasons. First, it would seem that experimental studies such as those cited thus far falsify his complaint by producing empirical evidence of something like the disturbances posited by the phenomenologists in question. It is not clear that the kind of evidence provided falls short of "proof" in any way meaningfully different from the conclusions of other kinds of experiments. Second, Jaspers takes empirical proof of these disturbances to be impossible partly due to his interpretation of these kinds of analyses (as in Minkowski, Binswanger, and Straus) as making claims about purely formal (transcendental) aspects of experience. If the claim of these psychiatrists is that basic disturbances in depression are located within the most basic syntheses of intrinsic temporality, analyzable independent of any particular content, then this part of Jaspers' objection may be right. We have suggested, however, that interpretations of classical phenomenological psychopathology as positing a disturbance at the most foundational level of the intrinsic temporality of primary passivity are somewhat ambiguous, perhaps conflating different aspects of temporal experience, and are at any rate not the only interpretations possible. Specifically, on our interpretation, and we think also for most contemporary phenomenological thinkers, form and content are thought to be inseparable from one another, and our interpretation in particular strives to be unambiguous about the relationship between these aspects. Accounts that locate the disturbances within syntheses that bridge form and content, that is, syntheses that irreducibly involve content, even at the level of abstract consideration, would be immune to Jaspers' complaint.

We have shown that classical phenomenological psychopathologists generally agree that depressive experience involves temporal alterations in the *how* of experience, though the specific accounts of these alterations and their take-up of Husserl differ in detail. In the next section, we explore the relation between the fundamental form of intrinsic temporality and the temporality in which pathological disturbances are purportedly manifest. The transition from one to the other is mediated by, and, as such, experience of a meaningful world depends on, *affectivity*.

Rejecting the idea that the temporal changes in depression, or psychopathology more generally, occur at the level of primary passive temporal synthesis makes it possible to account for the conditioning of those temporal changes by contents of experience taken in a wide sense to include, hypothetically, things that range from childhood trauma to capitalist alienation. Affectivity depends on the ways in which what we encounter in the world pull, push, or, in general, affect us. As such, the contents of experience introduce an element of contingency into the way in which we experience ourselves and the world. The hypothetical explanations just cited become coherent on such an account, and, as will now be shown, an affectivity-based approach also allows us to demonstrate a deeper consensus than is typically recognized between phenomenological psychopathology, 4E approaches, Gibsonian psychology, and recent work on psychopathology and narrative.

Affectivity

It is generally agreed that depression involves not only temporal but affective alterations (see, e.g., Aho, 2013; De Haan, Rietveld, Stokhof, & Denys, 2013; Gallagher & Daly, 2018; Ratcliffe, 2008, 2015; Rottenberg, 2005). Indeed, there is a growing consensus that temporality and affect are intimately related to one another, as well as to our sense of agency, what Gibson (1979/1986) calls "affordances," and sense-making in general. Here, we begin by exploring some relevant work by Husserl, developing the insights of the first section and demonstrate how a Husserlian phenomenological conception of affection broadly agrees with Gibsonian and 4E approaches. Doing so lays a foundation for considering narrative aspects of depressive experience in the final section.

From Husserl's analysis of primary passive temporality in his *Analyses Concerning Passive and Active Synthesis* (2001), he goes on to analyze two other forms of primary passive syntheses: association and affection. Associative syntheses operate on the contents of experience in terms of similarity and contrast – what is similar becomes grouped together, apart from what is dissimilar. We can think of this grouping in terms of intentionality, and reference to Hume would not be entirely misleading: When we experience something, the way in which it appears depends in part on other experiences we currently undergo or have already had of similar and dissimilar phenomena. A table, for instance, is like a chair or a counter or a couch, but tables and counters, in another way, are also dissimilar from chairs and couches. Since similarity and contrast function not only at a time but over time, association thus depends on primary passive temporality. The most important element of associative synthesis for our explication of affection here is the notion of *prominence*: Something that we experience can be experienced as prominent insofar as it is relevantly different from the rest of what is experienced, that is, insofar as it is in some way separated from the background.

"By affection," Husserl writes, "we understand the allure given to consciousness, the peculiar pull that an object given to consciousness exercises on the ego … Affection presupposes prominence above all else" (Husserl, 2001, p. 196). That is, in order for something to *affect* us, it must be differentiated – though not necessarily attentively, explicitly – from other things that we are experiencing. Furthermore, if association depends on primary passive temporal synthesis and affection depends on association, then affection depends on primary passive temporal synthesis; affection presupposes temporality as that which undergirds relations of similarity and contrast and, accordingly, prominence. We will see, however, that it also feeds back on lived temporality and, correlatively, on the association process, involving something of a circular or spiraling process. First, however, a clarification is in order. Though emotion and mood are affective phenomena, insofar as they are ways of being affected by ourselves and the world, affection in Husserl is a broader category that includes any pull exercised on us by what is experienced. In this respect, affectivity in Husserl is already closely related to the enactivist concept of affectivity, which is a foundational moment of the sense-making activity of all organisms, including those that do not apparently undergo what we traditionally know as emotions or moods.[5]

The general idea we take from Husserl's theory of affectivity is that what we encounter exerts an affective pull on us, and this pull draws our attention. The way in which objects pull us depends on (a) our own capacities, that is, what we can do in general and, in particular, what we can do with or to the object, and also on (b) the powers of the object, that is, what the object can do with or to us. For instance, because of the specific kind of digestive system that we (typically) have, certain objects draw our attention as edible, and more so when we are hungry. This already supposes association of contents of experience over time and dependence on our own bodily capabilities – not just of our objective properties or characteristics, but (also) our possibilities of bodily action – as well as features or powers of the objects themselves.

Though affectivity depends on our own capacities, it is in the conceptually first instance a form of passivity, since it is a way of being affected by that which is, properly speaking, not oneself; furthermore, we are affected by what we experience prior to any activity or intervention on the part of the ego. Depraz (1994, p. 75, our translation) writes that "Affect is there before

[5] For an excellent discussion on this topic, see Giovanna Colombetti's *The Feeling Body: Affective Science Meets the Enactive Mind* (2014), especially Chapter 1.

being there for me in full consciousness: I am affected before knowing I am affected. It is in this sense that affect can be said to be primordial." We can also recall Heidegger's notion of *Befindlichkeit*, often translated as "disposition" and associated with "mood" but perhaps better understood as the constancy with which we are affected: We always find ourselves affected in some way or other, and even indifference is just one mode of affective "attunement," or *Stimmung* (Heidegger, 1927/1957). However, to characterize affection as strictly passive is one-sided, and in two ways. First, as stated, the ways in which things affect us depend on what we can do, that is, depend on our own action possibilities and thus on a form of agency. But second, recall that objects affect us so as to draw our attention, and in this way, affection is a bridge between passivity and activity. Husserl (2001, p. 277) writes: "By following the affection, a theme is made out of the identical object; I sidle up to it, as it were, in order to get to know it better, to determine it, to know it in its true being." By consciously tending to what we experience, we thematize the object and discover new relations of similarity and contrast, which in turn alters the way in which we are affected. This attentive engagement with what we experience is the first moment of active synthesis, which then conditions what Husserl calls "secondary passivity," the level of sedimentation and habit. Secondary passive syntheses are shaped by, but no longer require, egoic engagement, or activity proper, and subsequently feed back on how we experience the world. Notice the temporal structure involved here: We are experientially pulled by some object in our present environment with which we actively engage, and as it comes to be retained as part of our past experience exerts an influence on our anticipated future action. In this sense, *how* we are affected also depends on our own activity – we are not only affected but self-affected – and in this sense, affectivity involves passivity (both primary and secondary) as well as activity: Affectivity is dynamic.

The last relevant feature of Husserlian affectivity for our purposes is the concept of *awakening*. The allure that objects exercise on consciousness institutes intentional awakening, which can be thought of as a kind of prereflective intentional direction from what affects us now to other things in the environment, such that the latter gain their own (derivative) affective force. For Husserl, everything that we experience affects us to some degree of intensity, and if that intensity reaches a certain threshold, then other aspects of what we currently, have already, or could soon experience also become experienced with a certain attention-drawing intensity, as separated out from the background. In relation to the past, what we have already experienced generally diminishes in affective force over time, and if nothing at the present moment pertaining to a particular object prominently affects us, then this object itself fades into not only an impressional but also a retentional background.[6] In regard to this temporality, Husserl writes "What else can awakening mean here than this: What is implicit becomes explicit once more?" (2001, p. 223). This process is what he calls "the first form of a disclosive awakening," in which "more 'emerges' from out of the 'fog'" (2001, p. 224).

In relation to the future, affection awakens intentional acts toward what I may soon experience, and due to occurrent affection, those possibilities come to affect me with their own intensity; this is conditioned by and conditions agency and underlies motivational phenomena. What shows up as a relevant course of action depends on the ways in which future possibilities affect me, in relation to the affective force of current actualities. Husserl calls those possibilities that exert a particularly strong affective pull on me "enticing possibilities," or "enticements," but we could also call them, in Gibsonian terminology, "salient" (Ramstead, Veissière, & Kirmayer, 2016) or "relevant" (e.g., Bruineberg & Rietveld, 2014; Rietveld, 2008; Rietveld & Kiverstein, 2014) affordances. Indeed, affectivity as depending on what the experiencing agent (or ego) and the object can do *with* or *to* or *for* one another can already be understood in terms of affordances.[7] And since these affordances depend on our own bodies and bodily possibilities, affectivity is inherently embodied, not only in a primary or intrinsic fashion but also in a secondary, action-oriented way. Moreover, since affectivity always takes place in an affordance-generating situation (of body-environment), affectivity is embedded; and since what we can do with objects depends on our access to other objects, affectivity extends or is extensively distributed; and since this is all ultimately a matter of making sense of objects and our environment in terms of our possible and actual actions – "What is constituted for consciousness exists for the ego only insofar as it affects me, the ego" (Husserl, 2001, p. 210) – affectivity is enactive.

We are now in a position to consider the affective and temporal alterations seemingly at play in depressive experience. By directing our

[6] He sometimes refers to this retentional background as "nightfall" (Husserl, 2001, p. 221).

[7] The following example may be illustrative of affective awakening. Music plays in your environment while you read. You attend to the text at hand and are inattentive to the song. The words on the page affect you strongly – they draw you away from your surroundings and toward themselves. The song is given weakly and is not at all thematized or attended to. Then, you find yourself humming in time to a familiar chorus. Such an event requires that you were indeed aware of how the song you were inattentive to would continue, and the way in which the chorus now affects you awakens your retention of the earlier segments of the song. You have been peripherally aware of it for some time, foot tapping and head nodding without your explicit volition. The question then becomes: "Do I return to work, or 'rock out' with the music?" This possibility was not salient before, but due to the way in which the song affects you, it is now an enticing possibility – a salient affordance.

attention and awakening intentional relations, affectivity undergirds phenomena of duration and temporal ordering. If our attention is keenly fixed on some aspect of experience, this can alter our perceived duration of it by awakening those things experienced as relevantly preceding or following it: It is plausible that what affects us most strongly, or what corresponds to a far-reaching awakening of intentional contents of experience, will be given as enduring longer than something that, while perhaps objectively persisting for a longer period, fails to awaken such a distant past or future. In this way, a particularly intense experience can come to be all-encompassing, and the future could be experienced as highly constrained in virtue of an excess of past determinations, as for example, in the case of regret where a feeling of regret for a past action dominates one's present state and constrains the appearance of future possibilities. What is awakened exerts a pull on our attention, and so that which is already past can reorient our temporal perspective. This can help us to understand certain aspects of depressive experience, such as the past being perceived as infinite and as replacing the future; what comes next affects one less than what has already occurred. Again, an example of this would be the prevalence of guilt and guilt narratives in depression, in which a person's attention is drawn away from the future toward the past, as the more salient, relevant, or even defining temporal dimension. Affection can also affect our ordering of events in time, such that what does not affect us in salient ways, or what does not affect us *immediately* (i.e., what affects us without us explicitly taking notice, or attending to it) does not become, at that time, thematically and explicitly situated among other events. At the time of recalling the seemingly irrelevant event, its objective ordinality may remain obscured, but this obscurity may make it difficult even to order relevant events, since the temporal position of one event always depends on its relation to others. All of this is closely related to the ways in which affectivity undergirds memory and anticipation, as what we attend to informs what we recall and what we can relevantly expect, and accordingly illustrates ways in which affectivity may modulate experience such that it is conceivable to become "pathologically" surprised or forgetful.

This account agrees with Gibsonian and enactive approaches to depression. Rottenberg (2005) argues that "Depression flattens the emotional landscape, greatly constricting the range of emotional reactions to differing emotional contexts." As depression flattens the emotional landscape, it also flattens the field of affordances (De Haan et al., 2013; see Figure 13.1). For the phenomenologist/enactivist, the issue is about meaning. In depression, things lose significance – everything just passes by and agency is diminished. And

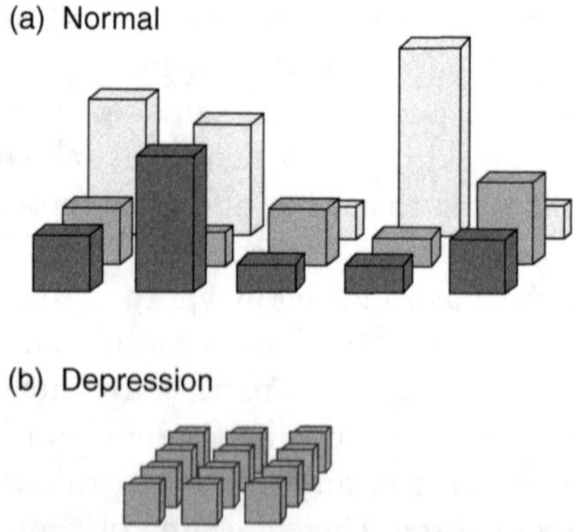

Figure 13.1 Sketch of different fields of relevant affordances (De Haan et al., 2013, p. 7). © De Haan, Rietveld, Stokhof, and Denys. Creative Commons license applies.

insofar as possibilities become affectively flattened, unenticing, nonsalient, this alters the way in which the future appears: It becomes an inert, dead, already settled realm, in which nothing changes, or even in which nothing can change (Ratcliffe, 2013). This does justice to Minkowski's claim (1970, p. 303) that "It is in the orientation of our life towards the future which gives it a meaning, a direction: when this orientation is missing, everything seems to amount to the same thing, seems stupid, without rhyme or reason," which is just what the depressed patient describes.

This account does not require a generative disruption at the most fundamental level of passive synthesis – it does not require a disruption of intrinsic temporality as a generating disorder. Rather, if our experience of temporality is disrupted (which appears to be the consensus among phenomenologists, enactivists, clinicians, and empirical scientists), it is generated as a disorder of affectivity.

The account is reinforced by insights from enactivist thinkers. Evan Thompson (2007, p. 161) helps us to understand how affect generates "vital significance" and shapes our ability to cope with the surrounding world. Giovanna Colombetti shows that sense-making is deeply affective: "[T]he world takes on significance and value precisely in relation to what the organism is concerned about and striving for" (2014, p. 19). Matthew Ratcliffe (2010, p. 603), likewise emphasizing the affective background, indicates that "all of the ways in which things and people matter to us are at the same time kinds of possibility that the world presents us with." Similarly, Michelle Maiese (2016, p. 4) contends: "A shift in affective framing changes not just how one perceives the world, but also what someone remembers, how one engages in practical reasoning, and how one relates to other people." The deep connection between temporality and affectivity has also been emphasized by phenomenologically inspired enactivist accounts (see Depraz, Varela, & Vermersch, 2000; Gallagher & Varela, 2003; Gallagher & Zahavi, 2014).

We have shown that an understanding of affectivity grounded in Husserl is in broad agreement with enactivist and Gibsonian approaches to depression. Such approaches can help us to understand the temporal alterations at play in depressive experience without positing a disruption of fundamental primary passive temporal synthesis. As such, affectivity has an effect on the "how" of experience, which often is referred to as "form" but which, we hope to have demonstrated, involves the *filling of form*, the integration or gestalt of form and content (understood widely).

Narrative

We want to conclude with some brief comments on how narrative reflects disruptions related to both temporality and affectivity in depression. In the case of psychopathology generally, self-narratives can provide a forensic measure, a linguistic fingerprint, of different conditions (Gallagher & Cole, 2011; Junghaenel, Smyth, & Santner, 2008). Narrative may not provide evidence concerning etiological order, but it can provide correlational evidence of anomalies in both temporal and affective experiences.

Generally speaking, narrative has a temporal structure in the sense that it typically follows a time line of the events or actions being narrated. For example, Delafield-Butt and Trevarthen (2015) consider the structure of narrative as involving a temporal sequence of introduction, development,

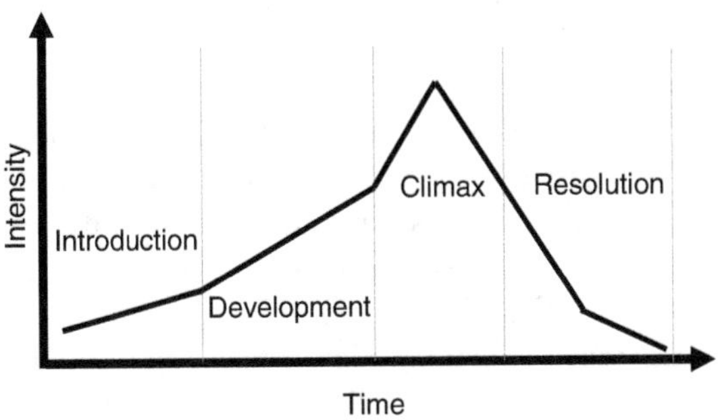

Figure 13.2 Four phases of narrative (from Trevarthen & Delafield-Butt, 2013).

climax, and resolution (in Figure 13.2), reflecting a serial organization of events or actions into complex expressions. A similar fourfold structure is found in semiotic accounts of narrative, which identify the four canonical stages as follows: contract, competence, performance, and sanction (Greimas, 1970; Paolucci, 2019). The temporal structure of narrative, however, is even more complex; it involves both an internal and external time frame. The internal time frame reflects serial order within the narrative. One can think of this in terms of McTaggart's (1908) notion of the B-series, where events are arranged as earlier or later than other events. In contrast, external time frame refers to temporal perspective (McTaggart's A-series, cast in relative terms of past–present–future). Specifically, from the narrator's viewpoint, events are either past, future, or present relative to the narrator's own present time. Such temporal structures, as well as syntactical structures, can be disrupted in different pathologies.

Qualitative analysis of spontaneous speech has indicated that individuals with depression, when attempting to recapitulate past events, were "rambling, repetitious, and vague" and had "difficulty in connecting … topics" (Bucci & Freedman, 1981, p. 348). Recovery from psychological distress, in turn, seems to be associated with the development of a coherent "story" about distressing events (Pennebaker & Seagal, 1999). Likewise, syntactical structures in narratives by persons with depression are disrupted. Pennebaker, Mehl, and Niederhoffer (2003) show that the increased use of the first-person pronoun in self-narratives predicts both depression and mania. Stirman and Pennebaker (2001), in a study of artists who committed suicide compared with those who did not, found relatively higher frequencies of self-reference words (e.g., I, me, my) as compared with other reference words (e.g., we, them, they).

Temporal structure as well as syntactic structure and semantic content represented in the narrative all get pushed and pulled or rearranged in different ways. Arguably, in cases of depression, the pushing and pulling are connected with affectivity. The narrative reports of a patient with depression may reveal patterns that reflect disorders in mood and affective processing as well as disrupted processes connected to the sense of agency and identity. Persons with depression may report feelings of helplessness, desperation, self-loathing, as well as the incapacity to work, to act, to think clearly (O'Brien, 2004; Solomon, 2001). In various depression narratives, alterations in existential feelings (Ratcliffe, 2015) can be mapped in bodily and experiential changes (Fuchs, 2005; Fuchs & Schlimme, 2009; Paskaleva, 2011; Slaby & Stephan, 2008).

It's not that the affective experiences of individuals with depression[8] are neatly or stably represented in the narrative timescale, but rather that this affectivity can disrupt the underlying dynamics at more basic integrative timescales that involve the intrinsic temporality of the living present. Such disruptions, however, do not amount to complete dysnarrativa. Temporal structure persists even if the content represented in the narrative gets pushed and pulled or rearranged in different ways. And intrinsic temporality persists even if it is modulated by affective processes.

Acknowledgment

The authors wish to thank an anonymous referee and the editor for helpful comments on this chapter. Edward A. Lenzo also wishes to thank Philip Turetzky for helpful discussions on these topics.

References

Aho, K. A. (2013). Depression and embodiment: Phenomenological reflections on motility, affectivity, and transcendence. *Medicine, Health Care and Philosophy*, 16(4), 751–759. doi:10.1007/s11019-013-9470-8

Binswanger, L. (2005). *Mélancolie et manie: Etudes phénoménologiques* [Melancholy and mania: Phenomenological studies]. Paris, France: Presses Universitaires de France. (Original work published 1960)

Blewett, A. E. (1992). Abnormal subjective time experience in depression. *The British Journal of Psychiatry*, 161(2), 195–200. doi:10.1192/bjp.161.2.195

Bloc, L., Souza, C., & Moreira, V. (2016). Phenomenology of depression: Contributions of Minkowski, Binswanger, Tellenbach and Tatossian. *Estudos de Psicologia (Campinas)*, 33(1), 107–116. doi:10.1590/1982-02752016000100011

Bruineberg, J., & Rietveld, E. (2014). Self-organization, free energy minimization, and optimal grip on a field of affordances. *Frontiers in Human Neuroscience*, 8, 1–14. doi:10.3389/fnhum.2014.00599

Bschor, T., Ising, M., Bauer, M., Lewitzka, U., Skerstupeit, M., Mueller-Oerlinghausen, B., & Baethge, C. (2004). Time experience and time judgment in major depression, mania and healthy subjects. A controlled study of 93 subjects. *Acta Psychiatrica Scandinavica*, 109(3), 222–229. doi:10.1046/j.0001-690X.2003.00244.x

Bucci, W., & Freedman, N. (1981). The language of depression. *Bulletin of the Menninger Clinic*, 45(4), 334–358.

[8] Listed in the DSM-V as including depressed mood, sadness, emptiness, hopelessness, diminished interest, feelings of worthlessness, or guilt, and in various other clinical reports based on self-narratives as including loss of empathic resonance with others, loneliness, self-loathing or low self-esteem, pervasive sense of dread, unaccountable fears, feeling that one's experience is absolutely private and absolutely isolating, despair, feeling of being excluded, not understood, underappreciated, self-alienation, and a sense of diminished engagement with the world – that things and surroundings are experienced as less salient. See Gallagher and Daly (2018) for complete references.

Cardinalli, I. E. (2012). *Daseinsanalyse e esquizofrenia: um estudo da obra de Medard Boss* [Daseinsanalyse and schizophrenia: A study of Medard Boss' work]. São Paulo, Brasil: Escuta.

Colombetti, G. (2014). *The feeling body: Affective science meets the enactive mind.* Cambridge, MA: Massachusetts Institute of Technology Press.

De Haan, S., Rietveld, E., Stokhof, M., & Denys, D. (2013). The phenomenology of deep brain stimulation-induced changes in OCD: An enactive affordance-based model. *Frontiers in Human Neuroscience*, 7(653), 1–14. doi:10.3389/fnhum.2013.00653

Delafield-Butt, J. T., & Trevarthen, C. (2015). The ontogenesis of narrative: From moving to meaning. *Frontiers in Psychology*, 6, 1–16. doi:10.3389/fpsyg.2015.01157

Depraz, N. (1994). Temporalité et affection dans les manuscrits tardifs sur la temporalité (1929–1935) de Husserl [Temporality and affection in Husserl's late manuscripts on temporality (1929–1935)]. *Alter*, 2, 63–86.

Depraz, N., Varela, F. J., & Vermersch, P. (2000). The gesture of awareness: An account of its structural dynamics. In M. Velmans (Ed.), *Investigating phenomenal consciousness: New methodologies and maps* (pp. 121–136). Amsterdam, Netherlands: John Benjamins.

Droit-Volet, S. (2013). Time perception, emotions and mood disorders. *Journal of Physiology – Paris*, 107(4), 255–264. doi:10.1016/j.jphysparis.2013.03.005

Fingelkurts, A. A., & Fingelkurts, A. A. (2017). Three-dimensional components of selfhood in treatment-naive patients with major depressive disorder: A resting-state qEEG imaging study. *Neuropsychologia*, 99, 30–36. doi:10.1016/j.neuropsychologia.2017.02.020

Fuchs, T. (2001). Melancholia as a desynchronization: Towards a psychopathology of interpersonal time. *Psychopathology*, 34(4), 179–186. doi:10.1159/000049304

Fuchs, T. (2005). Corporealized and disembodied minds: A phenomenological view of the body in melancholia and schizophrenia. *Philosophy, Psychiatry, & Psychology*, 12(2), 95–107. doi:10.1353/ppp.2005.0040

Fuchs, T. (2013). Temporality and psychopathology. *Phenomenology and the Cognitive Sciences*, 12(1), 75–104. doi:10.1007/s11097-010-9189-4

Fuchs, T., & Schlimme, J. E. (2009). Embodiment and psychopathology: A phenomenological perspective. *Current Opinion in Psychiatry*, 22(6), 570–575. doi:10.1097/YCO.0b013e3283318e5c

Gallagher, S., & Cole, J. (2011). Dissociation in self-narrative. *Consciousness and Cognition*, 20(1), 149–155. doi:10.1016/j.concog.2010.10.003

Gallagher, S., & Daly, A. (2018). Dynamical relations in the self-pattern. *Frontiers in Psychology*, 9, 1–13. doi:10.3389/fpsyg.2018.00664

Gallagher, S., & Varela, F. J. (2003). Redrawing the map and resetting the time: Phenomenology and the cognitive sciences. *Canadian Journal of Philosophy*, 33(Suppl. 1), 93–132. doi:10.1080/00455091.2003.10717596

Gallagher, S., & Zahavi, D. (2014). Primal impression and enactive perception. In D. Lloyd & V. Arstila (Eds.), *Subjective time: The philosophy, psychology, and neuroscience of temporality* (pp. 83–99). Cambridge, MA: Massachusetts Institute of Technology Press.

Gibson, J. J. (1986). *The ecological approach to visual perception.* Hillsdale, NJ: Erlbaum. (Original work published 1979)

Greimas, A. J. (1970). *Du sens II. Essais sémiotiques* [Meaning II. Essays on semiotic theory]. Paris, France: Seuil.

Heidegger, M. (1957). *Sein und Zeit* [Being and Time]. Tübingen, Germany: Max Niemeyer Verlag. (Original work published 1927)

Hsu, T. Y., Lee, H. C., Lane, T. J., & Missal, M. (2019). Temporal preparation and short-term temporal memory in depression. *Frontiers in Behavioral Neuroscience*, 13, 1–12. doi:10.3389/fnbeh.2019.00258

Husserl, E. (1970). *Logical investigations* (J. N. Findlay, Trans.). London, UK: Routledge & Kegan Paul. (Original work published 1900–1901)

Husserl, E. (1991). *On the phenomenology of the consciousness of internal time* (J. B. Brough, Trans.). Dordrecht, Netherlands: Kluwer Academic.

Husserl, E. (2001). *Analyses concerning passive and active synthesis* (A. J. Steinbock, Trans.). Dordrecht, Netherlands: Kluwer Academic.

Jaspers, K. (1997). *General psychopathology: Volume I and volume II* (J. Hoenig & M. W. Hamilton, Trans.). Baltimore, MD: The Johns Hopkins University Press. (Original work published 1913)

Junghaenel, D., Smyth, J. M., & Santner, L. (2008). Linguistic dimensions of psychopathology: A quantitative analysis. *Journal of Social and Clinical Psychology*, 27(1), 36–55. doi:10.1521/jscp.2008.27.1.3

Luft, S. (2008). Zur phänomenologischen Methode in Karl Jaspers' Allgemeine Psychopathologie [On the phenomenological method in Karl Jaspers' General Psychopathology]. In S. Rinofner-Kreidl & H. A. Wiltsche (Eds.), *Karl Jaspers' Allgemeine Psychopathologie zwischen Wissenschaft, Philosophie und Praxis* [Karl Jaspers' general psychopathology between science, philosophy, and practice] (pp. 31–51). Würzburg, Germany: Königshausen & Neumann.

Mahlberg, R., Kienast, T., Bschor, T., & Adli, M. (2008). Evaluation of time memory in acutely depressed patients, manic patients, and healthy controls using a time reproduction task. *European Psychiatry*, 23(6), 430–433. doi:10.1016/j.eurpsy.2007.07.001

Maiese, M. (2016). Affective scaffolds, expressive arts, and cognition. *Frontiers in Psychology*, 7, 1–11. doi:10.3389/fpsyg.2016.00359

McTaggart, J. E. (1908). The unreality of time. *Mind*, 17, 457–474. doi:10.1093/mind/XVII.4.457

Minkowski, E. (1970). *Lived time: Phenomenological and psychopathological studies* (N. Metzel, Trans.). Evanston, IL: Northwestern University Press.

Moskalewicz, M. (2018). Toward a unified view of time: Erwin W. Straus' phenomenological psychopathology of temporal experience. *Phenomenology and the Cognitive Sciences*, 17(1), 65–80. doi:10.1007/s11097-016-9494-7

O'Brien, S. (2004). *The family silver: A memoir of depression and inheritance*. Chicago, IL: University of Chicago Press.

Paolucci, C. (2019). Social cognition, mindreading and narratives. A cognitive semiotics perspective on narrative practices from early mindreading to autism spectrum disorder. *Phenomenology and the Cognitive Sciences*, 18(2), 375–400. doi:10.1007/s11097-018-9575-x

Paskaleva, A. (2011). *A phenomenological assessment of depression narratives. PICS – Publications of the Institute of Cognitive Science* (Vol. 3, Master's thesis, University of Osnabrück, Germany). Retrieved from https://portal.ikw.uni-osnabrueck.de/en/system/files/03-2011.pdf

Pennebaker, J. W., Mehl, M. R., & Niederhoffer, K. G. (2003). Psychological aspects of natural language use: Our words, our selves. *Annual Review of Psychology*, 54, 547–577. doi:10.1146/annurev.psych.54.101601.145041

Pennebaker, J. W., & Seagal, J. D. (1999). Forming a story: The health benefits of narrative. *Journal of Clinical Psychology*, 55(10), 1243–1254. doi:10.1002/(SICI)1097-4679(199910)55:10%3C1243::AID-JCLP6%3E3.0.CO;2-N

Ramstead, M. J. D., Veissière, S. P. L., & Kirmayer, L. J. (2016). Cultural affordances: Scaffolding local worlds through shared intentionality and regimes of attention. *Frontiers in Psychology*, 7, 1–21. doi:10.3389/fpsyg.2016.01090

Ratcliffe, M. (2008). *Feelings of being: Phenomenology, psychiatry, and the sense of reality*. New York, NY: Oxford University Press.

Ratcliffe, M. (2010). Depression, guilt and emotional depth. *Inquiry*, 53(6), 602–626. doi:10.1080/0020174X.2010.526324

Ratcliffe, M. (2012). Varieties of temporal experience in depression. *The Journal of Medicine and Philosophy*, 37(2), 114–138. doi:10.1093/jmp/jhs010

Ratcliffe, M. (2013). *The world of depression*. Unpublished manuscript. Retrieved from www.academia.edu/6054108/The_World_of_Depression

Ratcliffe, M. (2015). *Experiences of depression: A study in phenomenology*. Oxford, UK: Oxford University Press.

Rietveld, E. (2008). Situated normativity: The normative aspect of embodied cognition in unreflective action. *Mind*, 117(468), 973–1001. doi:10.1093/mind/fzn050

Rietveld, E., & Kiverstein, J. (2014). A rich landscape of affordances. *Ecological Psychology*, 26(4), 325–352. doi:10.1080/10407413.2014.958035

Rottenberg, J. (2005). Mood and emotion in major depression. *Current Directions in Psychological Science*, 14(3), 167–170. doi:10.1111/j.0963-7214.2005.00354.x

Slaby, J., & Stephan, A. (2008). Affective intentionality and self-consciousness. *Consciousness and Cognition*, 17(2), 506–513. doi:10.1016/j.concog.2008.03.007

Solomon, A. (2001). *The noonday demon: An atlas of depression*. New York, NY: Scribner.

Stirman, S. W., & Pennebaker, J. W. (2001). Word use in the poetry of suicidal and non-suicidal poets. *Psychosomatic Medicine*, 63(4), 517–522. doi:10.1097/00006842-200107000-00001

Straus, E. W. (1947). Disorders of personal time in depressive states. *Southern Medical Journal*, 40(3), 254–259. doi:10.1097/00007611-194703000-00011

Tatossian, A. (1979). *La phénoménologie des psychoses* [The phenomenology of psychoses]. Paris, France: Masson.

Thoma, S. (2014). Karl Jaspers' criticism of anthropological and phenomenological psychiatry. In T. Fuchs, T. Breyer, & C. Mundt (Eds.), *Karl Jaspers' philosophy and psychopathology* (pp. 85–98). New York, NY: Springer.

Thompson, E. (2007). *Mind in life*. Cambridge, MA: Harvard University Press.

Trevarthen, C., & Delafield-Butt, J. T. (2013). Biology of shared meaning and language development: Regulating the life of narratives. In M. Legerstee, D. Haley, & M. Bornstein (Eds.), *The infant mind: Origins of the social brain* (pp. 167–199). New York, NY: Guildford Press.

Wyrick, R. A., & Wyrick, L. C. (1977). Time experience during depression. *Archives of General Psychiatry*, 34(12), 1441–1443. doi:10.1001/archpsyc.1977.01770240067005

13.1

Commentary on "Intrinsic Temporality in Depression: Classical Phenomenological Psychiatry, Affectivity, and Narrative"

Temporality and Affectivity in Depression and Schizophrenia

Tom Froese

Introduction

Temporality is a foundational topic in phenomenological psychopathology, and it plays an especially important role in its analysis of depression and melancholia (e.g., Fuchs, 2001, 2013; Gallagher, 2012; Ratcliffe, 2015). An intuitive strategy is to explain abnormal experiences of time by appealing to a fundamental disruption of the temporal structure of consciousness, yet Lenzo and Gallagher (2021) highlight that this strategy is problematic. Let us consider the following autobiographical account of time experience in depression, which is cited as a paradigmatic example by Ratcliffe (2012): "I am in a time-locked place, where the moment I am in will stretch on, agonizingly, for ever. There is no possibility of redemption or hope. It is a final giving up on everything. It is death" (Lott, 1996, p. 247).

It is tempting to hypothesize that the structure of time-consciousness underlying this kind of abnormal experience is similarly abnormal, that is, dominated by the past without any forward-looking element. In a separate context, Gallagher imagines that kind of situation as follows: "If there were only retentions, everything I experience would already have just happened; we would be pure witnesses without the potential to engage" (2017b, p. 97). This hypothetical experience does capture key aspects of the phenomenology of depression, but there are reasons for concern.

Specifically, it seems more accurate to identify the moment when only retentions remain in someone's stream of consciousness with the moment that stream comes to an end. In other words, it is the onset of death, and we therefore have reached a basic limit of thought experimentation. As Shakespeare once pointed out, we simply do not know what dreams – if any – may come. To be fair, as exemplified by the autobiographical quote given earlier, people with severe depression often report being trapped inside a dying body (Fuchs, 2005). And yet they continue to live and to experience, which means that they did not suffer a total disintegration of the diachronic structure of temporality (Fuchs, 2017).

Lenzo and Gallagher suggest that we need to more clearly distinguish between (a) the flow of experience and (b) the experience of flow. In addition, they propose to reorient the focus of analysis to some of the other structural syntheses that are necessary for the constitution of subjectivity and objectivity. More specifically, they suggest that the locus of depression is not a disruption of the primary passive *temporal* synthesis, but rather of the primary passive *associative* and *affective* syntheses.

I agree with Lenzo and Gallagher about the diagnosis of the theoretical problem, and I also partially agree with their proposed remedy, although I will suggest that, in the end, we will need a more radical treatment. In the rest of this commentary, I will therefore complement their contribution in three respects:

(1) I extend their critical discussion to schizophrenia, where we find the same problematic appeals to a disruption of fundamental temporal structure;
(2) I radicalize their positive proposal by showing that once we distinguish between the experience of flow and the flow of experience, we can also envision a more general distinction between phenomenality and structure of consciousness; and
(3) I highlight that this more general distinction has important implications for the naturalization of phenomenology, in particular by supporting growing calls for a reconceptualization of the scientific concept of nature.

From Temporality to Affectivity

Since the late 1990s, the insights of phenomenological philosophy and embodied cognitive science have been brought together in a mutually informing manner. An important point of contact was the structure of time-consciousness, and this has been explored in quite some detail (Varela, 1999), including with respect to abnormal experience in schizophrenia.

For example, Gallagher applied this interdisciplinary approach to the characteristic symptom of thought insertion (Gallagher, 2005, pp. 173–205; Gallagher & Varela, 2003). While it is normal to occasionally experience unbidden thoughts, memories, and fantasies, there is still a sense that these experiences are originating within one's stream of consciousness. But it is argued that this lingering sense of passive generation disappears along with protention: "Without protention, thought continues, but it appears already made, not generated in my own stream of consciousness" (Gallagher & Varela, 2003, p. 117). However, in line with Lenzo and Gallagher's recommendation, we should refrain from positing such a fundamental disruption of temporality. Protention is inseparable from the stream of consciousness: The now, as the present phase of consciousness, is constituted by way of fulfillment of an otherwise empty protention (Gallagher & Zahavi, 2014). It is questionable to what extent a subject's thoughts, or even experience more generally, can continue without protention.

Again, the key problem is that the fundamental structural level of consciousness is an all-or-nothing affair: Either there is a continuous stream of consciousness or there is not. There is no middle way. As the work of Husserl and of later phenomenologists revealed, the basic unit of time-consciousness, that is, the present moment, has a concrete duration; it is not an abstract point on a line, but a temporal field that dynamically gives rise to the now ("primal impression") on the basis of the nearly present ("protention") continuously slipping into the just-past ("retention"). Given that this recursive slippage results in a nested, or even fractal-like temporal organization, the present moments become structurally linked into an internally unified whole, and thereby constitute the foundation for subjectivity and its meaningful engagement with the objective world (Gallagher & Zahavi, 2014). But this foundation in a tripartite temporality is precarious: Remove any of the parts, and the whole subject disappears.

Gallagher and Varela (2003, p. 120) seem to have sensed this tension because later on they emphasize that "the schizophrenic phenomenology is not simply a structural or logical problem." Accordingly, they moved from an abstract structural explication of protention to a process of protention that is always already suffused by an affective tone determined by the past, and is rooted in and constrained by distributed patterns of neurobiological dynamics, in line with Varela's (1999) neurophenomenology research program.

From Affectivity to Phenomenality

Lenzo and Gallagher build on this work on the deep connection between temporality and affectivity to show how there can be temporal alterations in depressive experience without a disruption of the most fundamental level of temporal synthesis. Their proposal is to shift the disruption from the primary temporal synthesis to a less fundamental level of structural synthesis, and thereby preserve the unity of time-consciousness.

They argue that a moment of experience that affects us strongly will attract our attention in such a way that it evokes far-reaching chains of associations of experiences that relevantly precede and follow it, and the moment will therefore appear as longer. This alteration can assume pathological proportions: an intensely affecting past experience, say a trauma, can be so prominent that it consistently reorients attention to that past moment, while the concomitantly evoked past associations overwhelm what is happening now. This is a plausible account of how differences in affectivity can give rise to differences in lived duration. However, it is not clear whether this account can also explain why it seems like time itself has ceased to flow. For example, occasionally I may feel overwhelmed by associations evoked by a prominent moment in my past, but I experience these unwanted associations in the present moment as part of my normal stream of consciousness.

I think the way forward is to radicalize Lenzo and Gallagher's proposal and further bracket the general strategy of appealing to structural differences to understand phenomenal differences. There are hints in their analysis that an alternative strategy could appeal to the feeling of prominence, relevance, or salience directly: What makes the key difference is not a prominent moment's quantity of associations, but rather the personal significance of its felt quality. This strategic reorientation involves a subtle but significant shift in the roles played by affectivity, which ambiguously refers both to being passively affected and to felt affect (Sass, 2004). I propose to replace Lenzo and Gallagher's focus on the former role with an emphasis on the latter role, which is at the core of the subject's "lived self-acquaintance" (Zahavi, 2005, p. 80) or "affective self-familiarity" (Fuchs, 2017) across time.

For example, we can imagine that an ordinary experience, like being lost in thoughts and spontaneously deciding to cross the street on the way home, can go nearly unnoticed if it has no further significant consequences, and yet become a target for obsessive attention if it leads to traumatic consequences. The fundamental structural differences between the moments surrounding the decision are the same in both scenarios, and yet the valence of those differences is incomparable: In the ordinary case, the moment of decision retains the same level of valence as the preceding and subsequent moments, while in the traumatic case, there is a shocking increase in the significance of the decision such that the valence of differences between the preceding and the subsequent moments pales in comparison. And without any appreciation of meaningful differences between the moments flowing through awareness, time itself may well seem to have stopped flowing altogether. We can compare this with the phenomenology of perception: Research into inattentional blindness, change blindness, and categorical perception have revealed that we often remain unaware of large structural changes in the visual scene, and this is facilitated if the changes do not impact the meaning of what is perceived (Froese & Leavens, 2014). Similarly, people with depression may suffer from disordered affect, which hides structural differences between moments in time by blanketing those differences with indifference, thereby making time itself appear stagnant. This disordered affect may have various origins, but trauma can certainly make the valence of all other changes in life pale in comparison.

New Horizons for the Naturalization of Phenomenology

This shift in analysis of affectivity from structural self-affection to phenomenally felt quality has broader implications. It points more generally to the relative independence of structural dynamics from phenomenology. This is presumably what made the structure of time-consciousness an appealing starting point for Varela's naturalization of phenomenology in the first place, but it also means that this strategy will not go far. First of all, whereas naturalization has mainly focused on how to relate the structures of consciousness with the structures of the brain, we also need to relate feelings being alive with our organismic embodiment (Fuchs, 2012). But even if the structures of consciousness could be explained in terms of whole brain–body–world structures, this would still fail to account for the felt quality. It would miss the fundamental subjective dimension of affectivity:

> It is an unmediated feeling or sense of aliveness, a sense of certain tonality or luminosity of consciousness that founds our existence and is a necessary condition for more elaborate levels of self-awareness and for our encountering of the world. (Sass, 2004, p. 138)

The only way forward is to bite the bullet and accept the phenomenal as an irreducible element of our existence, and one that can make an important difference in our lives. Yet this confronts us head-on with the hardest version of the mind-body problem, which is tied with a specific concept of nature:

> Anything that could count as a solution to the hard problem would have to buy into the assumptions of classic naturalism, since those assumptions define precisely the framework within which the hard problem is defined, namely, that a complete scientific description of the brain will be deterministic, and completely independent of first-person experience. (Gallagher, 2017a, p. 111)

The proposal by Lenzo and Gallagher that "affectivity can disrupt the underlying dynamics," therefore, must ultimately be considered in the context of the "ongoing theoretical struggle between the task of remaining scientific (which Varela certainly wanted to do) and reconceiving nature (and therefore reconceiving what science actually is)" (Gallagher, 2017a, p. 111). I suggest that the new "remedy" – not the solution – of the hard problem, that is, of how subjective affect could make a difference to objective dynamics, needs to involve two interdependent tasks: (1) develop an alternative theory of the brain, and of the whole organism more generally, which takes incompleteness and nondeterminism as its starting point, and (2) develop an account of how first-person experience could make a difference to the brain's or organism's activity.

Task (1) is slowly taking shape; it does not contradict any empirical evidence, and there is evidence that can be interpreted in its support (Froese & Taguchi, 2019). Task (2) is a much harder nut to crack, but crack it we must if we want to retain room for the subjective in an objective world (Fuchs, 2018). Lenzo and Gallagher's reference to Jaspers' *General Psychopathology* is useful here, especially his claim that both scientific explanation and phenomenological understanding are limited. It is tempting to see the objectively inexplicable and the subjectively unintelligible as complementary gaps through which the intertwinement of the living and lived body takes place, where each side can reach into the other, but without violating the defining essence of the other domain (Froese, 2018).

References

Froese, T. (2018). [Review of the book *Ecology of the brain: The phenomenology and biology of the embodied mind*, by T. Fuchs]. *Frontiers in Psychology*, 9, 1–3. doi:10.3389/fpsyg.2018.02174

Froese, T., & Leavens, D. A. (2014). The direct perception hypothesis: Perceiving the intention of another's action hinders its precise imitation. *Frontiers in Psychology*, 5, 1–15. doi:10.3389/fpsyg.2014.00065

Froese, T., & Taguchi, S. (2019). The problem of meaning in AI and robotics: Still with us after all these years. *Philosophies*, 4(2), 14. doi:10.3390/philosophies4020014

Fuchs, T. (2001). Melancholia as a desynchronization: Towards a psychopathology of interpersonal time. *Psychopathology*, 34(4), 179–186. doi:10.1159/000049304

Fuchs, T. (2005). Corporealized and disembodied minds: A phenomenological view of the body in melancholia and schizophrenia. *Philosophy, Psychiatry & Psychology*, 12(2), 95–107.

Fuchs, T. (2012). The feeling of being alive: Organic foundations of self-awareness. In J. Fingerhut & S. Marienberg (Eds.), *Feelings of being alive* (pp. 149–165). Berlin, Germany: De Gruyter.

Fuchs, T. (2013). Temporality and psychopathology. *Phenomenology and the Cognitive Sciences*, 12(1), 75–104. doi:10.1007/s11097-010-9189-4

Fuchs, T. (2017). Self across time: The diachronic unity of bodily existence. *Phenomenology and the Cognitive Sciences*, 16, 291–315. doi:10.1007/s11097-015-9449-4

Fuchs, T. (2018). *Ecology of the brain: The phenomenology and biology of the embodied mind*. Oxford, UK: Oxford University Press.

Gallagher, S. (2005). *How the body shapes the mind*. New York, NY: Oxford University Press.

Gallagher, S. (2012). Time, emotion, and depression. *Emotion Review*, 4(2), 127–132. doi:10.1177/1754073911430142

Gallagher, S. (2017a). Author's response: Internatural relations. *Constructivist Foundations*, 13(1), 110–113.

Gallagher, S. (2017b). The past, present and future of time-consciousness: From Husserl to Varela and beyond. *Constructivist Foundations*, 13(1), 91–97.

Gallagher, S., & Varela, F. J. (2003). Redrawing the map and setting the time: Phenomenology and the cognitive sciences. *Canadian Journal of Philosophy*, 29, 93–132. doi:10.1080/00455091.2003.10717596

Gallagher, S., & Zahavi, D. (2014). Primal impression and enactive perception. In V. Arstila & D. Lloyd (Eds.), *Subjective time: The philosophy, psychology, and neuroscience of temporality* (pp. 83–100). Cambridge, MA: Massachusetts Institute of Technology Press.

Jaspers, K. (1997). *General psychopathology: Volume I and volume II* (J. Hoenig & M. W. Hamilton, Trans.). Baltimore, MD: The Johns Hopkins University Press. (Original work published 1913).

Lenzo, E., & Gallagher, S. (2021). Intrinsic temporality in depression: Classical phenomenological psychiatry, affectivity and narrative. In C. Tewes & G. Stanghellini (Eds.), *Time and body: Phenomenological and psychopathological approaches* (pp. 289–310). Cambridge, UK: Cambridge University Press.

Lott, T. (1996). *The scent of dried roses*. London, UK: Viking.

Ratcliffe, M. (2012). Varieties of temporal experience in depression. *The Journal of Medicine and Philosophy*, 37(2), 114–138. doi:10.1093/jmp/jhs010

Ratcliffe, M. (2015). *Experiences of depression: A study in phenomenology*. Oxford, UK: Oxford University Press.

Sass, L. A. (2004). Affectivity in schizophrenia: A phenomenological view. *Journal of Consciousness Studies*, 11(10–11), 127–147.

Varela, F. J. (1999). Present-time consciousness. *Journal of Consciousness Studies*, 6(2–3), 111–140.

Zahavi, D. (2005). *Subjectivity and selfhood: Investigating the first-person perspective*. Cambridge, MA: The Massachusetts Institute of Technology Press.

14

Lost in the Socially Extended Mind
Genuine Intersubjectivity and Disturbed Self-Other Demarcation in Schizophrenia

Tom Froese and Joel Krueger

Introduction

Much of the characteristic symptomatology of schizophrenia can be understood as resulting from a pervasive sense of disembodiment. The body is experienced as an external machine that needs to be controlled with explicit intentional commands, which in turn leads to severe difficulties in interacting with the world in a fluid and intuitive manner. In consequence, there is a characteristic dissociality: Others become problems to be solved by intellectual effort and no longer present opportunities for spontaneous interpersonal alignment. This dissociality goes hand in hand with a progressive loss of the socially extended mind, which normally affords opportunities for co-regulation of cognitive and affective processes. However, at times people with schizophrenia report that they are confronted by the opposite of this dissociality, namely, an unusual fluidity of the self-other boundary as expressed in experiences of ambiguous body boundaries, intrusions, and even merging with others. Here, the person has not lost access to the socially extended mind but has instead become lost in it, possibly due to a weakened sense of self. We argue that this neglected aspect of schizophrenic social dysfunction can be usefully approached via the concept of *genuine intersubjectivity*: We normally participate in a shared experience with another person by implicitly co-regulating how our interaction unfolds. This co-regulation integrates our respective experience's dynamical bases into one interpersonal process and gives the interaction an ambiguous second-person character. The upshot is that reports of abnormal self-other fluidity are not indicative of hallucinations without any basis in reality, but of a heightened sensitivity and vulnerability to processes of interpersonal alignment and mutual incorporation that form the normal basis of social life. We conclude by discussing implications of this view for both the science of consciousness as well as approaches to intervention and therapy.

Genuine Intersubjectivity

Cognitive science has traditionally approached social cognition from the perspective of methodological individualism, whereby our whole experience of social life could in principle be realized by a single brain-in-a-vat (Searle, 1990). More recently, there is a growing interest in the role of social interaction for social cognition, but often the contribution of others is still relegated to merely external or contextual factors, such as sources of information or as triggers for neural activations or cognitive processes that are ultimately realizable in individual brains (Gallotti & Frith, 2013; Goldman & de Vignemont, 2009; Herschbach, 2012). In other words, recognition of the importance of social interaction generally stops short of treating that interaction process itself as part of the cognitive.

Yet in recent theoretical developments toward greater recognition of embodied, embedded, extended, and enactive approaches to cognitive science, so-called 4E cognition (Newen, de Bruin, & Gallagher, 2018), there is also increasing acceptance of the possibility that interaction with others, in itself, is an essential part of cognitive processes (De Jaegher, Di Paolo, & Gallagher, 2010; Di Paolo, Cuffari, & De Jaegher, 2018; Fuchs, 2018; Gallagher, 2013; Krueger, 2013). This theoretical development has been applied to qualitative and cultural studies of intercorporeal practices (Durt, Fuchs, & Tewes, 2017; Meyer, Streeck, & Jordan, 2017), and is starting to be cashed out in experimental terms. There is growing evidence from a variety of fields that social cognition is fundamentally different when we are in interaction with others rather than merely observing them (Schilbach et al., 2013). For instance, some of our work on social interaction using agent-based simulation modeling (Candadai, Setzler, Izquierdo, & Froese, 2019) and human real-time interaction paradigms (Froese, Iizuka, & Ikegami, 2014) has demonstrated that two interacting agents can form larger, coupled systems with new properties and processes at the collective level. These results are in line with theoretical developments that imply that social interaction can give rise to cognitive processes that could not be realized by the individuals in the absence of that social coupling, such as forms of collective memory (Sutton, 2008), patterns of interpersonally distributed emotion regulation (Varga & Krueger, 2013), and even aspects of phenomenal consciousness (Kirchhoff & Kiverstein, 2019).

We will refer to experience with a shared, social interactive basis as *genuine intersubjectivity* (Froese, 2018). This concept is loosely inspired by phenomenological research into intersubjectivity, social groups, and the "we" (for a review of the classical authors on these topics, see Zahavi, 2001), but it is formulated in the context of recent developments in 4E cognition. Specifically, genuine intersubjectivity refers to a subset of the phenomena captured by the notion of the socially extended mind (Krueger, 2011, 2013), namely, the subset that has to do with the socially extended *lived experience* that is associated with the co-regulated real-time interaction taking place between two or more persons. The concept therefore explicitly pursues a middle way between two radical positions: On the one hand, by being tied to concrete social encounters, the notion of genuine intersubjectivity can be distinguished from transcendental interpretations of intersubjectivity (like the phenomenological concept of open intersubjectivity), which refer to the a priori constitutive impact of other subjects regardless of their actual presence (e.g., Varga, 2013). On the other hand, the qualifier "genuine" is also intended to highlight that this concept contrasts with the prevalent theories of social cognition in cognitive science that categorically reject any constitutive role of others for a person's social cognition, even during concrete social interaction (e.g., Gallotti & Frith, 2013). In other words, the concept usefully accepts a broader constitutive basis of lived experience than traditional cognitive science, and yet not as broad as the constitutive basis assumed by transcendental intersubjectivity.

Genuine intersubjectivity is nothing mysterious; it simply means that social interaction makes a difference to lived experience: How we relate to the world in each moment of our experience is not independent from how we interact with others in that moment. For instance, think of two people engaged in a spontaneous dance: The fluid and tightly coordinated movements would be impossible to make in isolation, that is, without the mutually responsive co-regulation of the unfolding embodied interaction. Moreover, it is precisely this shared participation in the dance that transforms the experience into something that "we" do together. Thus, by making genuine intersubjectivity the starting point of our investigation into social cognition, it arguably brings the science of social cognition much closer to our normal experience of the embodied and interactive basis of social life, especially when compared with traditional, supposedly "folk" psychological approaches (Ratcliffe, 2007).

This premise also helps us to make better sense of the disorders of social cognition. Traditional approaches tend to over-narrowly look for the causes of these disorders in the cognitive malfunctioning of detached social observation, such as theory of mind or mental simulation (Gerrans & McGeer, 2003). However, paradoxically, people on the schizophrenic spectrum often intentionally employ sophisticated mindreading strategies and in a pervasive manner, yet without being able to properly compensate for the lack of common sense social understanding (Froese, Stanghellini, & Bertelli, 2013). Genuine intersubjectivity helps us to rethink this social dysfunction as resulting instead from disordered embodied interaction, as already highlighted in the field of phenomenological psychopathology (Fuchs, 2005; Stanghellini, 2004). When the body is no longer implicitly lived through, it awkwardly stands out in experience almost like an object or machine to be explicitly controlled (de Haan & Fuchs, 2010). Accordingly, the function of embodied interaction to disclose the world to perceptual experience becomes impaired and there is a progressive loss of the scaffolding provided by the socially extended mind, which also has disruptive consequences for social perception and social cognition (Krueger & Aiken, 2016), affect regulation (Krueger, 2020), and eventually for thought (Ratcliffe, 2017a).

However, at times people with schizophrenia report that they experience the opposite of dissociality, namely, an unusual fluidity of the self-other boundary as expressed in unpleasant experiences of ambiguous body boundaries, intrusions, and even merging with others (Lysaker, Johannesen, & Lysaker, 2005). Here, the person has not lost access to the socially extended mind, but has instead become lost in it, possibly due to a weakened sense of self. This anomaly was only briefly summarized in the *Examination of Anomalous Self-Experience* (EASE) under the heading "4.1 Confusion with the Other" (Parnas et al., 2005):

> The patient experiences himself and his interlocutor as if being mixed up or interpenetrated, in the sense that he loses his sense of whose thoughts, feelings, or expressions originate in whom. He may describe it as a feeling of being invaded, intruded upon in a nonspecific but unpleasant or anxiety-provoking way. (Parnas et al., 2005, p. 254)

Recently, this neglected anomaly received a more elaborate treatment in the *Examination of Anomalous World Experience* (EAWE) as part of Domain 3 "Other Persons" (Sass et al., 2017), specifically under heading "3.7 Disturbance of Self-Other Demarcation."

> The subject feels that *the basic sense of independence or separateness of self and other persons has broken down or become much more fluid than normal*. This may involve feelings of unusual empathy, openness, control, fusion, or confusion between self and others—whether experienced physically, psychologically, or concerning identity. (Sass et al., 2017, p. 28)

Despite the growing interest in analyzing the intersubjective dimension of schizophrenia (e.g., Fuchs, 2015; Henriksen & Nilsson, 2017; Van Duppen, 2017), this disturbance of self-other demarcation has so far received little attention.

We argue that this neglected aspect of the social dimension of schizophrenia can also be usefully approached via the concept of genuine intersubjectivity: We normally participate in a shared experience with another person by implicitly co-regulating how our interaction unfolds (Froese, 2018). This integrates our respective experience's dynamical bases into an extended body and gives the interaction an ambiguous second-person character (Froese & Fuchs, 2012; Fuchs & De Jaegher, 2009). The upshot is that reports of abnormal self-other fluidity are not indicative of hallucinations without any basis in reality, but of a heightened sensitivity and vulnerability to processes of interpersonal alignment and mutual incorporation that form the normal basis of social life. As in the case of other symptoms of schizophrenia, it is arguably such a fundamental alteration of self-awareness that is at the core of later developing delusions (Fuchs, 2013).

We conclude by discussing implications of this view for both approaches to intervention and therapy as well as the science of consciousness more generally. Specifically, we consider how body-focused therapeutic strategies such as yoga, music, and dance/movement therapies may help individuals develop the skills and sensitivities needed to more comfortably negotiate everyday processes of interpersonal alignment and mutual incorporation. We also show how disturbances of genuine intersubjectivity and the socially extended mind in schizophrenia challenge some prominent individualistic assumptions about the developmental origins of self-consciousness and about the phenomenology of the minimal self.

The Socially Extended Mind

The idea that the basis of cognition can extend outside the head and into interactions with other people has gained increased acceptance as part of the ongoing conceptual developments of embodied, embedded, extended, and enactive cognition (e.g., Gallagher, 2013; Krueger, 2011; Sutton, Harris, Keil, & Barnier, 2010). However, whether the same is true of consciousness remains a much more contentious topic (Clark, 2009). And yet, genuine intersubjectivity is not a mysterious nor elusive phenomenon.

Examples are already present from birth. Infants are born with a limited ability to self-regulate their attention, emotion, and behavior. Accordingly, they are deeply dependent upon the ongoing input of caregivers to physically "scaffold" their limited endogenous capacities and help them realize forms of self-regulation they could not realize in the absence of this social coupling. In this context, the notion of "scaffolding" refers to environmental (i.e., social and material) resources that drive and regulate human cognitive capacities.

To see an early instance of social scaffolding in action, consider breastfeeding, arguably the infant's first complex form of social interaction. Within breastfeeding episodes, mother and infant form a coupled social system via the rhythmic cycles and back-and-forth interplay of short feeding bursts. Via touch and gentle movements, mothers provide physical scaffolding (e.g., cradling the infant; gently "jiggling" them as a prompt to resume feeding) that organizes the infant's attention and guides their responsive behavior. However, this is not just a one-way process. Rather, mothers are, in turn, responsive to their infants: They adapt to the bout-pause rhythms of the infant's sucking behavior, which allows the infant to play a participatory role in structuring the dynamics of this exchange and, in so doing, realize feats of attention and emotion regulation that would otherwise elude them (Alberts, Kalverboer, & Hopkins, 1983; Kaye, 1982).

As children grow and develop, they remain deeply dependent upon the scaffolding provided by the ongoing input of caregivers – primarily comprised of direct bodily contact and vocal exchanges – to extend their self-regulative abilities. There is ample developmental evidence indicating that, beyond the expressive cues distinctive of breastfeeding, caregivers use a range of different strategies to regulate infant attention – for example, smiling, vocalizations, singing, caressing, diverting attention away from objects of distress – and, within these exchanges, infants and caregivers tightly integrate their expressive displays and realize attentional and affective convergence (Krueger, 2013; Taipale, 2016). When the infant becomes distressed by some object or event, for instance, caregivers will redirect their attention and downregulate their emotional disturbance by singing a soothing lullaby; likewise, when they become fussy or overly intrusive in adult contexts, sharp vocalizations and gestural manipulations from caregivers (e.g., emphatic hand waving, leaning in to crowd the infant's visual field) function as external mechanisms that guide and control the infant's experience (Spurrett & Cowley, 2004).

The key point is that within these early instances of genuine intersubjectivity, new cognitive processes and forms of self-regulative control emerge that would not otherwise exist outside of this coupled system. When part of a socially extended mind, infants can temporarily realize qualitatively new forms of attentional focusing, affective stability, and behavioral organization that exceeds their current phase of development (Tronick, 2005). Moreover, these exchanges enable infants to learn not simply *from* others but also *through* them, that is, to broaden their cognitive horizons as they begin to explore the external world (Tomasello, 1999). To be involved with others in instances of genuine intersubjectivity – even in its earliest forms – is to identity *affectively* with others. This is a shared process that "assimilates another person's bodily anchored psychological stance …, in such a way that the stance becomes a potential way of the observer relating to the world from his or her own position" (Hobson & Hobson, 2007, p. 411). The horizon-expanding character is a central epistemic function of genuine intersubjectivity.

Of course, instances of genuine intersubjectivity within socially extended minds are not confined to early infancy. They continue to develop and take shape throughout our lives. This is because the people we interact with, and the contexts in which we interact with them, provide rich forms of social and material scaffolding that drive and regulate our cognitive practices and patterns of interpersonal engagement. This scaffolding works at both local dyadic levels and at more encompassing group-level dynamics.

Within dyadic interactions, the gestures, facial expressions, intonation patterns, postural adjustments, and movements of others function as kinds of social scaffolding. That is, these expressive actions directly regulate the development and character of *our own* bodily responses. If someone smiles at us and makes a friendly gesture, for instance, these expressive actions will elicit similar responses from us and motivate an array of further friendly expressions; conversely, aggressive movements or threatening gestures compel us to tense up and prepare for our own aggressive response. Within the dynamics of face-to-face interaction, individuals spontaneously mimic others' facial expressions, gestures, and intonation patterns; they also coordinate and synchronize speech rhythms and bodily movements, which leads to affective convergence and heightened feelings of rapport (Bernieri & Rosenthal, 1991; Wiltermuth & Heath, 2009).

This socially distributed feedback loop regulates the affective dynamics of group-level engagements, too. When we are drawn into the exuberance of a lively party, for example, or swept along by the collective rage of a political protest or the euphoria of a live concert with thousands of other enthusiastic listeners, the expressions of others literally take hold of *our* bodily responses. They pull responsive movements and affective responses out of us that diachronically integrate with those of the crowd (Chartrand & Bargh, 1999; Slaby, 2014). As with the coupling processes that characterize our dyadic engagements, these group-level processes create "a circular interplay of expressions and reactions running in split seconds and constantly modifying each partner's bodily state, in a process that becomes highly autonomous and is not directly controlled by the partners" (Froese & Fuchs, 2012, p. 213). In other words, we are drawn into socially distributed co-regulatory systems that are partially comprised of scaffolding beyond our individual head. The ability to become active participants within such systems is crucial for prosocial behavior and shared experience. In addition to providing important resources for regulating our own affective experiences, socially distributed feedback loops enhance feelings of rapport, connectedness, and cooperation with others (Lakin & Chartrand, 2003; Van Baaren, Holland, Kawakami, & Van Knippenberg, 2004). These shared feelings are what drive instances of genuine intersubjectivity. They are at the core of our ability to perceive and respond to affordances found in others and social contexts more generally, coordinate joint actions, and remain sensitive to the often unspoken "rules of the game" (e.g., what to say, how to act, how to express and manage emotions, etc.) governing the social contexts we negotiate on a day-to-day basis. As we will see in more detail later, the ability to enter into socially extended systems such as these is compromised in schizophrenia, leading to breakdowns and disruptions of social cognition.

Loss of the Socially Extended Mind

Within phenomenological psychopathology, much recent work has focused on qualitative transformations of experience that appear to be distinctive of schizophrenia. In particular, many of these approaches argue that qualitative transformations in schizophrenia are rooted in a disturbance of the minimal or core sense of self (Parnas & Henriksen, 2016; Sass & Parnas, 2003).

According to these "ipseity-disturbance models" – *ipseity* is Latin for "self" or "itself" – this core self is a prereflective form of self-awareness: the enduring feeling of being a subject of experience from one moment to the next. From this perspective, all experiences – for example, visually savoring a particularly colorful sunset; feeling a twinge of pain in your lower back; being gripped by a bout of melancholy; and smiling at the memory of your deceased grandmother – occur in a first-personal mode of presentation. This first-person dimension marks that experience as belonging to a subject (i.e., the subject or owner *of* that experience); it is a necessary structural feature of experience that is inextricable from "the distinct manner, or *how*, of experiencing" (Zahavi, 2014, p. 22).

According to ipseity-disturbance approaches, there is evidence that this first-person dimension can become disturbed in schizophrenia, particularly during the prodromal phase. Such disturbances are indicated by patient reports in which individuals say that they have somehow lost a felt sense of connection or immediacy with respect to their own experience. They say things like, "My I-feeling is diminished"; "My I is disappearing for me" (Parnas & Handest, 2003, p. 125); "I am disconnected, disintegrated, diminished … I feel that my real self has left me" (Kean, 2009, p. 1034). This self-splitting in schizophrenic self-experience can be understood as a pathological exaggeration of the alterity that is normally implicit in the structure of subjectivity, and which thereby reveals a "vulnerability in the functioning of auto-affection, which normally assures the feeling of self-coincidence in the constant differentiation and reintegration of the subject" (Stephensen & Parnas, 2018, p. 639). Often, this "diminished self-affection," as it is sometimes called, is framed primarily as a disturbance of phenomenal self-consciousness. However, it is becoming increasingly recognized that self-disturbances in schizophrenia frequently harbor a pronounced bodily and social dimension as well. We will return to a deeper consideration of the social dimension of experience toward the end of this chapter, and will now focus on the bodily dimension.

Many of the negative symptoms of schizophrenia can be usefully approached as symptoms of specific kind of disembodiment (Fuchs, 2005; Stanghellini, 2004). Reports from individuals with schizophrenia spectrum disorders indicate that they often experience their bodies more like deanimated objects.

> Many of these reports indicate a diminishment or loss of bodily *self-intimacy*, which is often a consequence of *depersonalization*. Instead of living transparently *through* their body as a unified center of agency and experience—that is, the body-as-subject—they describe feeling disconnected or alienated from their bodies. (Krueger & Aiken, 2016, p. 131)

This kind of disembodiment – which involves a kind of hyperreflective self-monitoring (Fuchs, 2010) – not only makes it difficult to act spontaneously and flexibly in the world but it also has negative consequences for the capacity to feel related to others and to access shared meaning (Sass, 2017). Within this hyperreflective stance, habitual styles of thinking, moving, acting, perceiving, speaking, expressing emotions, and interacting with the world come to the foreground and become objects of intense scrutiny. Some patients report that thinking becomes difficult because thoughts develop spatial or object-like qualities (Parnas & Handest, 2003). Others say that performing normally spontaneous actions like gesturing, falling asleep, putting a book on a shelf, or brushing their teeth becomes very difficult or even impossible due to the individuals' excessive attention to every aspect of the performance (Fuchs, 2010). This disruption is also manifest in how individuals bodily engage with the social world. Making small talk, gesturing naturally while speaking, laughing at appropriate moments in the flow of conversation, or simply knowing when and how to enter into spontaneous social exchanges with others becomes difficult due to this experience of disembodiment. The experience of disembodiment in this way leads to a kind of "attunement crisis": an inability "to attune with the current situation, to intuitively get a grasp on the thinking of the person you are talking to, and above all their emotional plane, to match it" (Stanghellini, 2004, p. 22).

The disruptions of embodiment and of social cognition are thus closely related. Faced with a progressive loss of intuitive, common-sense understanding of social life, and a diminished capacity for direct social perception of others' intentions, individuals are forced to increasingly rely on detached observation and theorizing, but without being able to fully compensate for the lack of self-evidence (Froese et al., 2013). Individuals who feel disembodied, and hence end up disembedded from the social world, also have difficulties in taking advantage of the cognitive scaffolding that is normally afforded by interacting with others, that is, when becoming entrained into a socially extended mind (Krueger, 2020). Alongside the disaffection from one's own body and the estrangement from others, there develop more fundamental cognitive disruptions as the integrity of human experience is consistently undermined, ultimately giving rise to positive symptoms such as auditory verbal hallucinations and thought insertion (Ratcliffe, 2017a).

Lost in the Socially Extended Mind

The concept of genuine intersubjectivity allows us to appreciate how interacting with others makes a difference to our cognitive capacities, empowering us to do things we could not do on our own. And it also helps us to make sense of how a breakdown of the capacity for fluid embodied interaction can give rise to disruptions in social cognition, and even undermine the integrity of the intentional structure of consciousness, giving rise to hallucinations. But there is another characteristic anomaly often found in reports of individuals with schizophrenia spectrum disorder that has so far received less attention, namely, confusions of self and other, which can also be illuminated by the concept of genuine intersubjectivity.

From the perspective of traditional cognitive science, according to which the self is inside the head and hence fundamentally separated from others, this disturbance of self-other demarcation must logically be approached as a category of positive symptoms, that is, as hallucinations without basis in reality. However, the concept of genuine intersubjectivity provides an alternative perspective because it follows the enactive approach in accepting that a certain amount of self-other fluidity is a normal part of the human condition. For instance, the concept of participatory sense-making highlights that people's sense-making processes can become intertwined while they engage in interaction (De Jaegher & Di Paolo, 2007), and this typically involves dynamical processes of mutual incorporation leading to what might be called an extended body (Froese & Fuchs, 2012; Fuchs & De Jaegher, 2009). The presence of others can move us both physically and affectively; we are moved by movement and moved to move in a reciprocal manner (Fuchs & Koch, 2014). And yet despite this irreducible ambiguity between self and other during social interaction, we normally do not worry about who is ultimately responsible for our cognitive processes, and we do not feel that our bodies are invaded by or merged into others' bodies. If so, then what goes wrong with this kind of genuine intersubjectivity for people on the schizophrenic disorder spectrum?

The key here is to note that the disturbance has to do with feelings of "unusual" self-other fluidity. We can get a better sense of the different forms of this disturbance by considering the items listed under EAWE heading 3.7:

3.7.1 Hyperattunement
3.7.2 Unusual Influence over Others
3.7.3 Pathological Openness
3.7.4 Experiences of Being Controlled
3.7.5 Merging or Fluid Psychological Boundaries
3.7.6 Universal Merging with Others
3.7.7 Uncertain Personal Identity/Attitudes
3.7.8 Uncertain Physical Boundaries
3.7.9 Experience of Being Imitated

What is immediately striking is that this list of items reads almost like the direct opposite of the dissociality caused by schizophrenic disembodiment we discussed in the previous section. This suggests that we might need a broader view of anomalous social experience that is associated with the schizophrenia spectrum. However, in the ancillary article to EAWE

Domain 3, only a couple of items listed under heading 3.7 are mentioned, and without any attempt at conceptually integrating them with the other characteristic disruptions of this domain (Stanghellini, Ballerini, & Mancini, 2017). Most of the discussion of the specific anomalies of this domain continues to be focused on forms of *dissociality*, a concept which builds on and extends the concept of autism. There is therefore an unresolved tension in current accounts of the social dimension of schizophrenia.

The concept of genuine intersubjectivity provides us with an intuitive way of understanding this two-sided nature of social dysfunction in schizophrenia. We normally form coupled systems during social interaction, in which the interactors become integrated into a larger, collective process that shapes their individual cognitive capacities, including their social cognitive capacities. Simply put, skillful embodied social interaction facilitates direct social perception (Krueger, 2012, in press; McGann & De Jaegher, 2009), so schizophrenic disembodiment will impair this direct access and thus feed into the characteristic symptoms of dissociality. But if the individual is not strongly rooted in their body, this weakened ego-pole could also create a vulnerability to the intermingling and entraining effects of social coupling. Cases of genuine intersubjectivity would then no longer present themselves as opportunities for taking advantage of the new affordances unleashed by the socially extended mind, but as a danger of becoming lost in the ensuing coupled social system. Accordingly, from our perspective, the disturbance of self-other demarcation is no longer seen as a type of hallucination, but rather as rooted in an ambiguity that is part of the normal human condition:

> For phenomenologists, the fluid oscillation between the body-as-subject and the body-as-object highlights a "bodily ambiguity" at the heart of our embodied experience: as embodied subjects, we are neither wholly subjects nor wholly objects, but somehow always both. (Krueger & Henriksen, 2016, p. 263)

The role of an unusually fluid or unstable sense of self-presence, self-intimacy, or ipseity in giving rise to schizophrenic dissociality has already been recognized (Krueger & Henriksen, 2016; Stephensen & Parnas, 2018), and what remains to be explored is the other side of the bodily ambiguity, that is, when the lived distance between the self and the body becomes too attenuated. Indeed, it has been observed that some patients not only report a progressive loss of their sense of embodiment but also problems of getting lost in their embodiment to the extent that they become completely absorbed in manual activities such that they can no longer maintain a sense of self at all (de Haan & Fuchs, 2010).

> Everything I do, I do with logic and reconsideration. Almost nothing works naturally, of its own accord … However, I can also do things without even noticing. I get up, I brush my teeth, I get back, and I cannot even remember what I have done in between. That also happens. It is a combination of both: either complete automatism, or complete control. (de Haan & Fuchs, 2010, p. 330)

Putting these different strands together, we arrive at a more general concept of affective instability that includes both hypofamiliarity and hyperfamiliarity: Most frequently, the affective pendulum swings toward an extreme disaffection from the body and from others, leading to hyperreflectivity, but occasionally the pendulum swings the other way toward an extreme identification with one's body and with others, leading to what de Haan and Fuchs termed "hyperautomaticity" (2010, p. 330). We suggest that in the latter case, persons on the schizophrenia disorder spectrum come to closely coincide with the alterity, that is, intrinsic to subjectivity (Zahavi, 1999), thereby losing (or at least weakening) the self-distance that is required for adopting a distinct first-person perspective on the world. The result is that they are uncomfortably "open" to the world, and thereby also unusually sensitive to the spontaneously entraining effects of the presence of others. Absorbed by the self-organized actions of their own objective bodies, they are vulnerable to becoming completely lost in the interactively extended body, too (Gozé, Grohmann, Naudin, & Cermolacce, 2017). The person with schizophrenia is unable to maintain the existential balance between independence (distinction) and openness (participation), and temporary collapses into the latter side lead to "a loss of boundaries and an experienced immersion with others" (Kyselo, 2016, p. 612).

It is an open question how being lost in the socially extended mind manifests itself from the point of view of others, or how it could be measured during social interactions. One possibility is that the lost individual becomes abnormally entrained with the others' movements, which should be reflected in significantly increased nonverbal interpersonal synchrony. Nevertheless, the experimental consensus is that there is a notable decrease in motion synchrony, at least in individuals who are stabilized and who are typically medicated (Galbusera, Finn, & Fuchs, 2018; Kupper, Ramseyer, Hoffmann, & Tschacher, 2015). It would be interesting to investigate whether there is abnormal interpersonal synchrony at the level of brain and physiological activity. Alternatively, it may be the case that the lost individual's sense of self is already sufficiently weakened that even normal levels of entrainment feel too confusing, intrusive, and threatening. In this case, becoming lost in self-other confusion may instead express itself as a withdrawal from social interaction in the attempt to preserve a sense of self. This interpretation is consistent with a number of studies showing that patients in social interaction display fewer nonverbal behaviors inviting further interaction from their counterparts (Lavelle, Healey, & McCabe, 2014).

Accordingly, what has been described as dissociality may actually encompass two distinct phenomena. On the one hand, there is an involuntary impairment of fluid social interaction capabilities arising from hypopermeable self-other boundaries, and on the other hand, there is voluntary avoidance of fluid social interaction in response to hyperpermeable self-other boundaries (Van Duppen, 2017, p. 408). We can also easily imagine that the latter compensatory strategy, while permitting the individual to confront the social world on their own terms for some time, in the long term ultimately feeds into the former phenomenon, that is, a degradation of social skills that becomes the basis of their more characteristic involuntary social decoupling.

If this interpretation is on the right track, then it could also help to make sense of the otherwise seemingly paradoxical finding that, whereas patients comparatively gesture less when speaking, when they do gesture more, this is associated with others experiencing poorer patient rapport (Lavelle, Healey, & McCabe, 2013). For while one strategy to avoid becoming lost in self-other interaction is complete social withdrawal, another, less drastic response is to continue engaging socially, but to do so in a desynchronized manner that counteracts the spontaneous tendencies for mutual entrainment that would otherwise threaten to overwhelm the weakened sense of self. From the interlocutor's perspective, this alternative compensatory strategy would result in the strange experience of interacting with a person and yet their presence simultaneously hides, withdraws, and undermines itself. Accordingly, this perspective could support the development of an enactive explanation of the sense of unease or "praecox-feeling" felt by the interviewer when diagnosing patients (Varga, 2013).

Finally, this perspective also sheds new light on findings that individuals with schizophrenia exhibit normal levels of interpersonal synchrony and imitation when confronted by virtual agents or videos of others (Raffard et al., 2018; Simonsen et al., 2019). These virtual situations permit "social" interactions that do not actually involve other people, and hence there is in principle no possibility for genuine intersubjectivity nor for its characteristic self-other ambiguities. The upshot is that even if such experimental paradigms are ecologically more valid than completely passive paradigms that lack any possibility for interaction, such as viewing photos of emotional expressions, we should still be careful to generalize from artificial interactive scenarios to those involving genuine intersubjectivity.

Conclusions and Further Implications

The hypothesis of the socially extended mind has been usefully applied to make sense of schizophrenic dissociality as arising from the condition's characteristic sense of disembodiment, and the challenge of interacting with others in the fluid manner required for effective social coupling. Consequently, the condition also involves reduced access to the various forms of scaffolding normally provided by the socially extended mind. Here, we have applied this hypothesis to a neglected aspect of the condition, namely, the disturbance of self-other demarcation. We have argued that the concept of genuine intersubjectivity, that is, that interaction with others makes a difference to individual experience in its own right, enables us to sharpen our understanding of this disturbance. It turns out that it is not the self-other ambiguity as such that is the problem, given that this ambiguity is a normal part of social interaction, but rather that there is a heightened sensitivity or vulnerability to this ambiguity. It is no longer a transparent or implicit aspect of social experience and hence can be felt as threatening and overwhelming.

There are implications for therapy: If a patient reports being disturbed by a felt ambiguity regarding self-other boundaries, a traditional internalist approach would tend to discount the disturbing experience as a delusion or hallucination without basis in reality and would try to find ways of eliminating it. Alternatively, from the perspective we have been developing here, this unusual experience is reconceived as a heightened sensitivity and vulnerability to a self-other ambiguity that is a normal, albeit usually transparently lived through, aspect of social interaction. In other words, while it agrees that it is desirable to develop ways of helping patients avoid getting lost in the socially extended mind, it also suggests that the aim should not be to eliminate experience of self-other ambiguity altogether. Given the essential role assigned to this ambiguity in the constitution of genuine intersubjectivity, interventions that completely suppress it could inadvertently contribute to symptoms of dissociality. A better approach would be to find ways of helping patients to cope and live with the self-other ambiguity that is at the core of human embodiment and intersubjectivity (Kyselo, 2016).

While they are not yet mainstream, there are nevertheless existing therapeutic approaches that may help individuals to develop the bodily, perceptual, and affective skills needed to negotiate aspects of self-other ambiguities that constitute genuine intersubjectivity. For example, Maiese (2015) convincingly argues for the need to develop and further explore "bottom-up treatment methods," as she terms them. Such bottom-up methods include yoga, music, and dance/movement therapies. These methods may be particularly effective in the context of schizophrenia because they directly address the dynamics of bodily movement, affective expression, and interpersonal coordination and entrainment. Specifically, these are body-focused therapeutic strategies that can help individuals deepen their felt sense of bodily ownership and agency, feel more at home and engaged with their social and material environment, and develop more effective and refined ways of expressing, sharing, and regulating their emotions both alone and with others (see Galbusera et al., 2018).

For example, musical activities such as listening, singing, and joint music-making provide regulative contexts in which individuals can enhance social skills like eye contact, joint attention, mimicry, and turn-taking (this is why music therapy can also be effective for children and adults with autism [Srinivasan & Bhat, 2013]). These activities furnish rich, multimodal environments for individuals with schizophrenia to strengthen their ability to perceive fine-grained social cues in others and develop their capacity for "body-reading." In musical contexts, subjects rely on bodily expressions to communicate with one another – but expressive movements, eye contact, and mimicry tend to be more exaggerated than in nonmusical interactions, which creates more opportunities for subjects to develop their perceptual sensitivity to these things.

Additionally, musical environments provide opportunities to become experientially acquainted with what it *feels like* to negotiate fluctuations of agency, control, and self-other ambiguities within genuine intersubjectivity. This is because musically generated auditory and rhythmic signals scaffold attention, movement, and experience in a number of ways. Dynamic changes in the quality and tempo of tones and rhythm regulate participants' attention, pull bodily and affective responses out of them, and punctuate the timing and quality of both individual movements and patterns of joint music-making that unfold over time. Individuals in this way experience themselves voluntarily "letting go" with the music. However, they also exert some degree of control over this process: Via their own movements, they directly shape the responsive movements and experiences of others. Music can thus serve as scaffolding for the development of selective attention and strengthen individuals' sense of embodied intersubjectivity (Krueger, 2014; Maiese, 2016). While research in this area is still emerging, there is some evidence that improvised sessions creating music with a therapist can lead to at least a short-term reduction in general symptoms (e.g., depression) and negative symptoms in schizophrenic patients (Talwar et al., 2006).

There are also implications for the science of consciousness: While phenomenological approaches have long argued that lived experience is necessarily characterized by a first-person givenness, known as the minimal self (Zahavi, 2005), this characterization sits uneasily with its deeply social dimension, as revealed by the experiential effects of social disorder in conditions such as schizophrenia (Kyselo, 2016; Ratcliffe, 2017b). Neither does the premise of a minimal self make a good fit with hyperautomaticity: Patients report a complete loss of self, but presumably they continue to experience the flow of consciousness albeit from an apparently egoless vantage point. In such cases, it might be more appropriate to say that there is ongoing experience, but not an experience for or given to "me"; or at least there is significantly weakened sense of ownership (almost, at times, to the point of disappearance) with respect to the experience. Similarly, if first-personal givenness is a necessary component of all experiences, it becomes difficult to accept at face value patients' reports of being confused about the ownership of thoughts and other experiences. Here, the structural integration of these experiences into a patient's stream of consciousness evidently remains intact, since they are indeed undergone as lived experiences and can later be recalled, but they seem to lack the quality of first-personal perspectival ownership.

If so, it would be more parsimonious to agree that all experience is necessarily perspectival; it structurally belongs to a distinct perspective. However, a specifically *first-person* perspective from which "I" live through experiences "for me" is an additional achievement that depends on sociocultural capacities (Hutto & Ilundáin-Agurruza, 2020), and these capacities are acquired via social interaction during development (Fuchs, 2013). So, a refinement of the ipseity-disturbance model is to say that the distinctive perspectivalness of experience remains intact, but that the additional capacities needed for a stable first-person perspective are disrupted in schizophrenia.

More generally, this turns the science of self-consciousness on its head: Rather than starting with the assumption of self-awareness emerging from a single brain and then trying to overcome the problem of other minds, we start with genuine intersubjectivity emerging from the socially extended mind and then investigate how a stable sense of self can arise from such an ambiguous self-other demarcation.

Acknowledgment

Tom Froese thanks the organizers of the *Time, the Body, and the Other* conference for the opportunity to test out some of these ideas in front of a lively audience at Heidelberg University.

References

Alberts, E., Kalverboer, A. F., & Hopkins, B. (1983). Mother-infant dialogue in the first days of life: An observational study during breast-feeding. *Journal of Child Psychology and Psychiatry*, 24(1), 145–161. doi: 10.1111/j.1469-7610.1983.tb00111.x

Bernieri, F. J., & Rosenthal, R. (1991). Interpersonal coordination: Behavior matching and interactional synchrony. In R. S. Feldman & B. Rimé (Eds.), *Studies in emotion & social interaction. Fundamentals of nonverbal behavior* (pp. 401–432). Cambridge, UK: Cambridge University Press.

Candadai, M., Setzler, M., Izquierdo, E. J., & Froese, T. (2019). Embodied dyadic interaction increases complexity of neural dynamics: A minimal agent-based simulation model. *Frontiers in Psychology*, 10, 1–5. doi: 10.3389/fpsyg.2019.00540

Chartrand, T., & Bargh, J. A. (1999). The chameleon effect: The perception-behavior link and social interaction. *Journal of Personality and Social Psychology*, 76(6), 893–910. doi: 10.1037//0022-3514.76.6.893

Clark, A. (2009). Spreading the joy? Why the machinery of consciousness is (probably) still in the head. *Mind*, 118(472), 963–993. doi: 10.1093/mind/fzp110

de Haan, S., & Fuchs, T. (2010). The ghost in the machine: Disembodiment in schizophrenia – Two case studies. *Psychopathology*, 43, 327–333. doi: 10.1159/000319402

De Jaegher, H., & Di Paolo, E. A. (2007). Participatory sense-making: An enactive approach to social cognition. *Phenomenology and the Cognitive Sciences*, 6(4), 485–507. doi: 10.1007/s11097-007-9076-9

De Jaegher, H., Di Paolo, E. A., & Gallagher, S. (2010). Can social interaction constitute social cognition? *Trends in Cognitive Sciences*, 14(10), 441–447. doi: 10.1016/j.tics.2010.06.009

Di Paolo, E. A., Cuffari, E. C., & De Jaegher, H. (2018). *Linguistic bodies: The continuity between life and language*. Cambridge, MA: Massachusetts Institute of Technology Press.

Durt, C., Fuchs, T., & Tewes, C. (Eds.). (2017). *Embodiment, enaction, and culture: Investigating the constitution of the shared world*. Cambridge, MA: Massachusetts Institute of Technology Press.

Froese, T. (2018). Searching for the conditions of genuine intersubjectivity: From agent-based models to perceptual crossing experiments. In A. Newen, L. de Bruin, & S. Gallagher (Eds.), *The Oxford handbook of 4e cognition* (pp. 163–186). Oxford, UK: Oxford University Press.

Froese, T., & Fuchs, T. (2012). The extended body: A case study in the neurophenomenology of social interaction. *Phenomenology and the Cognitive Sciences*, 11(2), 205–235. doi: 10.1007/s11097-012-9254-2

Froese, T., Iizuka, H., & Ikegami, T. (2014). Embodied social interaction constitutes social cognition in pairs of humans: A minimalist virtual reality experiment. *Scientific Reports*, 4, 1–10. doi: 10.1038/srep03672

Froese, T., Stanghellini, G., & Bertelli, M. O. (2013). Is it normal to be a principal mindreader? Revising theories of social cognition on the basis of schizophrenia and high functioning autism-spectrum disorders. *Research in Developmental Disabilities*, 34(5), 1376–1387. doi: 10.1016/j.ridd.2013.01.005

Fuchs, T. (2005). Corporealized and disembodied minds: A phenomenological view of the body in melancholia and schizophrenia. *Philosophy, Psychiatry & Psychology*, 12(2), 95–107. doi: 10.1353/ppp.2005.0040

Fuchs, T. (2010). The psychopathology of hyperreflexivity. *The Journal of Speculative Philosophy*, 24(3), 239–255. doi: 10.1353/jsp.2010.0010

Fuchs, T. (2013). The phenomenology and development of social perspectives. *Phenomenology and the Cognitive Sciences*, 12(4), 655–683. doi: 10.1007/s11097-012-9267-x

Fuchs, T. (2015). Pathologies of intersubjectivity in autism and schizophrenia. *Journal of Consciousness Studies*, 22(1–2), 191–214.

Fuchs, T. (2018). *Ecology of the brain: The phenomenology and biology of the embodied mind.* Oxford, UK: Oxford University Press.

Fuchs, T., & De Jaegher, H. (2009). Enacting intersubjectivity: Participatory sense-making and mutual incorporation. *Phenomenology and the Cognitive Sciences*, 8(4), 465–486. doi: 10.1007/s11097-009-9136-4

Fuchs, T., & Koch, S. C. (2014). Embodied affectivity: On moving and being moved. *Frontiers in Psychology*, 5, 1–12. doi: 10.3389/fpsyg.2014.00508

Galbusera, L., Finn, M. T., & Fuchs, T. (2018). Interactional synchrony and negative symptoms: An outcome study of body-oriented psychotherapy for schizophrenia. *Psychotherapy Research*, 28(3), 457–469. doi: 10.1080/10503307.2016.1216624

Gallagher, S. (2013). The socially extended mind. *Cognitive Systems Research*, 25–26, 4–12. doi: 10.1016/j.cogsys.2013.03.008

Gallotti, M., & Frith, C. D. (2013). Social cognition in the we-mode. *Trends in Cognitive Sciences*, 17(4), 160–165. doi: 10.1016/j.tics.2013.02.002

Gerrans, P., & McGeer, V. (2003). Theory of mind in autism and schizophrenia: A case of over-optimistic reverse engineering. In B. Repacholi & V. Slaughter (Eds.), *Individual differences in theory of mind: Implications for typical and atypical development* (pp. 271–304). New York, NY: Psychology Press.

Goldman, A., & de Vignemont, F. (2009). Is social cognition embodied? *Trends in Cognitive Sciences*, 13(4), 154–159. doi: 10.1016/j.tics.2009.01.007

Gozé, T., Grohmann, T., Naudin, J., & Cermolacce, M. (2017). New insight into affectivity in schizophrenia: From the phenomenology of Marc Richir. *Psychopathology*, 50(6), 401–407. doi: 10.1159/000481516

Henriksen, M. G., & Nilsson, L. S. (2017). Intersubjectivity and psychopathology in the schizophrenia spectrum: Complicated we, compensatory strategies, and self-disorders. *Psychopathology*, 50(5), 321–333. doi: 10.1159/000479702

Herschbach, M. (2012). On the role of social interaction in social cognition: A mechanistic alternative to enactivism. *Phenomenology and the Cognitive Sciences*, 11(4), 467–486. doi: 10.1007/s11097-011-9209-z

Hobson, J. A., & Hobson, R. P. (2007). Identification: The missing link between joint attention and imitation? *Development and Psychopathology*, 19(2), 411–431. doi: 10.1017/S0954579407070204

Hutto, D. D., & Ilundáin-Agurruza, J. (2020). Selfless activity and experience: Radicalizing minimal self-awareness. *Topoi*, 39, 509–20. doi: 10.1007/s11245-018-9573-1

Kaye, K. (1982). *The mental and social life of babies: How parents create persons*. Chicago, IL: The University of Chicago Press.

Kean, C. (2009). Silencing the self: Schizophrenia as a self-disturbance. *Schizophrenia Bulletin*, 35(6), 1034–1036. doi: 10.1093/schbul/sbp043

Kirchhoff, M., & Kiverstein, J. (2019). *Extended consciousness and predictive processing: A third wave view*. Abingdon, UK: Routledge.

Krueger, J. (2011). Extended cognition and the space of social interaction. *Consciousness and Cognition*, 20(3), 643–657. doi: 10.1016/j.concog.2010.09.022

Krueger, J. (2012). Seeing mind in action. *Phenomenology and the Cognitive Sciences*, 11(2), 149–173. doi: 10.1007/s11097-011-9226-y

Krueger, J. (2013). Ontogenesis of the socially extended mind. *Cognitive Systems Research*, 25–26, 40–46. doi: 10.1016/j.cogsys.2013.03.001

Krueger, J. (2014). Affordances and the musically extended mind. *Frontiers in Psychology*, 4, 1–13. doi: 10.3389/fpsyg.2013.01003

Krueger, J. (in press). Enactivism, other minds, and mental disorders. *Synthese*.

Krueger, J. (2020). Schizophrenia and the scaffolded self. *Topoi*, 39, 597–609. doi: 10.1007/s11245-018-9547-3.

Krueger, J., & Aiken, A. T. (2016). Losing social space: Phenomenological disruptions of spatiality and embodiment in Moebius syndrome and schizophrenia. In J. Reynolds & R. Sebold (Eds.), *Phenomenology and science* (pp. 121–139). New York, NY: Palgrave Macmillan.

Krueger, J., & Henriksen, M. G. (2016). Embodiment and affectivity in Moebius syndrome and schizophrenia: A phenomenological analysis. In J. A. Simmons & J. E. Hackett (Eds.), *Phenomenology for the twenty-first century* (pp. 249–267). London, UK: Palgrave Macmillan.

Kupper, Z., Ramseyer, F., Hoffmann, H., & Tschacher, W. (2015). Nonverbal synchrony in social interactions of patients with schizophrenia indicates socio-communicative deficits. *PLoS ONE*, 10, 1–18. doi: 10.1371/journal.pone.0145882

Kyselo, M. (2016). The enactive approach and disorders of the self – The case of schizophrenia. *Phenomenology and the Cognitive Sciences*, 15(4), 591–616. doi: 10.1007/s11097-015-9441-z

Lakin, J. L., & Chartrand, T. L. (2003). Using nonconscious behavioral mimicry to create affiliation and rapport. *Psychological Science*, 14(4), 334–339. doi: 10.1111/1467-9280.14481

Lavelle, M., Healey, P. G. T., & McCabe, R. (2013). Is nonverbal communication disrupted in interactions involving patients with schizophrenia? *Schizophrenia Bulletin*, 39(5), 1150–1158. doi: 10.1093/schbul/sbs091

Lavelle, M., Healey, P. G. T., & McCabe, R. (2014). Nonverbal behavior during face-to-face social interaction in schizophrenia: A review. *The Journal of Nervous and Mental Disease*, 202(1), 47–54. doi: 10.1097/NMD.0000000000000031

Lysaker, P. H., Johannesen, J. K., & Lysaker, J. T. (2005). Schizophrenia and the experience of intersubjectivity as threat. *Phenomenology and the Cognitive Sciences*, 4(3), 335–352. doi: 10.1007/s11097-005-4067-1

Maiese, M. (2015). *Embodied selves and divided minds*. New York, NY: Oxford University Press.

Maiese, M. (2016). Affective scaffolds, expressive arts, and cognition. *Frontiers in Psychology*, 7, 1–11. doi: 10.3389/fpsyg.2016.00359

McGann, M., & De Jaegher, H. (2009). Self-other contingencies: Enacting social perception. *Phenomenology and the Cognitive Sciences*, 8(4), 417–437. doi: 10.1007/s11097-009-9141-7

Meyer, C., Streeck, J., & Jordan, J. S. (Eds.). (2017). *Intercorporeality: Emerging socialities in interaction*. New York, NY: Oxford University Press.

Newen, A., de Bruin, L., & Gallagher, S. (Eds.). (2018). *The Oxford handbook of 4e cognition*. Oxford, UK: Oxford University Press.

Parnas, J., & Handest, P. (2003). Phenomenology of anomalous self-experience in early schizophrenia. *Comprehensive Psychiatry*, 44(2), 121–134. doi: 10.1053/comp.2003.50017

Parnas, J., & Henriksen, M. G. (2016). Mysticism and schizophrenia: A phenomenological exploration of the structure of consciousness in the schizophrenia spectrum disorders. *Consciousness and Cognition*, 43, 75–88. doi: 10.1016/j.concog.2016.05.010

Parnas, J., Møller, P., Kircher, T., Thalbitzer, J., Jansson, L., Handest, P., & Zahavi, D. (2005). EASE: Examination of Anomalous Self-Experience. *Psychopathology*, 38(5), 236–258. doi: 10.1159/000088441

Raffard, S., Salesse, R. N., Bortolon, C., Bardy, B. G., Henriques, J., Marin, L., … Capdeville, D. (2018). Using mimicry of body movements by a virtual agent to increase synchronization behavior and rapport in individuals with schizophrenia. *Scientific Reports*, 8, 1–10. doi: 10.1038/s41598-018-35813-6

Ratcliffe, M. (2007). *Rethinking commonsense psychology: A critique of folk psychology, theory of mind and simulation*. New York, NY: Palgrave Macmillan.

Ratcliffe, M. (2017a). *Real hallucinations: Psychiatric illness, intentionality, and the interpersonal world*. Cambridge, MA: Massachusetts Institute of Technology Press.

Ratcliffe, M. (2017b). Selfhood, schizophrenia, and the interpersonal regulation of experience. In C. Durt, T. Fuchs, & C. Tewes (Eds.), *Embodiment, enaction, and culture: Investigating the constitution of the shared world* (pp. 149–171). Cambridge, MA: Massachusetts Institute of Technology Press.

Sass, L. (2017). *Madness and modernism: Insanity in the light of modern art, literature, and thought*. Oxford, UK: Oxford University Press.

Sass, L., Pienkos, E., Škodlar, B., Stanghellini, G., Fuchs, T., Parnas, J., & Jones, N. (2017). EAWE: Examination of Anomalous World Experience. *Psychopathology*, 50(1), 10–54. doi: 10.1159/000454928

Sass, L. A., & Parnas, J. (2003). Schizophrenia, consciousness, and the self. *Schizophrenia Bulletin*, 29(3), 427–444. doi: 10.1093/oxfordjournals.schbul.a007017

Schilbach, L., Timmermans, B., Reddy, V., Costall, A., Bente, G., Schlicht, T., & Vogeley, K. (2013). Toward a second-person neuroscience. *Behavioral and Brain Sciences*, 36(4), 393–462. doi: 10.1017/S0140525X12000660

Searle, J. R. (1990). Collective intentions and actions. In P. Cohen, J. Morgan, & M. E. Pollack (Eds.), *Intentions in communication* (pp. 401–415). Cambridge, MA: Massachusetts Institute of Technology Press.

Simonsen, A., Fusaroli, R., Skewes, J. C., Roepstorff, A., Campbell-Meiklejohn, D., Mors, O., & Bliksted, V. (2019). Enhanced automatic action imitation and intact imitation-inhibition in schizophrenia. *Schizophrenia Bulletin*, 45(1), 87–95. doi: 10.1093/schbul/sby006

Slaby, J. (2014). Emotions and the extended mind. In C. von Scheve & M. Salmela (Eds.), *Collective emotions: Perspectives from psychology, philosophy, and sociology* (pp. 32–46). Oxford, UK: Oxford University Press.

Spurrett, D., & Cowley, S. J. (2004). How to do things without words: Infants, utterance-activity and distributed cognition. *Language Sciences*, 26(5), 443–466. doi: 10.1016/j.langsci.2003.09.008

Srinivasan, S. M., & Bhat, A. N. (2013). A review of "music and movement" therapies for children with autism: Embodied interventions for multisystem development. *Frontiers in Integrative Neuroscience*, 7, 1–15. doi: 10.3389/fnint.2013.00022

Stanghellini, G. (2004). *Disembodied spirits and deanimated bodies: The psychopathology of common sense*. New York, NY: Oxford University Press.

Stanghellini, G., Ballerini, M., & Mancini, M. (2017). Other persons: On the phenomenology of interpersonal experience in schizophrenia (ancillary article to EAWE Domain 3). *Psychopathology*, 50(1), 75–82. doi: 10.1159/000456037

Stephensen, H., & Parnas, J. (2018). What can self-disorders in schizophrenia tell us about the nature of subjectivity? A psychopathological investigation. *Phenomenology and the Cognitive Sciences*, 17, 629–642. doi: 10.1007/s11097-017-9532-0

Sutton, J. (2008). Between individual and collective memory: Coordination, interaction, distribution. *Social Research*, 75(1), 23–48.

Sutton, J., Harris, C. B., Keil, P. G., & Barnier, A. J. (2010). The psychology of memory, extended cognition, and socially distributed remembering. *Phenomenology and the Cognitive Sciences*, 9(4), 521–560. doi: 10.1007/s11097-010-9182-y

Taipale, J. (2016). Self-regulation and beyond: Affect regulation and the infant-caregiver dyad. *Frontiers in Psychology*, 7, 1–13. doi: 10.3389/fpsyg.2016.00889

Talwar, N., Crawford, M. J., Maratos, A., Nur, U., McDermott, O., & Procter, S. (2006). Music therapy for in-patients with schizophrenia: Exploratory randomised controlled trial. *The British Journal of Psychiatry*, 189, 405–409. doi: 10.1192/bjp.bp.105.015073

Tomasello, M. (1999). *The cultural origins of human cognition*. Cambridge, MA: Harvard University Press.

Tronick, E. (2005). Why is connection with others so critical? The formation of dyadic states of consciousness and the expansion of individuals' states of consciousness: Coherence governed selection and the co-creation of meaning out of messy meaning making. In J. Nadel & D. Muir (Eds.), *Emotional development: Recent research advances* (pp. 293–316). New York, NY: Oxford University Press.

Van Baaren, R. B., Holland, R. W., Kawakami, K., & Van Knippenberg, A. (2004). Mimicry and prosocial behavior. *Psychological Science*, 15(1), 71–74. doi: 10.1111/j.0963-7214.2004.01501012.x

Van Duppen, Z. (2017). The intersubjective dimension of schizophrenia. *Philosophy, Psychiatry & Psychology*, 24(4), 399–418. doi: 10.1353/ppp.2017.0058

Varga, S. (2013). Vulnerability to psychosis, I-thou intersubjectivity and the praecox-feeling. *Phenomenology and the Cognitive Sciences*, 12(1), 131–143. doi: 10.1007/s11097-010-9173-z

Varga, S., & Krueger, J. (2013). Background emotions, proximity and distributed emotion regulation. *Review of Philosophy and Psychology*, 4(2), 271–292. doi: 10.1007/s13164-013-0134-7

Wiltermuth, S. S., & Heath, C. (2009). Synchrony and cooperation. *Psychological Science*, 20(1), 1–5. doi: 10.1111/j.1467-9280.2008.02253.x

Zahavi, D. (1999). *Self-awareness and alterity: A phenomenological investigation.* Evanston, IL: Northwestern University Press.

Zahavi, D. (2001). *Husserl and transcendental intersubjectivity: A response to the linguistic-pragmatic critique.* Athens, OH: Ohio University Press.

Zahavi, D. (2005). *Subjectivity and selfhood: Investigating the first-person perspective.* Cambridge, MA: Massachusetts Institute of Technology Press.

Zahavi, D. (2014). *Self and other: Exploring subjectivity, empathy, and shame.* Oxford, UK: Oxford University Press.

14.1

Commentary on "Lost in the Socially Extended Mind: Genuine Intersubjectivity and Disturbed Self-Other Demarcation in Schizophrenia"

Mimicry and Normativity

Edward A. Lenzo and Shaun Gallagher

As Froese and Krueger indicate, much attention has been paid to negative symptomology of schizophrenia known as "dissociality." Persons with schizophrenia commonly report a detachment from themselves, a kind of disembodiment and depersonalization of the body; and "others become problems to be solved by intellectual effort and no longer present opportunities for spontaneous interpersonal alignment" (Froese & Krueger, 2021, p. 318). Froese and Krueger note, however, that a closely related yet seemingly opposed set of phenomena have been relatively neglected by researchers: Persons with schizophrenia commonly experience disturbances of self-other demarcation, reporting an "unusual fluidity" (2021, p. 318) between self and other. Sass et al. write:

> The subject feels that the basic sense of independence or separateness of self and other persons has broken down or become much more fluid than normal. This may involve feelings of unusual empathy, openness, control, fusion, or confusion between self and others—whether experienced physically, psychologically, or concerning identity. (2017, p. 28)

In order to address this aspect of schizophrenia experience, Froese and Krueger situate themselves in line with the "4E" (embodied, embedded, extended, and enactive) approaches to cognitive research, and leverage a notion of *genuine intersubjectivity* developed by Froese (2018). According to this concept, "how we relate to the world in each moment of our experience is not independent from how we interact with others in that moment" (Froese & Krueger, 2021, p. 320). That is, we co-regulate our experience with others, such that what we do, think, feel, etc. stands in a dynamical relation to the acts and experiences of others. An important aspect to this claim is that some of what we experience is possible only in virtue of genuine intersubjectivity: Dynamical co-regulation with others allows for certain kinds of experience.

The concept of genuine intersubjectivity, Froese and Krueger rightly claim, helps us to recognize a certain ambiguity between self and other at the heart of experience: What we experience normally depends on an intermingling of self and other, such that it is not always clear, not always relevant, and often not even possible to separate out one's own contributions from those of others. They then reinterpret reports and literature on dissociality through the lens of this concept, arguing that disembodiment can lead to a breakdown of genuine intersubjectivity and thus to disturbances of a form of sociality foundational for everyday, normal experience; dissociality refers to a "loss of the socially extended mind" (Froese & Krueger, 2021, p. 318). Next, they apply this concept to the aforementioned, neglected problems of self-other demarcation. They critique the traditional view that unusual fluidity is a matter of "hallucination without basis in reality" (Froese & Krueger, 2021, p. 328), arguing instead that such phenomena indicate "a heightened sensitivity or vulnerability" to the self-other ambiguity inherent to experience. Unusual fluidity refers to being "lost in the socially extended mind" (Froese & Krueger, 2021).

Not only does their approach promise a new interpretation of certain reports by persons with schizophrenia, as well as offer some useful speculation for future experiments and research, it also has implications for therapeutic intervention and for the "science of consciousness" more generally. Regarding therapy, Froese and Krueger's position entails that we should not aim to eliminate the ambiguity to which some schizophrenic persons are hypersensitive, but rather to foster the skills needed to negotiate this ambiguity in a healthy way. This insight pivots into an endorsement of "bottom-up treatment methods," such as those endorsed by Maiese (2015), which emphasize embodiment and/or interpersonal synchrony, for example, "yoga, music, and dance/movement therapy" (Froese & Krueger, 2021, p. 333). Regarding the science of consciousness generally, Froese and Krueger challenge the centrality of "ipseity" models, which analyze consciousness by reference to the cluster of concepts including self, self-disturbance, minimal self, and so on. They offer a refinement of ipseity models, arguing that the concept of genuine intersubjectivity demonstrates the need for a social dimension neglected by ipseity models, and that the pathology phenomena in question undermine the often definitive characteristic attributed to the self, that is, first-personal givenness.

Froese and Krueger recognize and begin to account for an often neglected aspect of schizophrenia experience. Doing so is difficult and admirable: Often, for a given psychopathological condition, there will exist comorbidities and seemingly contradictory symptomologies, and theorists will often have little choice but to focus on that one side that appears most pertinent to their position. Froese and Krueger begin to address this tension, and offer a more general concept that promises to resolve it. While genuine intersubjectivity potentially brings these aspects theoretically closer together than before, it is left somewhat unclear what makes the difference, for a particular person at a particular time, between a "loss of" and being "lost in" the socially extended mind. They refer to a kind of pendulum swing, but it would be interesting and useful to determine the basis according to which the pendulum swings, in any particular case, one way rather than the other.

The authors also provide compelling examples in explication and support of the thesis of the socially extended mind, ranging from the dyad that forms between infant and mother during breastfeeding, to getting swept up in the group-level dynamics involved in an exciting party, or an enraging political protest.

Froese and Krueger propose genuine intersubjectivity as an alternative to traditional cognitive science approaches, such as theory of mind or simulation approaches. However, their approach as presented seemingly inherits at least one contentious and problematic aspect of the latter: from simulation theory, in particular, an emphasis on similarity and mimicry. They write that "to be involved with others in instances of genuine intersubjectivity – even in its earliest forms – is to identify *affectively* with others. This is a shared process that 'assimilates another person's bodily anchored psychological stance'" (Froese & Krueger, 2021, p. 324),[1] such that

> If someone smiles at us and makes a friendly gesture, for instance, these expressive actions will elicit *similar* [emphasis added] responses from us and *motivate an array of further friendly expressions* [emphasis added]; conversely, aggressive movements or threatening gestures compel us to tense up and prepare for our own *aggressive* [emphasis added] response. Within the dynamics of face-to-face interaction, individuals spontaneously mimic others' facial expressions, gestures, and intonation patterns; they also coordinate and synchronize speech rhythms and bodily movements, which leads to affective convergence and heightened feelings of rapport. (Froese & Krueger, 2021, p. 324)

A disruption of genuine intersubjectivity is the disruption of this dynamic process of identification, assimilation, motivation of similar expressions from similar expressions, spontaneous mimicry, coordination and synchrony, and convergence. This reliance on mimicry – the term we can use to capture this cluster of processes – is troubling for two reasons.

[1] The quote within this quote is taken from Hobson and Hobson (2007, p. 411).

First, this betrays some of the examples employed earlier, such as that of breastfeeding, in which it does not seem that co-regulation depends on identification or similar expression. As Zahavi convincingly reminds us, mimicry is not necessary for either social cognition or direct social perception, and so also not necessary for the co-regulation specified by "genuine intersubjectivity." He notes that "we might of course encounter a furious neighbor and become furious ourselves, but our empathetic understanding of our neighbor's emotion might also elicit a quite different response, namely the feeling of fear" (Zahavi, 2010, p. 7). Admittedly, this is perhaps an innocuous concern: We might think that what is necessary is not a strict mimicry or matching between oneself and others but rather a kind of appropriate reaction; fear might not be aggressive, but is nevertheless an appropriate reaction to fury, and so we could say that the neighbor's fury and my fear are "in sync" or co-regulated. Here, one could explore different concepts of intersubjective alignment, not all of which involve simple matching, imitation, or entrainment processes (e.g., Rothwell, Shalin, & Romigh, 2017), but perhaps something more complex (e.g., Tollefsen, Dale, & Paxton, 2013).

But there is a second, more worrisome concern. By suggesting that participation in genuine intersubjectivity depends on affective identity, with an emphasis on similarity and mimicry, Froese and Krueger run the risk of defining social interaction in terms of simple adherence to societal norms: That is, in reacting to others in appropriate ways, be it strict mimicry or the kind of co-regulation just noted. Conversely, pathology is conceptualized as a break in participation, conceived in terms of identification. Froese and Krueger ask "what goes wrong [?]" in schizophrenia (Froese & Krueger, 2021, p. 328). If pathology is a breakage from participation with societal norms, however, and if it is "desirable" to prevent such a divergence, then this raises questions about the status of such norms, cultural diversity, nonconformity, and precisely when we should think that behavior becomes pathological.

References

Froese, T. (2018). Searching for the conditions of genuine intersubjectivity: From agent-based models to perceptual crossing experiments. In A. Newen, L. de Bruin, & S. Gallagher (Eds.), *The Oxford handbook of 4e cognition* (pp. 163–186). Oxford, UK: Oxford University Press.

Froese, T., & Krueger, J. (2021). Lost in the socially extended mind: Genuine intersubjectivity and disturbed self-other demarcation in schizophrenia. In C. Tewes & G. Stanghellini (Eds.), *Time and body: Phenomenological and psychopathological approaches* (pp. 318–340). Cambridge, UK: Cambridge University Press.

Hobson, J. A., & Hobson, R. P. (2007). Identification: The missing link between joint attention and imitation? *Development and Psychopathology*, 19(2), 411–431. doi: 10.1017/S0954579407070204

Maiese, M. (2015). *Embodied selves and divided minds*. New York, NY: Oxford University Press.

Rothwell, C. D., Shalin, V. L., & Romigh, G. D. (2017). Quantitative models of human-human conversational grounding processes. In G. Gunzelmann, A. Howes, T. Tebrink, & E. J. Davelaar (Eds.), *Proceedings of the 39th annual conference of the cognitive science society* (pp. 1016–1021). Austin, TX: Cognitive Science Society. Retrieved from https://mindmodeling.org/cogsci2017/papers/0198/paper0198.pdf

Sass, L., Pienkos, E., Škodlar, B., Stanghellini, G., Fuchs, T., Parnas, J., & Jones, N. (2017). EAWE: Examination of Anomalous World Experience. *Psychopathology*, 50(1), 10–54. doi: 10.1159/000454928

Tollefsen, D. P., Dale, R., & Paxton, A. (2013). Alignment, transactive memory, and collective cognitive systems. *Review of Philosophy and Psychology*, 4(1), 49–64. doi: 10.1007/s13164-012-0126-z

Zahavi, D. (2010). Empathy, embodiment and interpersonal understanding: From Lipps to Schutz. *Inquiry*, 53(3), 285–306. doi: 10.1080/0020174X.2010.484663

15

Closing Up
The Phenomenology of Catatonia

Zeno Van Duppen and Pascal Sienaert

Introduction

Since its introduction by Karl Jaspers at the beginning of the twentieth century, phenomenological psychopathology has shown how focus on subjective experience can help to increase our understanding of psychiatric conditions, symptoms, and phenomena (Jaspers, 1913). Schizophrenia, for example, has famously been analyzed by early psychopathologists like Jaspers, Minkowski, Blankenburg, and Kimura. These investigations have shown how schizophrenia is not just a disorder of objectifiable psychotic and negative symptoms, as contemporary views often hold it, but includes fundamental changes to subjectivity, including self-experience, intersubjectivity, and embodiment. These insights have inspired both theoretical work on schizophrenia and empirical research (Parnas et al., 2005; Sass et al., 2017). Phenomenological psychopathology thereby contributes to the general understanding of schizophrenia, in times where most attention is given to objective measurements, making way for phenomenology-informed psychiatric research. This comes at a good time, given the fact that questions on the scientific validity and the clinical use of the *Diagnostic and Statistical Manual* (DSM) have stimulated debate on what psychiatric conditions actually are, how one should diagnose them, and how they should consequently be treated. Today, hope has slowly vanished that neurobiological or neuroimaging research will discover underlying mechanisms or biomarkers able to identify the DSM's disorders as discrete disease entities (Linden, 2012; Van Praag, 2000). More realist approaches propose the integration of different forms of knowledge into psychiatric research, including first-person experience and phenomenology (Parnas, Sass, & Zahavi, 2013). Phenomenological research has already contributed to our knowledge and understanding of many disorders, including mood, anxiety, and psychotic disorders (Fuchs, 2010). One of the psychiatric conditions that has, however, received only little phenomenological attention is catatonia. We will therefore present a case of catatonia and investigate it phenomenologically, with particular emphasis on fear, embodiment, and temporality. This phenomenological analysis could, on the one hand, contribute to our understanding of the condition; while it can, on the other, be of interest to phenomenological theory on (inter)subjectivity, temporality, and embodiment.

Clinical Vignette: A Woman in the Hallway

One day, I, the first author, was on call in the psychiatric hospital. I received a phone call from a receptionist, late in the afternoon. A woman was standing in one of the long hallways of the hospital where usually nobody comes. She did not react, the receptionist said, and no one she had asked knew who this woman was.

When I arrived, I saw a woman at the end of the hallway, right in front of an emergency exit leading to the hospital's garden. She was standing there all by herself. When I approached her, she did not move, as if she did not notice me at all. I estimated that she was in her forties. Her jacket and a shopping trolley were lying next to her on the floor. She was leaning forward with her head against the glass of the emergency door. Her arms were raised half-way in the air, her hands cramped up like claws. I started talking to her. I explained her who I was. She did not react. Her eyes shut, I could notice minor movements of her eyeballs. I then noticed that she was not actually leaning her head against the glass door, but instead, there was about a centimeter of space between her head and the door. She was standing on the external sides of her feet, with her toes inverted. She must have been standing there for over half an hour. There was no way to contact her, and I felt I was talking to an object. It seemed clear that she was catatonic.

I did not touch her, but told her I would try to search for someone who knew her and that I would contact nurses from some of the wards I expected her to be hospitalized in. I mentioned some of the names of these wards, hoping she would somehow react when hearing the correct one. I was thinking of the closed ward for intensive care, where people with catatonia are usually treated. I also thought of the ward for patients with chronic psychosis and schizophrenia. Although I did not know who she was, I was convinced she suffered from a severe mental illness, and particularly because of the catatonic state I was thinking of bipolar disorder or schizophrenia.

After calling different wards, nurses, and therapists, I finally found someone who told me it was probably K., who had had an outpatient appointment with her therapist earlier. It was apparently not the first time K. had become lost in the hospital after a psychotherapy session. When I contacted her therapist, he told me she was not simulating, she was not psychotic, nor was she known with schizophrenia or bipolar disorder. She was, in fact, not chronically ill. She had a job, a family, and she led a normal life.

As a matter of fact, right before I found her in a catatonic state in the hallway, she had a session of trauma therapy. During these sessions, K. relived parts of past traumatic experiences. The therapist told me that normally, certain nurses kept an eye on her for a few hours after each session. There was a room where she could stay after therapy, before returning home.

I was baffled to find out that this woman I had seen as an object-like figure at the end of the hallway actually led a normal life, had a job, a family, and so on, while I saw her as having lost her way, her fluidity and mobility, as well as her connection with others. Her body had shut down and closed up. With her clawed hands half-way raised, standing on the side of her feet, and her body leaning forward in the air, it seemed the laws of gravity or physiology did not apply to her body. At that moment, she was unreachable.

Catatonia

Catatonia is a severe psychiatric syndrome, characterized by specific motor abnormalities. These include stupor, catalepsy, waxy flexibility, mutism, negativism, posturing, mannerism, stereotypy, agitation, grimacing, echolalia, and echopraxia. Stupor is a temporary reduction or obliteration of reactive and spontaneous relation functions, namely, action and speech (Berrios, 1981). Catalepsy and posturing are probably the best-known catatonic symptoms, characterized by rigidity and fixity of posture, often in unusual or unlikely positions, as described in the clinical vignette and evoked by Figure 15.1.

Stereotypy refers to repetitive, senseless movements, while mannerism describes repetitive movements or postures that are purposeful, albeit awkward or inadequate. Negativism and mutism describe the behavior where patients do or say exactly the opposite of what is asked or withhold talking altogether. In ambitendency, patients seem to struggle with opposing options (e.g., hesitatingly giving a hand while being told not to), while automatic obedience describes the phenomenon when patients cooperate in an exaggerated way to instructed moves, or only slight pressure (*mitgehen*). It is severe and can be life threatening when patients stop eating and drinking, leading to renal failure and possibly death.

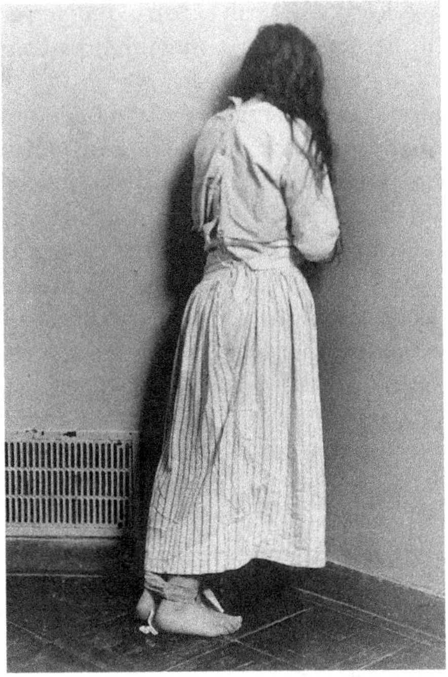

Figure 15.1 Frederik Salomon Meijers, patient in Wilhelmina Hospital, Amsterdam, about 1906. Collection Dolhuys, Haarlem, The Netherlands

According to the DSM-5 (American Psychiatric Association, 2013), at least 3 of 12 symptoms need to be present. If this is the case, clinicians will need to specify whether catatonia is associated with another mental disorder, for example, bipolar disorder or schizophrenia, whether it is due to a medical condition, or whether it is unspecified, meaning it stands on its own. This last type of catatonia is a new and remarkable addition to the DSM-5 classification, as we will see further on. The large symptom variety and the possibility to make symptom combinations of at least 3 of 12 symptoms imply a high variability of the clinical presentation, but motor abnormality constitutes the common core. Attempts have been made to differentiate forms of catatonia based on clinical presentation, for example, chronic versus acute, retarded versus excited, progressive versus benign (Fink & Taylor, 2001; Kay, Kanofsky, Lindemayer, & Opler, 1987; Pfuhlmann & Stöber, 2001; Taylor & Fink, 2003). Because catatonia is – as every psychiatric condition – a clinical diagnosis, rating scales have been developed to guide the diagnostic process. The Bush-Francis Rating Scale is most known and clinically used (Bush, Fink, Petrides, Dowling, & Francis,

1996; Sienaert, Rooseleer, & de Fruyt, 2011). The prevalence of catatonia is remarkably high, particularly in hospitalized patients. Several reports of systematic screening found an incidence of 7–17 percent of admitted patients (Francis, 2006, 2010). From the earliest descriptions of catatonic states, it was noted that prognosis was extremely variable, ranging from good recovery to progression to death (Penland, Weder, & Tampi, 2006). Although severe and life threatening, catatonia today has a good prognosis.

A number of pharmacological agents have been tried successfully in catatonia, but the effect is rarely as immediate and dramatic as seen with benzodiazepines. Lorazepam can be used as a diagnostic probe and as a treatment. If the response is inadequate or transient, Sienaert, Dhossche, Vancampfort, de Hert, and Gazdag (2014) have argued that electroconvulsive therapy (ECT) should be started without delay. If the underlying condition warrants ECT, or in life-threatening situations like malignant catatonia or neuroleptic malignant syndrome (NMS), ECT is the treatment of first choice (Sienaert et al., 2014).

Despite recent renewed interest and research in the pathology and treatment of catatonia, it remains surrounded by mystery. The recent changes to the DSM classification did not alter this. In fact, the concept of catatonia has been the topic of an ongoing debate ever since its first introduction. It was the German psychiatrist Karl Kahlbaum in 1874 who first used the term, although earlier reports mention symptoms that would today be called catatonic (Shorter & Fink, 2018). For example, in 1583, the English physician Philip Barrough described "congelation" or "taking": "It is a sodaine detention & taking both of mind and body, both sense and moving being lost, the sicke remaining in the same figure of bodie wherin he was taken, whither he sit or lye, or stand, or whiter his eyes be open or shut" (Barrough, 1590/1624). Kahlbaum was, however, the first to describe how a variety of often strange motor alterations or changed behavior all fit together in one disease concept. Yet, what is catatonia really? Is it an organic, medical condition, or should we consider it psychiatric or even psychological in nature? Is it a symptom, part of an underlying disease or a broader syndrome, or is it an independent disease entity? Should we diagnose associated disorders as schizophrenia or bipolar disorder based on catatonic symptoms, or the other way around? And lastly, after acute catatonia has disappeared, should treatment be continued depending on whether catatonia stands alone or whether it is part of, say, a mood or a psychotic disorder, and should it then be treated accordingly?

For Kahlbaum, catatonia was an independent or primary illness (Kahlbaum, 1874). The presence of associated mood or psychotic symptoms would thus be secondary. Psychiatry has, however, long maintained that catatonia is a symptom: an expression of an underlying primary illness, like schizophrenia. Historically, this is at least partly due to the immense impact of Emil Kraepelin's work on psychopathology. Kraepelin famously distinguished the mood disorders (cyclic disorders) from dementia praecox, or what would later be called schizophrenia (Kraepelin, 1904). In his view, dementia praecox could further be differentiated into different subtypes, including the catatonic subtype. Since then, a variety of authors have argued for and against this position (see Hirjak, Kubera, Wolf, & Northoff, 2019). The changes to the DSM-5 are thus meaningful in this historical context, because it integrates Kahlbaum's view of catatonia as a primary illness.

In phenomenological psychopathology, catatonia has received little attention. It was Jaspers himself who remarked in the *General Psychopathology*, not long after Kraepelin's redefinition of catatonia as a subtype of dementia praecox, that the phenomenology of catatonia touches on the very heart of his distinction between explanation (*erklären*) and understanding (*verstehen*). He wrote: "Their movements are situated between motor inhibitions on the one side, which may be investigated neurologically; and on the other side we have meaningful emotional expression that one might approach empathically" (Jaspers, 1913, p. 114; see Van Duppen, 2016).[1] Could it be that the phenomenology of catatonia does prove to be understandable, or do we indeed reach the limits of comprehensibility, and encounter the need for explanation? In the next section, we return to the clinical vignette and attempt to elaborate the phenomenology of catatonia by clarifying the subjective and intersubjective dimensions with regards to fear, temporality, and embodiment.[2]

Phenomenological Analysis

Fear

The woman in the vignette went through a session of trauma therapy, minutes before freezing at the end of the hallway. It was not the first time,

[1] Besides Jaspers, Conrad (1958), Binswanger (1956/2012), and Wulff (1995) have elaborated on phenomena one could describe as catatonic.

[2] Due to the particular therapeutic relationship and the privacy involved, we were not able to integrate the first-person experience of the patient into the vignette. This is a major limitation to our approach, and one that phenomenological studies often struggle with. See Van Duppen and Sips (2018) for an illustration of how fruitful this can be. The case was, however, discussed with her therapist.

and precautions were taken so that she could go home safely afterward. During such sessions, patients are asked to remember moments before and during traumatic events. Several times before, she had dissociated afterward and had difficulties finding her way out of the hospital. There were marks of her hands on the glass windows of the door, so we could assume that she did try to open the door. What would it be like to reexperience trauma, albeit in a safe and controlled environment, and then not be able to leave? It seems probable that she was trying to get out, could not, and ended up freezing into catatonia. All discussion about causes of catatonic symptoms left aside, it seems clear that the therapy session and the intense emotions arising there must had some causal influence.

It is remarkable that in their recent study on the history of catatonia, Shorter and Fink (2018) used the expression "madness of fear" to typify what catatonia according to them actually is or may be. Notice that "fear" is a different emotional state, a different affect than anxiety. Anxiety can be called a mood, while fear is an intentional (i.e., directed to) and often bodily experienced reaction to a possible threat. Fear is not just an emotion, it is equally the stimulation of the sympathetic nervous system, raising the heartbeat and the depth and speed of breathing, and it is at the same time the strong urge one can feel to break free, to flee, or to hide (Fuchs, 2013a). According to Shorter and Fink, catatonic patients are frequently overwhelmed by fear, dread, and anxiety. Fear has always played a cardinal role in the concept of stupor and catatonia (Fink & Shorter, 2017; Perkins, 1982; Shorter & Fink, 2018). Fear could be causing catatonia, but it can equally be the emotion most present in the catatonic state itself. Moskowitz (2004) argued that the motor symptoms of catatonia are in fact inbuilt evolutionary reactions to threat, like animals reacting to carnivores with tonic immobility ("playing possum"). It is closer to being "scared stiff" and to an unconscious "death feint" than to a neuromotor dysfunction. The immediate and dramatic effect of benzodiazepines, as also witnessed in the treatment of anxiety and panic, is an extra argument to consider catatonia a form or consequence of extreme fear. Yet, the embodied expression of this fear is so extreme and deviates so strongly from reality and from the concrete situation people are in that many have called it psychotic. Parnas (2013, p. 213), for example, described it as a dislocation from intersubjectivity, and referred to it as nonpropositional psychosis. Others report the unexpressed feeling of imminent doom accompanying catatonia, as seen in melancholic or psychotic depression (Moskowitz, 2004).

There are only a few studies, however, on the actual first-person experience of catatonic patients. In one study, comparing akinetic catatonic and Parkinson patients, the catatonic patients reported being overwhelmed by feelings of anxiety, and by the blockade of their movements by emotions and feelings of isolation from their environment (Northoff, Krill, Wenke, Travers, & Pflug, 1996; Northoff et al., 1998). Furthermore, "the patients' greatest fears were their inability to control intense anxiety. They felt threatened and feared dying and were less concerned about their lack of control of body movement or of self-care" (Shorter & Fink, 2018, p. 90). Fear could thus be a cause for, as well as a result from a catatonic state. In traumatic events, like being the victim of rape or violent assault, it is well known that people can react with dissociation or even paralysis (Marx, Forsyth, Gallup, Fusé, & Lexington, 2008). For the woman in the vignette, the experience of reliving her traumatic life events could be so intense that fear arose, urging her to leave, "to break free, to flee," and the threat of not being able to due to disorientation and a locked door could have been the last straw for her body to close up into catatonia.

Embodiment

What happens to the body in catatonia? We have seen how the core of catatonic symptoms is motor abnormality, ergo the body is primarily involved. The result of untreated catatonia equally impacts the body directly: people stop eating and drinking, with fatal consequences. But the body transforms in a different way as well. In fact, we need the phenomenological distinction between the lived-body and the object-body to account for this transformation (Fuchs & Schlimme, 2009; Plessner, 1970). The lived-body (German: *Leib*) is the subjective body that we prereflectively live, while the object-body is the body we become aware of, we can point our attention to, and which we can experience as object-like. Fuchs and Schlimme (2009) described how our experience of the world is constituted by an ongoing oscillation between these two bodily modes.

The woman in the hallway was object-like. To be object-like means to have (partially) lost subjectivity. Her body was positioned in an unfamiliar way, and it was kept that way for a prolonged time. There seemed to be no person involved, only this human-shaped object. The scene, with her trolley and her jacket lying on the ground, suggested the transformation must have happened suddenly. Suddenly, as Barrough had described in 1583, she was "taken," she became an object: The oscillation Fuchs and Schlimme (2009) described was halted at the far extreme of being an object-body. But what was it about her that made me see her as object-like, and not as the woman she actually was – which afterward baffled me? Clearly, her body itself did not change, although her hands, feet, and posture were in unusual positions. I only got a mere glimpse at something of a living-body, when I saw her eyeballs move behind her eyelids. Something more was in there, albeit covered and seemingly unreachable. Yet, apart from these subtle eye movements, the "meaningful emotional expressions that one might approach empathically" (*verständliche Ausdrucksbewegungen*), as Jaspers (1913, p. 114, our translation) referred to, were absent.

Unlike how one would normally behave with a disoriented person, I did not take her arm to lead her in the right direction, that is, the exit of the hospital. In fact, I did not dare to touch her at all. Touching her would feel like assaulting her in all her fragility, and at the same time, it could well be that I feared a sudden explosive response, the "fight" of the fight-flight reaction. Yet, she was not only physically untouchable: She was also emotionally disconnected. There was no communication at all. There was the mere assumption that she could maybe understand what I said, which made me try to comfort her in a neutral and distant way.

Although her body itself did not change, the unusual posture did transform something: There was no spontaneous bodily attunement to my presence, to my movements. Nothing I did or said seemed to influence her body – apart from her eyes. What Merleau-Ponty (1960, p. 167) described as intercorporeality, being part of a community of the flesh, and what later has been described in terms of developmental psychology as primary intersubjectivity (Trevarthen, 1998; Van Duppen, 2017), namely, the most fundamental embodied connection to others, seemed missing. Catatonic symptoms like "*Gegenhalten*," stereotypy, or catalepsy seem to refute intercorporeal connection. An arm passively raised in the air that remains there after the examining clinician pulls his hand away suggests the clinician's hand did not matter in the first place. In fact, catatonic phenomena express a dislocation from shared lived space (Minkowski, 1970, p. 403). Stereotypic movements of the hands or fingers are not only meaningless but incorporate a lack of attunement to the body of others. We encounter others as embodied beings, and we do part participate unconsciously in an embodied interaction, even if we explicitly refuse to do so. The shape, meaning, rhythmicity, or intensity of our movements are attuned to those of others. Even if some embodied being suddenly makes an unexpected move, we immediately attune by responding, moving away, or more subtle changes. A catatonic person becomes a body that does not attune and does not afford or invite the attunement by others. She closes up.

In phenomena like *mitgehen* and automatic obedience, we see how light touch can induce a forceful movement: An arm gently raised by the examiner continues to move strongly in the air. The external stimulus meets no resistance at all. The body shows with exaggeration what it lacks: a resistant and embodied self. It may be akin to what happens to a body under severe pressure and threat, as in physical and sexual abuse: disembodiment (Young, 1992).

The woman was standing all by herself. None of the people who had called me actually stayed to accompany her. And I, myself, went off after a few minutes to make phone calls. It is a body not open to the presence of others. Catatonia is a disruption of intercorporeality. And it could well be a disruption between the patient's body and her mind as well. Indeed, the body could be almost completely separated from the mind, as Leon Hirschel had already remarked on stupor in 1769 (cited in Shorter & Fink, 2018, p. 79). Only the subtle movement of her eyes suggested there was something "inside," protected and covered up by a body that would withstand communication, touch, or pain.

Temporality

We have seen how intense fear and the closing up of the body can transform a person into an object-like figure, disconnected from the movements and meanings of others. But, it remains unclear how this would actually happen. How could fear induce catatonic symptoms? And how could the body close up in ways we described as stupor, catalepsy, mutism, and the like. One possibility to answer this question is to review neurobiological processes from traumatic events and fear until the manifestation of catatonia (e.g., Hirjak et al., 2019). Here, we prefer to address these questions theoretically, turning to one of the cornerstones of the phenomenological approach to subjectivity: temporality. Fuchs (2006) distinguished explicit time and implicit time. Explicit time is the time of timetables and calendars: it is measured and objectified time. Catatonia, however, involves implicit or lived time. Implicit time is "to live time" (Kupke, 2006). It is the movement of life, implicit in our experience of being engaged in the world and oriented toward our immediate goals. It is present in our bodily commitment to our particular situation. This implicit time is the undercurrent of our experience (Fuchs, 2013b, p. 2). There are two components of implicit time. The first refers to what Husserl (1966), called "inner-time consciousness" corresponding to the basic form of prereflective consciousness. It is the constitutive or transcendental synthesis of experience: Husserl famously described this synthesis of three moments: protention, presentation, and retention (Husserl, 2012, p. 44). Protention is the open anticipation of the experiences that are to come. Presentation consists of the primal impression as given at every moment. Retention consists of retaining what has just been experienced as it slips away. Hearing a melody illustrates this clearly: We hear the current tone (presentation), while we are aware of the tones we just heard (retention) and we anticipate certain tones to come (protention). To be clear, the synthesis of these moments is a passive, transcendental process that the subject is not actively or reflectively "doing." It is not time as experienced, that is, explicit time, but it allows for experience to appear in a unified, dynamic, and fluid way in the first place.

Apart from this structural component of implicit time, there is a more conative and affective component. This includes drive, striving, urge, or affection. It functions as the root for spontaneity, affective directedness, attention, and the pursuit of goals. It corresponds to the temporal dimension of what Bergson (1970) and Minkowski meant with the "élan vital." It is related to a felt direction or a drive: "Lived time is connected with the experience of the embodied human subject as being driven and directed towards the world in terms of bodily potentiality and capability" (Wyllie, 2006, p. 173). These two components are only conceptually distinguishable. It has been argued that some of the core phenomenological disturbances in schizophrenia can be related to disturbances to implicit temporality (Fuchs, 2007; Fuchs & Van Duppen, 2017).

In catatonia, however, there may be an even more remarkable disruption on the transcendental level of lived-time and the lived-body. Indeed, one should recall that implicit or lived-time and the lived-body are essentially connected. "The lived body is … the concrete realization of lived time" (Wehrle, 2019, p. 8). When we are engaged in the world, with others, we forget explicit time and we live time; we forget our object-body and we are our living body (Fuchs, 2006). Crucially, what connects implicit or lived-timed and the lived-body is openness. The body is open to receive, to react, and to act. It is open to experience, to be affected. It keeps track of what it has experienced, what has affected it, what it has done (Fuchs, 2012; Van der Kolk, 1994). And it is capable of doing, reacting, of opening horizons of possibility. Implicit temporality, and particularly inner-time consciousness, has been said to be essentially open as well: Rodemeyer (2006) has argued that particularly protention is a necessary correlate of intersubjectivity and interaffectivity: To be with others, to affect others, and to be affected by others, we need a certain openness of passive anticipation of experiences to come. These possible experiences are essentially "other," including "the other." Van Duppen (2017) has argued for the concept of open subjectivity, based on this essential openness and structural connection between subjectivity and intersubjectivity. However, the openness of Protention is not unlimited, nor is it static. We therefore use the figure of the "cone of probability" to describe the changes to protentional openness (Fuchs, 2007). A central aspect thereof is that the protentional cone can widen and close. This means that temporal openness is dynamic and selective. Retention and impression fundamentally motivate protention: We emptily expect something rather than something else. We expect a certain tone in the melody, rather than another, based on the previous tones. Inner-time consciousness, and thus, implicit temporality is essentially open to experience in the first place and is connected to the openness of the body to be affected, to act, and to affect.

If we now recall how the woman in the hallway had just relived her past traumatic experiences in the therapy session, we can describe the progression toward the catatonic state as follows: These memories are accompanied by strong and often intense emotions, sometimes so intense that they are actually relived. Fear arises, and forces one to "to break free, to flee, or to hide," as the woman attempted when trying to open the emergency door. The threat of the inner danger combined with being stuck, not getting out at that moment may have been so immense that on the implicit temporal level, protentional openness, the open anticipation of what is to come, abruptly closes up. The conative-affective drive comes to a complete stop, literally, in that nothing moves anymore. The body, then, becomes an object-like figure, expressing the impossibility to experience – when the experience itself is unbearable. It expresses the impossibility to experience the other – when the threat of the other is unbearable. The body loses its abilities, its capability to open a new horizon of possibility. The door was locked, there was no way out.

Conclusion

This chapter aimed to expand the phenomenology of catatonia. In doing so, it became clear that fear, embodiment, and temporality could play a major role in the emergence of symptoms sometimes described as purely organic or incomprehensible. Clearly, not all forms of catatonia, whether stand-alone or associated with other disorders, will follow the same process described here. It may well be that only patients with "reactive catatonia" said to involve "massive affective dysregulation" (Hirjak et al., 2019) would go through this phenomenology, but it can make their motor symptoms more understandable. We have seen how catatonia is often associated to or termed psychotic, and in a sense our elaboration could explain why (apart from the epidemiological data, of course): like psychosis, catatonia affects a transcendental aspect of human life, and like psychosis, it is manifested on the level of embodiment and temporality, particularly the lived-body and lived-time. Unique to catatonia, however, is that it involves a sudden, momentary, but complete closing up of subjectivity (Van Duppen, 2017), of the interaction between self and others, of intercorporeality.[3] It is the experience of a reality so frightening and disturbing that the body shuts down and time closes up. Phenomenologically, this means that structural or transcendental disturbances ("closing of protention," Van Duppen (2017), or Ratcliffe's (2017) "altered modalities of intentionality" for that matter) should be considered essentially dynamic, and connected to the concrete world, to the trust we develop in relation to and with others. This allows for affective connection and communication, yet it equally implies fragility and vulnerability. Although psychologically we are not closer to understanding catatonia in general, we did clarify what can happen on the level of subjectivity, intersubjectivity, embodiment, and temporality. Yet, as Jaspers rightly remarked on catatonia: "In these puzzling conditions we are dealing with the most baffling mental states. They are just as baffling to the psychiatrist as to the laity." Despite over a century of research, clinical progress and effective treatment: "We have no idea what is in the patient's mind" (Jaspers, 1913, p. 281). Although phenomenology may get us closer, the mystery of catatonia remains.

Acknowledgment

Thanks firstly to Max Fink, MD, Departments of Psychiatry and Neurology, Stony Brook University School of Medicine, for his comments on an earlier version of this chapter, and to the two anonymous reviewers for their helpful remarks and suggestions.

References

American Psychiatric Association. (2013). *Diagnostic and statistical manual of mental disorders* (5th ed.). Washington, DC: Author.

Barrough, P. (1624). *The method of physick; containing the causes, signs, and cures, of inward diseases in man's body, from the head to the foot: Whereunto is added the forme and rule of making remedies and medicines, which our physitions commonly*

[3] It could be worthwhile to differentiate catatonic phenomena from other psychomotor phenomena, as in epilepsy or in certain dissociative phenomena. An overlap is certainly present, but its phenomenology, etiology, and psychodynamic would probably be different.

use at this day, with the proportion, quantity, and names of each medicine. London, UK: Imprinted by Richard Field. (Original work published 1590)

Bergson, H. (1970). *Essai sur les données immédiates de la conscience* [Essay on the immediate data of consciousness]. Paris, France: Presses Universitaires de France.

Berrios, G. E. (1981). Stupor: A conceptual history. *Psychological Medicine*, 11(4), 677–688. doi:10.1017/s0033291700041179

Binswanger, L. (2012). *Drei Formen missglückten Daseins: Verstiegenheit, Verschrobenheit, Manieriertheit* [Three forms of failed existence: Extravagance, crankiness, mannerism]. Berlin, Germany: Walter de Gruyter. (Original work published 1956)

Bush, G., Fink, M., Petrides, G., Dowling, F., & Francis, A. (1996). Catatonia. I. Rating scale and standardized examination. *Acta Psychiatrica Scandinavica*, 93(2), 129–136. doi:10.1111/j.1600-0447.1996.tb09814.x

Conrad, K. (1958). *Die beginnende Schizophrenie. Versuch einer Gestaltanalyse des Wahns* [The beginning schizophrenia. Attempt of a Gestalt analysis of the delusion]. Stuttgart, Germany: Thieme.

Fink, M., & Shorter, E. (2017). Does persisting fear sustain catatonia? *Acta Psychiatrica Scandinavica*, 136(5), 441–444. doi:10.1111/acps.12796

Fink, M., & Taylor, M. A. (2001). The many varieties of catatonia. *European Archives of Psychiatry and Clinical Neuroscience*, 251(Suppl. 1), 18–13. doi:10.1007/PL00014200

Francis, A. (2006). Update on catatonia. *Psychiatric Times*, 23(9), 85–86.

Francis, A. (2010). Catatonia: Diagnosis, classification, and treatment. *Current Psychiatry Reports*, 12(3), 180–185. doi:10.1007/s11920-010-0113-y

Fuchs, T. (2006). Implicit and explicit temporality. *Philosophy, Psychiatry & Psychology*, 12(3), 195–198. doi:10.1353/ppp.2006.0004

Fuchs, T. (2007). The temporal structure of intentionality and its disturbance in schizophrenia. *Psychopathology*, 40(4), 229–235. doi:10.1159/000101365

Fuchs, T. (2010). Phenomenology and psychopathology. In S. Gallagher & D. Schmicking (Eds.), *Handbook of phenomenology and the cognitive sciences* (pp. 546–573). Dordrecht, Netherlands: Springer.

Fuchs, T. (2012). The phenomenology of body memory. In S. C. Koch, T. Fuchs, M. Summa, & C. Müller (Eds.), *Body memory, metaphor and movement* (pp. 9–22). Amsterdam, Netherlands: John Benjamins.

Fuchs, T. (2013a). The phenomenology of affectivity. In B. Fulford, M. Davies, G. T. Gipps, G. Graham, J. Sadler, G. Stanghellini, & P. Thornton (Eds.), *The Oxford handbook of philosophy and psychiatry* (pp. 612–631). Oxford, UK: Oxford University Press. doi:10.1093/oxfordhb/9780199579563.013.0038

Fuchs, T. (2013b). Temporality and psychopathology. *Phenomenology and the Cognitive Sciences*, 12(1), 75–104. doi:10.1007/s11097-010-9189-4

Fuchs, T., & Schlimme, J. (2009). Embodiment and psychopathology: A phenomenological perspective. *Current Opinion in Psychiatry*, 22, 570–575. doi:10.1097/YCO.0b013e3283318e5c

Fuchs, T., & Van Duppen, Z. (2017). Time and events: On the phenomenology of temporal experience in schizophrenia (Ancillary article to EAWE Domain 2). *Psychopathology*, 50(1), 68–74. doi:10.1159/000452768

Hirjak, D., Kubera, K. M., Wolf, R. C., & Northoff, G. (2019). Going back to Kahlbaum's psychomotor (and GABAergic) origins: Is catatonia more than just a motor and dopaminergic syndrome? *Schizophrenia Bulletin*. Advance online publication, 46(2), 272–285. doi:10.1093/schbul/sbz074

Husserl, E. (1966). *Zur Phänomenologie des inneren Zeitbewusstseins* [On the phenomenology of inner time consciousness]. The Hague, Netherlands: Nijhoff.

Husserl, E. (2012). *Cartesikanische Meditationen* [Cartesian meditations]. Hamburg, Germany: Felix Meiner.

Jaspers, K. (1913). *Allgemeine Psychopathologie* [General psychopathology]. Berlin, Germany: Springer.

Kahlbaum, K. L. (1874). *Klinische Abhandlungen über psychische Krankheiten: Eine klinische Form psychischer Krankheit. Die Katatonie oder das Spannungsirresein* [Clinical treatise on mental diseases: A clinical form of mental illness. Catatonia or Spannungsirresein]. Berlin, Germany: Verlag von August Hirschwald.

Kay, S. R., Kanofsky, D., Lindemayer, J.-P., & Opler, L. A. (1987). The changing presentation of catatonia. *American Journal of Psychiatry*, 144(6), 834–835. doi:10.1176/ajp.144.6.aj1446834

Kraepelin, E. (1904). *Psychiatrie. Ein Lehrbuch für Studierende und Ärzte. 7., vielfach umgearbeitete Auflage. Band 2.* [Psychiatry. A textbook for students and doctors. 7th often revised edition. Volume 2]. Leipzig, Germany: Verlag von Johan Ambrosius Barth.

Kupke, C. (2006). Lived time and to live time: A critical comment on a paper by Martin Wyllie. *Philosophy, Psychiatry, & Psychology*, 12(3), 199–203. doi:10.1353/ppp.2006.0011

Linden, D. E. (2012). The challenges and promise of neuroimaging in psychiatry. *Neuron*, 73(1), 8–22. doi:10.1016/j.neuron.2011.12.014

Marx, B. P., Forsyth, J. P., Gallup, G. G., Fusé, T., & Lexington, J. M. (2008). Tonic immobility as an evolved predator defense: Implications for sexual assault survivors. *Clinical Psychology: Science and Practice*, 15(1), 74–90. doi:10.1111/j.1468-2850.2008.00112.x

Merleau-Ponty, M. (1960). *Signes* [Signs]. Paris, France: Les Éditions Gallimard.

Minkowski, E. (1970). *Lived time. Phenomenological and psychopathological studies* (N. Metzel, Trans.). Evanston, IL: Northwestern University Press.

Moskowitz, A. K. (2004). "Scared stiff": Catatonia as an evolutionary-based fear response. *Psychological Review*, 111(4), 984–1002. doi:10.1037/0033-295X.111.4.984

Northoff, G., Krill, W., Wenke, J., Gille, B., Russ, M., Eckert, J., … Pflug, B. (1998). Major differences in subjective experience of akinetic states in catatonic and Parkinsonian patients. *Cognitive Neuropsychiatry*, 3(3), 161–178. doi:10.1080/135468098396125

Northoff, G., Krill, W., Wenke, J., Travers, H., & Pflug, B. (1996). The subjective experience in catatonia: Systematic study of 24 catatonic patients. *Psychiatrische Praxis*, 23(2), 69–73.

Parnas, J. (2013). On psychosis: Karl Jaspers and beyond. In G. Stanghellini & T. Fuchs (Eds.), *One century of Karl Jaspers' general psychopathology* (pp. 208–228). Oxford, UK: Oxford University Press.

Parnas, J., Møller, P., Kircher, T., Thalbitzer, J., Jansson, L., Handest, P., & Zahavi, D. (2005). EASE-scale: Examination of Anomalous Self-Experience. *Psychopathology*, 38(5), 236–258. doi:10.1159/000088441

Parnas, J., Sass, L. A., & Zahavi, D. (2013). Rediscovering psychopathology: The epistemology and phenomenology of the psychiatric object. *Schizophrenia Bulletin*, 39(2), 270–277. doi:10.1093/schbul/sbs153

Penland, H. R., Weder, N., & Tampi, R. R. (2006). The catatonic dilemma expanded. *Annals of General Psychiatry*, 5, 14. doi:10.1186/1744-859X-5-14

Perkins, R. J. (1982). Catatonia: The ultimate response to fear? *Australian and New Zealand Journal of Psychiatry*, 16(4), 282–287. doi:10.3109/00048678209161268

Pfuhlmann, B., & Stöber, G. (2001). The different conceptions of catatonia: Historical overview and critical discussion. *European Archives of Psychiatry and Clinical Neuroscience*, 251(Suppl. 1), 14–17. doi:10.1007/PL00014199

Plessner, H. (1970). *Laughing and crying: A study of the limits of human behavior* (J. S. Churchill & M. Grene, Trans.). Evanston, IL: Northwestern University Press.

Ratcliffe, M. (2017). *Real hallucinations: Psychiatric illness, intentionality, and the interpersonal world.* Cambridge, MA: Massachusetts Institute of Technology Press.

Rodemeyer, L. (2006). *Intersubjective temporality: It's about time.* Dordrecht, Netherlands: Springer. doi:10.1007/1-4020-4214-0

Sass, L., Pienkos, E., Škodlar, B., Stanghellini, G., Fuchs, T., Parnas, J., & Jones, N. (2017). EAWE: Examination of Anomalous World Experience. *Psychopathology*, 50(1), 10–54. doi:10.1159/000454928

Shorter, E., & Fink, M. (2018). *The madness of fear: A history of catatonia*. Oxford, UK: Oxford University Press.

Sienaert, P., Dhossche, D. M., Vancampfort, D., de Hert, M., & Gazdag, G. (2014). A clinical review of the treatment of catatonia. *Frontiers in Psychiatry*, 5, 1–9. doi:10.3389/fpsyt.2014.00181

Sienaert, P., Rooseleer, J., & de Fruyt, J. (2011). Measuring catatonia: A systematic review of rating scales. *Journal of Affective Disorders*, 135(1–3), 1–9. doi:10.1016/j.jad.2011.02.012

Taylor, M. A., & Fink, M. (2003). Catatonia in psychiatric classification: A home of its own. *American Journal of Psychiatry*, 160(7), 1233–1241. doi:10.1176/appi.ajp.160.7.1233

Trevarthen, C. (1998). The concept and foundations of infant intersubjectivity. In S. Braten (Ed.), *Intersubjective communication and emotion in early ontogeny* (pp. 15–46). Cambridge, MA: Cambridge University Press.

Van der Kolk, B. A. (1994). The body keeps the score: Memory and the evolving psychobiology of posttraumatic stress. *Harvard Review of Psychiatry*, 1(5), 1253–265. doi:10.3109/10673229409017088

Van Duppen, Z. (2016). The phenomenology of hypo- and hyperreality in psychopathology. *Phenomenology and the Cognitive Sciences*, 15(3), 423–441. doi:10.1007/s11097-015-9429-8

Van Duppen, Z. (2017). The intersubjective dimension of schizophrenia. *Philosophy, Psychiatry & Psychology*, 4(24), 399–418. doi:10.1353/ppp.2017.0058

Van Duppen, Z., & Sips, R. (2018). Understanding the blind spots of psychosis: A Wittgensteinian and first-person approach. *Psychopathology*, 51(4), 276–284. doi:10.1159/000490257

Van Praag, H. M. (2000). Nosologomania: A disorder of psychiatry. *The World Journal of Biological Psychiatry*, 1(3), 151–158. doi:10.3109/15622970009150584

Wehrle, M. (2019). Being a body and having a body. The twofold temporality of embodied intentionality. *Phenomenology and the Cognitive Sciences*. Advance online publication. doi:10.1007/s11097-019-09610-z

Wulff, E. (1995). *Wahnsinnslogik. Von der Verstehbarkeit schizophrener Erfahrung* [Insane logic. The understandability of schizophrenic experience]. Bonn, Germany: Psychiatrie-Verlag.

Wyllie, M. (2006). Lived time and psychopathology. *Philosophy, Psychiatry & Psychology*, 12(3), 173–185. doi:10.1353/ppp.2006.0017

Young, L. (1992). Sexual abuse and the problem of embodiment. *Child Abuse & Neglect*, 16(1), 89–100. doi:10.1016/0145-2134(92)90010-O

15.1

Commentary on "Closing Up: The Phenomenology of Catatonia"

Catatonia, Intercorporeality, and the Question of Phenomenological Specificity

Matthew Ratcliffe

In their contribution to this volume, Zeno Van Duppen and Pascal Sienaert (2021) develop an interesting and original phenomenological account of catatonia, which they take to apply to some but perhaps not all cases. They suggest that an experience of interpersonally or socially directed fear, originating in traumatic events, leads to a partial or complete loss of "intercorporeality" (bodily responsiveness to the movements, expressions, and gestures of others). To illustrate this, they reflect on the first author's encounter in a hospital corridor, with a woman who was completely unresponsive to the interpersonal environment and maintained a fixed, rigid posture. It transpired that she had been to a trauma therapy session shortly beforehand, where she was asked to recall traumatic events. Consistent with this, Van Duppen and Sienaert hypothesize a causal link between intense fear that cannot find an outlet and the subsequent onset of catatonia. The latter, they suggest, sometimes consists in an extreme form of dissociation: One cannot escape the object of fear and instead disengages from the social world via an altered experience of one's body. Their account of the fear–catatonia relationship is both causal and constitutive: fear causes catatonia, and catatonia incorporates fear.

Van Duppen and Sienaert suggest that catatonia can involve a profound change in the structure of bodily experience, which also amounts to an altered sense of time:

> The threat of the inner danger combined with being stuck, not getting out at that moment may have been so immense that on the implicit temporal level, protentional awareness, the open anticipation of what is to come, abruptly closes up. The conative-affective drive comes to a complete stop, literally, in that nothing moves anymore. The body, then, becomes an object-like figure, expressing the impossibility to experience—when the experience itself is unbearable. It expresses the impossibility to experience the other—when the threat of the other is unbearable. (2020, p. 357)

However, on reading this, one might wonder whether such a predicament involves any phenomenology at all. Van Duppen and Sienaert appeal to a distinction between the lived-body and the object-body. Ordinarily, we experience the surrounding environment *through* our bodies rather than encountering our bodies principally as objects located in that environment. Through our lived-bodies, we experience things as mattering, in ways that solicit activities from us and thus facilitate purposive interaction with our surroundings. Experiencing the world in this way is also inextricable from our sense of time. A kind of practical, bodily immersion in the world is required in order to experience meaningful possibilities and their actualization, amounting to a sense of temporal unfolding.

Now, suppose this bodily immersion was altogether absent. What remains of experience, when the world no longer offers practically meaningful possibilities and there is no sense of transition from the possible to the actual? It is not enough to characterize the resultant phenomenology solely in terms of what is absent; some positive characterization is also required. Van Duppen and Sienaert speculate that catatonia involves disruption of the mind–body relationship and that the body "could be almost completely separated from the mind" (p. 355). However, there is a need for caution here. In drawing on the tradition of phenomenological psychopathology and emphasizing the role of the lived-body, they endorse an approach to the study of human experience that takes the mind to be phenomenologically inextricable from the body. Indeed, one might go so far as to say that the subject of experience simply *is* the lived-body. Hence, if catatonia sometimes involves a complete or near-complete shift from lived-body to object-body, it is not clear what kind of experiential subject survives the transformation.

This also raises issues concerning phenomenological method. How might we go about studying and further clarifying the form(s) of experience involved in catatonia? One approach would be to draw on the testimonies of those who have recovered from catatonic states and are able to recall their experiences. However, first-person reflection is likely to be unreliable here. If catatonia sometimes involves forms of experience that are radically different in structure from everyday experience, this may well interfere with the abilities to remember, reflect upon, interpret, and/or describe what catatonic experience is like. Another approach, evident throughout Van Duppen and Sienaert's discussion, is instead to reflect on one's own experience of encountering someone who is catatonic; one *feels* cut off from that person, in a way that indicates a profound disturbance of bodily intersubjectivity. As they write, "there was no spontaneous bodily attunement to my presence, to my movements." Thus, "primary intersubjectivity," "the most fundamental embodied connection to others," seemed absent (p. 354).

However, there is the objection that the catatonic person is unresponsive to other people as an inevitable consequence of her being largely or wholly unresponsive to everything around her. After all, the person described by Van Duppen was already standing motionless in a corridor, wholly unresponsive to her surroundings, before anyone else appeared on the scene. By analogy, it would be misleading to claim that a complete loss of sight consists principally in loss of visually guided interactions with other people. One cannot participate in these specific forms of interactions because one cannot engage with the world in *any* of those ways that depend on a functioning visual system.

So, why might one arrive at the view that catatonia relates more specifically to the interpersonal realm? One possibility to consider is that the apparent specificity is an artifact of how the *interpreter* experiences an unusual interpersonal situation. More usually, we experience the bodies of other people as receptive to our own movements, gestures, and expressions, in ways that distinguish them from inanimate objects and from the bodies of nonhuman organisms. This, perhaps more than anything else, is what renders them phenomenologically distinctive. Hence, when one comes across a human body that is unresponsive to its surroundings, but not in a state of sleep, what might appear to us as most salient, peculiar, and unsettling is the lack of specifically interpersonal responses. Van Duppen and Sienaert write that the body of the catatonic person somehow "expresses" the impossibility of experiencing the "other" (p. 357). But what, exactly, does this mean? Is the impossibility somehow integral to or symptomatic of the person's experience? Alternatively, is it all in the eye of the beholder? Suppose that one anticipates, in a prereflective, bodily way, a pattern of responses to one's own actions, gestures, expressions, and words. With the catatonic person's failure to respond, there is a pervasive experience of negated expectation, rendering the lack of interpersonal reciprocity more salient than a wider lack of responsiveness. One thus experiences a general deficit as a more specifically interpersonal deficit. This would seem entirely consistent with the observation that "a catatonic person becomes a body that does not attune and does not afford or invite the attunement by others. She closes up" (p. 354).

However, even if this objection proves sound, there may be a way of reconciling it with Van Duppen and Sienaert's approach. Experiencing another person as awake, but at the same time motionless and disengaged from her surroundings, interferes with the ability to experience and interact with her *as* a person. Given this, it will also interfere more specifically with the ability to direct certain kinds of hostile actions toward her, insofar as those actions involve relating to her in a distinctively personal way. Thus, even if catatonia (or, at least, a certain form of catatonia) does involve a wider disengagement from the world, it could still have a *purposive* structure that relates more specifically to interpersonal threat. Such a structure could be conceived of in phenomenological and/or nonphenomenological terms. Van Duppen and Sienaert develop an interesting and insightful case for the former, but I suggest that it requires further clarification and support: How, if at all, is the interpersonal structure of catatonia integral to its phenomenology, and which phenomenological methods are best equipped to investigate this?

Reference

Van Duppen, Z., & Sienaert, P. (2021). Closing up: The phenomenology of catatonia. In C. Tewes & G. Stanghellini (Eds.), *Time and body: Phenomenological and psychopathological approaches* (pp. 346–362). Cambridge, UK: Cambridge University Press.

16

Embodied Selfhood and Personal Identity in Dementia

Christian Tewes

Introduction

In recent decades, the embodiment paradigm has gained increasing influence on how we regard the interrelationship between selfhood, personality, body, and Alzheimer's disease. While there is a strong tendency in public discourse and science today to regard the late stages of Alzheimer's disease as a complete loss of the patient's personality, leading proponents of a phenomenologically oriented embodied approach call for a reevaluation of this view. They point to the need for a radical improvement in how we organize care in residential and nursing homes for patients with dementia by taking into consideration insights from embodied research and ethical debates (Kontos & Martin, 2013). In support of their arguments, they draw not only on classical phenomenological works by Edmund Husserl or Maurice Merleau-Ponty but also on detailed empirical research: Recent studies underscore the significance of gestures in communicative processes, of emotional expressions, embodied, and extended memories, as well as the capacity of dance and music to increase the well-being of people living with dementia (Hameed et al., 2018; Hydén, 2018; Kontos & Martin, 2013).

A question remains, however, as to how far reaching these insights are concerning the constitution of personal identity in the case of Alzheimer's disease. There is a strong philosophical tradition – going back in important respects to John Locke – that explains personhood and diachronic identity in terms of reflexivity, explicit memory capacities (declarative memory), narrative capacities, and mechanisms of psychological continuity and responsibility.

If one follows this tradition and accepts these properties as vital for any fully fledged manifestation of personhood, as embodied approaches often do, then the onus is on them to clarify how and indeed whether the embodied approach can avoid the same conclusion as the cognitivist picture: that Alzheimer's patients turn from persons into *nonpersons*. In what follows, I attempt exactly this task. I begin with an explication of how proponents of the cognitivist picture of personal identity justify their conclusions and an exploration of the assumptions they rely upon. In the second section, I reconstruct insights from phenomenologically oriented embodied research that challenge the cognitivist's one-sided anthropological view and its problematic ethical implications. After evaluating these claims, I argue in the third section that the strongly embodied characteristics of selfhood, agency, and consciousness have a constitutive function for the creation of *personal selfhood*, which I suggest is present even in the later stages of Alzheimer's disease.

The Cognitivist Challenge to the Interpretation of Alzheimer's Disease

When we consider the historical roots of the concept of personhood, it is already apparent in medieval theological discourse that the term "person" is not confined to human beings but can be applied to other entities, such as God and angels. Whereas in theological discourse, the attribute of personhood extends beyond the human species, the contemporary debate on personal identity deals with a further possibility: that *not all* members of the human species are persons.

An ongoing debate today attempts to determine whether key symptoms of dementia – the loss of declarative memories, symbolic communication skills, and fluid orientations in time and space – entail the patient's loss of their *status as a person*. Those who maintain that this status *is* lost, I argue here, neglect crucial dimensions of deeply embodied human existence.

In the next section, I introduce two leading theories of personal identity, which are both sophisticated examples of the predominant "cognitivist stance" in research on personal identity. In a first step, I take a closer look at the "psychological continuity" theory of persons. Following that, the "narrative" account of personhood is introduced: here, the symbolic capacities of human beings are regarded as essential for personal identity. Having presented these approaches, I point out their shortcomings, which indicate the need to ground personal identity in strongly embodied features of human existence.

Declarative Memory Capacities and Psychological Continuity

Key ideas concerning the psychological continuity of personal existence have their roots, as already indicated, in John Locke's highly influential chapter on "identity and diversity" in his *Essay concerning human understanding* (Locke, 1690/2017). One crucial element for diachronic unity of personhood, according to Locke, is the capacity to reflect on past actions or ideas of the same consciousness:

> For it is by the consciousness he has of his present thoughts and actions that he is *self to himself* now, and so will be the same self as far as the same consciousness can extend to actions past or to come. (Locke, 1690/2017, XXVII, p. 116)

Several aspects in this quotation are highly significant for the subsequent development of the discourse on personal identity. Locke's approach in this passage is concerned with "numerical identity" or identity over time (diachronic identity). Diachronic identity focuses on necessary and sufficient conditions for specifying that person S at t_1 is the same as the same person S at $t_2, t_3, \ldots, t_n$ (Noonan, 2019, pp. 84–85). Such an approach is differentiated in the literature from "qualitative identity," whereby the focus is on an identity that persists despite changing properties, for instance, we take an individual to be the same person over a lifespan despite changes in appearance (McMillan, 2006, pp. 63–64).

Both dimensions of personal identity are intertwined and have implications for how we understand Alzheimer's disease. The same is true of the role of consciousness, which Locke specifies in the quotation as the necessary bond relating past thoughts and actions (and those to come) to the present self and its mental activities. In today's terminology, the retrospective function of consciousness is called *declarative memory.* In the cognitive sciences, it is defined as comprising personal knowledge (episodic memories) and conceptual/factual knowledge (semantic memory) that can be voluntarily retrieved and verbally expressed (Tramoni et al., 2011, p. 817).

A question arises as to whether and how the existence of persons depends on the function of declarative memory capacities. In his early critique of Locke's personal identity theory, Thomas Reid pointed out that humans' power of recollecting past events is always limited. Our memory does not capture every experience that we have ever had and does not even capture everything that we have previously remembered. To define identity in terms of explicit memories or similar mental states/dispositions such as beliefs and desires thus undermines the required *transitivity relation* of personal identity (Reid, 1785/1975, p. 114).[1]

Proponents of the psychological continuity theory of personal identity such as Derek Parfit have added further criteria for psychological continuity, which do not violate the principle of transitivity. One major approach to

[1] Thus, at a late stage of her life, a person S might remember what she did twenty years before, and she might in turn have remembered *at that time* what she did in a specific situation F during her school days. However, S does not necessarily remember at her late stage of life what happened to her at the original situation F. This shows that the principle of transitivity is violated by Locke's criteria of personal identity.

understanding psychological continuity is the notion of "psychological connectedness." Parfit explains its relation to a well-functioning memory system in the following way:

> [T]he word "I" can be used to imply the greatest degree of psychological connectedness. When the connections are reduced, when there has been any marked change of character or style of life, or any marked loss of memory, our imagined beings would say, "It was not I who did that but an earlier self." (Parfit, 1971, p. 25)

The way Parfit defines "psychological connectedness" in this passage shows his kinship to Locke's approach, even if he speaks of "character" or "style of life" and not just memory capacities. In more formal terms, Parfit argues that the "greatest degree of psychological connectedness" is an explication of "direct psychological connections," that is, direct memories of earlier experiences or the formation of beliefs and desires thereof. That direct connections of mental states are only a matter of *degree* indicates that, for Parfit as for Locke, these connections do not by themselves satisfy the transitivity principle. For that reason, Parfit specifies "psychological connectedness" as a relation consisting of "the holding of overlapping chains of *strong* connectedness" (Parfit, 1984, p. 206). He then defines "psychological continuity" as requiring only *overlapping chains* of direct psychological relations, that is, connections (Parfit, 1971, p. 20). Defined in this much weaker way, his definition of psychological continuity satisfies the transitivity principle (Parfit, 1971, p. 20). Without going further into the complex issues Parfit raises, the question that must concern us here is what these approaches tell us about the status of personal identity in the case of dementia and Alzheimer's disease.[2]

Let us start with an assessment of Locke's original account. On the basis of the criteria he gives for identity in the earlier quotation, Locke cannot ascribe the status of persons to Alzheimer's patients at late stages of their disease. This is so because Alzheimer's disease – one of the most frequent forms of dementia – proceeds by way of a gradual but progressive loss of mental capacities, including autonomous orientation in time and space. Also symptomatic is the loss of symbolic communication skills, a change in socioemotional behavior, and the deterioration of (declarative) memory (Hughes, Louw, & Sabat, 2006, p. 2; Sabat & Harré, 1994). Such progressive destruction of mental, behavioral, and social skills is caused by

[2] For a thoroughgoing critique of Parfit's attempt to circumvent the transitivity problem, see Schechtman (1996, pp. 29–38).

an underlying neurodegenerative pathology of specific parts of the brain, such as plaques and tangles (Hughes et al., 2006, p. 3). If the decisive criterion for personal identity is that the "same consciousness can extend to actions past or to come," it is plain in the case of the progression of Alzheimer's disease that personhood diminishes to the point where the affected human being turns into a *nonperson*.

Does Parfit's theory of psychological continuity fare any better in avoiding this conclusion? I suggest that it does not. "Strongly overlapping psychological connections" are at the very least a vague basis for personal identity (how many connections are required for strong connectedness and how does one justify an answer to this question?). Parfit in effect faces the same ontological problem as Locke's original account. If we assume Parfit's definition, then the progressive deterioration of mental capacities in dementia implies that there are patients who, due to a lack of psychological continuity, are no longer persons at an ontological level of description. This conclusion holds despite the late Parfit augmenting his psychological continuity theory with an "embodied part view." The latter holds that the brain is the decisive organ where consciousness and personality are situated.[3] As Parfit puts it: "[W]e might be embodied heads. And most of us would believe that, for us to survive, it would be enough that our head survives, and continues to be the head of a conscious being" (Parfit, 2012, p. 17). Parfit's claim that we are "embodied heads" nicely reflects the underlying brain centrism of his theory (also a decisive feature of the wider debate on personal identity), but it does not solve the problem.

Jens Brockmeier has criticized such approaches, which frequently understand (declarative) memories in analogy with an organ or a part thereof "that can be affected by various dementia, such as AD, the 'memory killer', just like the lung can be affected by cancer" (Brockmeier, 2014, p. 72). One can formulate Brockmeier's point even more strongly. Cognitivist approaches to personal identity converge in the claim that the brain is the *central organ* for personal identity because it controls enduring memories and the character of the person. What this reveals is a kind of *internalism*, which conceives the brain as a self-contained organ separated from social interactions, from the living body, and from the experiential dimension

[3] Parfit takes the "embodied part view" from McMahan who originally called it the "embodied mind view" (2002). According to McMahan, we are essentially embodied minds. Physical and only minimal functional continuity of the brain is required to sustain personal identity over time especially with regard to *rational egoistic self-concern* (McMahan, 2002, p. 68ff.). I assess this position in comparison with other embodied approaches to personal identity and dementia in more detail in the next section.

of agency (Brockmeier, 2014, p. 73). There is, however, a different theory circulating in contemporary discourse that is highly relevant for evaluating the personal status of dementia patients. This is the "narrative" conception of selfhood and dementia.

Narrative Conceptions of Personality and Selfhood

It is a deeply rooted feature of thinking about dementia that the gradual loss of symbolic language capacities is related to a loss of personal identity. Hilde Lindemann, in a study of the difficult daily social situations faced by a person with dementia and her daughter Kate who is caring for her, observes that:

> In any progressive dementia, a point is reached when speech begins to misfire, becoming clumsy, then garbled, and finally vanishes altogether.... [Kate's mother] loses her understanding of who she herself is: the tissue of stories by which she has made sense of her own life gradually or suddenly come unraveled.... The disease destroys her second nature, and with it, her self. (Lindemann, 2014, p. 19)

This description of a severe case of advanced dementia captures essential ingredients of the narrative conception of selfhood. By losing her power of speech, Kate's mother is not only losing an important means for social communication and orientation; the *sense-dimensions* of her life are equally shrinking when she forfeits not only her symbolic communication skills but the "tissue of stories" that have become part of her second nature.[4] When we extend the Aristotelian concept of "second nature" to include incorporated habits, abilities, and expressive behavior, it remains a major empirical research question whether and in what sense Kate's mother's second nature is actually destroyed. But what this debate already indicates is that the narrative conception of personhood is not concerned with different (possible) dimensions of personality in the analysis of dementia patients. Rather, it is assumed from the outset that the defining features of personhood are *symbolic capacities* that enfold "centers of narrative gravity," to use Dennett's famous metaphor for the personal stance (Dennett, 1991).

[4] Lindemann rejects the conclusion that the destruction of Kate's mother's "second nature" also implies the loss of her self. She maintains that so long as infants and people with severe dementia are "held in personhood" by other people who take care of them, one can still ascribe to them the status of personhood (Lindemann, 2014, pp. 20–22). Lindemann touches here on very important dimensions of the social embeddedness of persons and questions of moral obligation in geriatric care. However, as will become clear in the following sections, I do not think that her approach is sufficient to allow an ascription of the ontological status of personhood to Kate's mother.

The following passage by Charles Taylor captures the typical justification for this view:

> I define who I am by defining where I speak from, in the family tree, in social space, in the geography of social status and functions, in my intimate relations to the ones I love, and also crucially in the space of moral and spiritual orientation within which my most important defining relations are lived out.... This obviously cannot be just a contingent matter. There is no way we could be inducted into personhood except by being initiated into a language. (Taylor, 1989, p. 35)

One cannot deny that Taylor here pinpoints significant features of the fully fledged concept of qualitative personal identity, such as its intertwinement with the "moral and spiritual space" of social interactions and institutions. Moreover, there are good conceptual and empirical reasons for believing that the emergence of these capacities depends on human beings' *symbolic enculturation* (Deacon, 2016). On this basis, proponents of the "narrative constitution view" have claimed that their position can explain our intuitions about "personal identity and survival," "moral responsibility," or "self-concern and compensation" (Schechtman, 1996, p. 93). However, narrative accounts of personhood still have important lacunae, for instance the question of how to specify the process of autobiographical self-production in the process of its narrative constitution. Is storytelling a fictitious enterprise, like a novelist's inventing a character, or does it also represent experiences by relating them to a form-finding unity (Strawson, 2004, pp. 444–446)? We will come back to this question in the next section.

Missing Phenomenal Dimensions of Selfhood in the Cognitive Approach

An early philosophical response to Locke's account of personal identity objected that it rests on a criterion of memory that is viciously circular (Butler, 1736/1975). Why is this so? When the explicit act of recollection is supposed to constitute the identity of persons, it already presupposes a form of prereflective self-acquaintance or self-familiarity that cannot be the result of an explicit act of reflection. This points to an insight that is still highly relevant to the current debate on personal identity: We experience selfhood from the *first-person perspective*, as an irreducible feature of numerical and qualitative identity.

Can psychological continuity theories such as Parfit's do justice to the significance of the first-person experience of selfhood? It is doubtful whether direct psychological connections between beliefs, desires, and memories (and their causal interrelationship) could ever explain the specific form of self-familiarity that characterizes the first-person dimension of recollected events. To reach a deeper understanding of the explanatory challenge contained in the circularity problem, it is necessary to explain in more detail the neglected dimensions of selfhood in the cognitivist accounts of personal identity. A good place to start is to specify how the "in-built" relation of selfhood is part of every phenomenal experience (Zahavi & Kriegel, 2016). Dan Zahavi in particular has shown that experience, even at the prereflective level, is not anonymous or unconscious but involves a basic self-manifesting *for-me-ness*, which one can also describe as a kind of basic "perspectival ownership" of experiences (Zahavi, 2017, p. 194).

But how is the sense of selfhood – beyond its minimal form of for-me-ness – related to personal continuity over time? Marya Schechtman has made an important contribution to answering this question. As her analysis makes clear, the simple addition of psychologically and causally connected memories, beliefs, desires, and intentions does not elucidate in any way how it could ever give rise to selfhood or personal identity over time (Schechtman, 2005, p. 15). Her alternative account is built on the concept of a "perceiver self." The basic idea is that we are constantly self-monitoring our stream of consciousness with the aim of detecting an underlying unity: "The 'perceiver-self' should be thought of as a stable observer who views and records the passing flux of experience, and recognizes it as part of a single life" (Schechtman, 2005, p. 19). In contrast to the causal connections between psychological events or dispositions, the stream of consciousness consists in an incessant temporal experience of phenomenal continuity (Dainton & Bayne, 2005, pp. 555–558), a continuity that is inseparably linked to a perceiver or monitoring self.

This phenomenal continuity has been further analyzed from the first-person perspective in its *implicit* "micro-temporal order" of time-consciousness by Edmund Husserl. Especially what he calls the "passive synthesis" of "original impression," "retention," and "protention" is based on the insight that every experience is temporally intertwined according to this structural order. Thus, the "retentional consciousness" refers to the experience that, for instance, parts of a melody are still present in consciousness when we already perceive the next tone or part of the succeeding musical event. "Protentential consciousness" points to the implicit anticipation of the melody or parts thereof that are not yet perceived (Husserl, 1966/1991). These considerations indicate that the self is both a foundational part of the stream of consciousness and simultaneously (prereflectively) the detector of the unified temporal flow of phenomenal experiences.

It might come as a surprise that a leading proponent of the "narrative constitution view" such as Schechtman claims an experiential or phenomenal foundation of selfhood and personal identity. Why does she include this foundation of personal identity and selfhood in her theory? The reason is that the concept of the perceiver self should bridge the gap between forgotten or irretrievable experiences that might have an ongoing impact on one's life, and the active *sense-making dimension* of the self as an actor who seeks an understanding of her own biography. Schechtman (2005) calls this dimension of personhood the "self-understanding view."

Several issues are in need of further clarification at this point. First, when the narrative self is not conceived – pace Dennett – as a fictitious entity, it requires a foundation in phenomenal experiences and a sense-making activity of selfhood/agency that is an essential *precondition* and no mere *result* of the narrative constitution of the self (Summa & Fuchs, 2015). This is also an important factor in any phenomenological analysis of the coherence of narrative structures in dementia research (McLean, 2006, p. 174). According to this view, the (re)integration of previously forgotten experiences into one's own biography is both a sense-making activity of the agent and a *detection* of earlier and still ongoing life-forming features (experiences) of one's own personality. Second, I suggest, the developments from the for-me-ness of the minimal self to the sense-making activity of the self-understanding agent are mere moments inseparable from the fully fledged phenomena of real selfhood where all these aspects are intertwined. Thus, there is not only a perceiver self who passively registers her own stream of consciousness but always an active self too, one who strives to generate sense-making "Gestalten" in the world and in her life (biography) (Bär, 2010). As will become clear in the following sections, this is also true of patients suffering from late-stage Alzheimer's; it sheds new light on the question of whether and how they actually lose their status as persons.

Embodied Theories of Dementia and Personal Identity

Within the field of embodied theories of cognition, perception, and emotion, an important distinction is to be made between those approaches that are committed to *weak* and to *strong* versions of embodiment theory. Thus, to give an example, the identity theory of the mind–body problem (all mental states or events are physical states but not vice versa) is a weak version, insofar as it argues that mental states are constituted by brain states. Stronger versions, by contrast, seek to show that "extracranial parts," bodily activities, or extended interactions can play a constitutional role in psychological capacities (Menary, 2015). In this section, I explore ways in which embodied-oriented research on dementia helps explain how qualitative and numerical personal identities are intertwined. This can help us answer the question of whether we are justified in ascribing both properties to patients at late stages of Alzheimer's disease. What makes these questions so complex is that any answer needs to explain how a human can be the *same person* over time despite the *qualitative changes* (development and decline) that are essential elements of human existence.

Weak Embodied Approaches to Dementia

Jeff McMahan's "embodied mind view" or "embodied part view" of personal identity demonstrates that using the term "embodied" for building an account of personal identity is not sufficient to overcome the cognitivist brain-centered view that conceives of the brain as the locus of memories and personality. He develops his account by rejecting the psychological continuity theory because it leads to the consequence that patients in severe cases of Alzheimer's disease are regarded as *nonpersons*. Assuming that psychological continuity is broadly destroyed in such cases, McMahan instead grounds personal identity on the continuing physical and (minimal) functional capacity of the brain to produce the same consciousness or mind (McMahan, 2002, p. 67). As he puts it, "[a]ccording to the Embodied Mind Account, the criterion of personal identity is physical and minimal functional continuity of the brain" (McMahan, 2002, p. 69).

As already indicated, this version of an embodied view is ill equipped to avoid the challenges faced by psychological continuity theories of personal identity. How the physical and minimal functional organization of the brain alone can generate and ground numerical personal identity and the qualitative dimensions of selfhood (perspectival ownership, monitoring self) remains unclear. The reference to brain states is not an appropriate foundation for specifying numerical and qualitative personal identity, because the "explanatory gap" created by explicating phenomenal consciousness in physicalist terms *re-appears* with regard to the qualitative dimensions of selfhood, personality, and the stream of consciousness (McMahan, 2002, p. 88). How can a specific minimal functional continuity of the brain be a sufficient foundation for personal identity over time? Why not extend this foundational base to further parts of the body and the social realm? What is missing in McMahan's internalistic account is an explication of why consciousness – realized or caused by minimal functional continuity of the brain – is appropriate for grounding personal identity (or egoistic concerns) in the first place. His reference to the continuing minimal functional capacity of the brain to produce the same consciousness or mind fails to answer the question of why we are entitled to ascribe to the brain this capacity in severe cases of dementia.

Strongly Embodied Approaches to Dementia

In contrast to the explicitly or implicitly cognitivist stances on dementia, strongly embodied and phenomenologically oriented approaches do not regard dementia patients as losing their self and status as a person (Hydén, 2018, p. 229). How do the proponents of a strongly embodied view justify this conviction?

As we have already seen, "personal identity" is a multifaceted term that refers to intertwined but also distinct dimensions of selfhood, properties of a person, and conditions of persistence over time. The currently dominant research questions about numerical identity (how does a person persist over time?) are important issues but hardly exhaust the underlying phenomena of personhood. Indeed, all persons undergo *constant changes*: They lose certain physical and mental properties and gain new ones, which means that any concept of qualitative identity needs to incorporate "growth and decline" as essential characteristics of selfhood and personal identity (Lesser, 2006, pp. 56–57). Focusing on these latter aspects, the strongly embodied approach does not deny that severe late-stage dementia (as the case of Kate's mother vividly illustrates) leads to momentous transformations and disruptions of qualitative aspects of their personality. Nevertheless, it stands opposed to the following view, which Richard Taylor, a former psychiatrist and himself living with dementia, ascribes to the public:

> I think that, for most people, Alzheimer's disease means certain death before your "natural time," preceded by a period of time during which you have been stripped of your personality and your memories and have become someone you cannot imagine. You have no dignity and no sense of self, and eventually you just sit around waiting for your body to forget how to keep itself alive. (Taylor, 2007, p. 114)

To admit that a disruptive qualitative change occurs in Alzheimer's patients does not (necessarily) entail that these patients "have been stripped of [their] personality." But why exactly does this conclusion not follow from the premise? For proponents of a strongly embodied mind view, it is because a patient's prereflective self-awareness and subjectivity remain intact even at a late stage of Alzheimer's disease (Hydén, 2018, p. 229). This is so despite the loss of symbolic language capacities, vanishing declarative memories, increasing limitations of orientation and emotional changes. As long as the phenomenal temporal continuity of the perceiver self is not interrupted, nothing speaks against the ascription of numerical identity. Furthermore, as the following reflections will show, an Alzheimer's patient is not only passively experiencing the ongoing activities in their vicinity. He or she retains the capacity of an active self that expresses itself in enacted body memories (skills and habits), emotional attunements, and sense-making actions. Taking these components together allows the ascription of personal identity even at late stages of Alzheimer's disease. Let me explain these claims in more detail.

Pia Kontos is a thinker who has – in her research on dementia and care – developed a phenomenological and strongly embodied-oriented concept of selfhood, which breaks with the cognitivist and brain-centered views on personal identity outlined earlier. Drawing in particular on Maurice Merleau-Ponty's work, she understands embodied selfhood as a primordial, nonrepresentational form of *intentionality*, which is deliberately but prereflectively directed toward the lifeworld (Kontos, 2004, pp. 837–841, 2005, pp. 559–560, 2012). Citing Merleau-Ponty, this kind of primordial intentionality is acted out in a "system of possible movements"; it "radiates from us to our environment" (Merleau-Ponty, 1964/1968, p. 5). The coordination of such movements has an inherently practical dimension: A pianist, for instance, knows how to play her instrument without any reflective knowledge of exactly where the keys of the piano are situated in objective physical space and exactly when the sounds of a melody are to be played. According to Kontos, such movements are not anonymous but are intimately related to "selfhood, at the most fundamental level [and] must be understood as inhering in the existential capacity of the body to engage with the world" (Kontos, 2012, p. 4). This basic concept of embodied selfhood brings together and deepens the different strands of the preceding sections. It shows that basic bodily movements and interactions are not necessarily the performance of an anonymous unconscious activity. Minimal selfhood (for-me-ness) and the perceiver self are already manifested in the intentional "system of movements" of the entire body in relation to the lifeworld.

Drawing upon a different discipline, that of biology, Thomas Fuchs has pointed to phenomena that complement this embodied theory of selfhood and personal identity. Fuchs explains how organisms demarcate in autopoetic terms their own boundaries from their environment in metabolic processes. A living organism does this by generating a semipermeable membrane that delimits it from its environment while simultaneously constituting the organism's own processual and dynamic self-identity over time (Fuchs, 2017, pp. 302–303; Thompson, 2007). In the human organism, it is above all the constant interaction between body, brain, and environment that leads to the *feeling of being alive*.

One can conceive the latter as a background feeling, rooted in homeostatic processes (Damasio, 1994). According to ecological and embodied approaches to affective neuroscience, the brain is therefore integrated into a larger network comprising the vascular, visceral, and motor system of the body, which manifests emotional valence and arousal as a (bidirectional) effect of dynamical environmental changes (Kiverstein & Miller, 2015, p. 7). At the same time, these processes are the foundation for an emerging self that develops and is enculturated in the extended interactions with the lifeworld.

Thus, Fuchs notes that these considerations at the level of the organism are consistent with the phenomenological concept of "primordial intentionality." We can add that they are consistent with strongly embodied-oriented concept of selfhood represented by Kontos and others too: "[S]entience and movement allow the living being to actively regulate its interaction with the environment, to adapt itself to changing circumstances, or in other words, to put itself in a relationship to what is other than self" (Fuchs, 2017, pp. 302–303). In the subset of strongly embodied approaches known as "enactivist" theories, such self and other-related activities are defined as *sense-making processes* due to their emotional valence and primordially intentional structure (Thompson, 2007).

These brief remarks indicate, on the one hand, the undeniable significance of the brain in the constitution of embodied selfhood. On the other hand, the first-person phenomenological and the more third-person-oriented autopoetic and affective neuroscientific account have the potential to go beyond McMahan's "embodied part view" and show that primordial intentionality (understood as "a system of potential movements") manifests *a self*. This self is realized in the expressivity of bodily acts, gestures, and social relationships and thus cannot be located solely inside the brain.[5] Or

[5] A further explanation of why the brain itself is not an agent with representational capacities but an indispensable meditating organ for relating the embodied self with the world can be found in Fuchs (2018).

to put it in another way, the self is an entity that manifests itself in the social realm too, an aspect that I elaborate in the next section in more detail.

Pia Kontos' phenomenologically inspired concept of embodied selfhood backs up these theories, presupposing the nonreflective but continuous stream of personal consciousness that is required, for instance, in the attention-based playing of the piano. Though dementia patients experience a disruptive psychological breakdown, it does not imply that their stream of consciousness is broken too. For embodied approaches to affective neuroscience, the phenomenal continuity and manifestation of selfhood are deeply rooted in the cyclical homeostatic processes of the whole organism in relation to its environment, even during sleep; it does not depend on the proper function of specific cognitive capacities (Fuchs, 2017, p. 305).[6]

Expressivity, Body Memory, and Intercorporeality

It is crucial to add that, though it has a pivotal foundation in organic processes, embodied selfhood is also co-constituted through social interactions. The concrete manifestation of selfhood and personality in human actions (system of intentionally performed movements) and *affective-emotional expressions* is the result of habitualized socially learned skills and styles of behavior. In recent phenomenological and embodied-oriented works, these phenomena are termed "body memories" (Casey, 1984/2000; Fuchs, 2012; Tewes & Fuchs, 2018). As already mentioned, one important facet of this memory type appears in skill-based learned behavior that forms a kind of implicit or procedural knowledge or "know-how" as exemplified before by playing a piano. Schacter defines implicit memory as operating when previous experience facilitates the performance of a task that does not require an explicit (reflective) conscious recollection (Schacter, 1987, p. 501). In addition to stereotyped routines or hard-wired stimulus-response contingencies, this memory type also allows flexible and adaptive interactions with objects and other persons (Casey, 1984/2000, p. 46). Taking this into consideration, one should not reduce the body memory to mere automatic sensorimotor functions because it is in many circumstances related to attention-based flexible behavior too (Sutton, McIlwain, Christensen, & Geeves, 2011; Tewes, 2018).

How does this memory type demonstrate that embodied selfhood and personality is also co-constituted in social interactions? Drawing on

[6] A thorough justification of phenomenal continuity, even during sleep, can be found in Fuchs (2017).

Merleau-Ponty's concept of "intercorporeality," which can be defined as a network of meaningful sets of body–object and body–body relations (Jordan & Mays, 2017, p. 364; Merleau-Ponty, 1964/1968, p. 180), we can shed light on the intersubjective foundation and dimension of selfhood and body memory. Research in developmental psychology on infants, for instance, has demonstrated the significance of primordial intercorporeal relations for the constitution of the self and body memories. From birth onward, children relate to their caregivers in recurrent schemas of interaction and emotional affect attunement, which then become habitualized as interactive patterns in the infant's body memory (Stern, 1985). Such patterns of shared intersubjective social practices are incorporated in the infant's implicit memory system long before they acquire the ability to communicate symbolically. These considerations also have far-reaching consequences for *collective embodied memories*, as research in sociology and anthropology has shown (Bourdieu, 1977; Csordas, 1990). The incorporating practices that occur in rituals and commemorations, for example, repeatedly performed social activities embodied in gestures, postures, or speech structure mnemonic systems, contribute in turn to differences in class, gender, and cultural identities in general (Connerton, 1989, p. 73). As we will see in the following sections, each of these phenomena plays a decisive role in the expressive behavior of people living with dementia and the enculturation of personality.

Expressivity, Embodied Memories, and Selfhood in Dementia

Pia Kontos has worked with people living with dementia in Chai Village, an Orthodox Jewish long-term care facility in Ontario, Canada. Her observations are valuable documents of the importance of these characteristics of embodied selfhood for research on (and the practical care of) people suffering from dementia. As Kontos remarks, interaffective relations among the care home residents are very important, especially when one perceives vulnerability in another. The following quotation describes an event where one care facility resident eases the anxiety of another through empathetic affection (compassion):

> After breakfast Dora was in her wheelchair in a line-up of residents against the wall in the hallway. The resident next to her was crying out, "nurse, nurse," and then started to weep and repeated the same phrase over and over—"I want to go home." Dora reached over and placed her hand gently on top of the resident's forearm. Holding her hand there, she sang Tumbalalayka, a Yiddish lullaby. (Kontos, 2005, p. 834)

This description is an intriguing example of the intertwinement of body memory, expressivity, and selfhood in embodied interactions. Dora obviously appreciates the anxiety of her coresident and tries to comfort her by first establishing a direct dyadic intercorporeal relationship ("reached over and placed her hand gently on top of the resident's forearm"). When she then starts to sing the lullaby, she is expressing deeply entrenched and habitualized body memories in a cross-cultural setting – music often elicits highly affective-emotional reactions because of the power of ritualized song in early childhood to establish a resonance of mutually shared emotional values. That Dora decides to sing the lullaby is thus a highly apt way to ease her coresident's discomfort, because it has the power to activate intercorporeal memory schemes via the attunement of listener and singer.

In a further respect, it is striking that Dora uses the *musical expressivity of her voice* to comfort her fellow resident after first establishing contact by a gentle touch. This is because what Kontos calls "musical embodied memories" often remain intact even in late stages of dementia when other abilities such as linguistic skills and fluid social orientation have been severely disrupted. This phenomenon is illustrated in filmmaker Paul Watson's documentary *Malcolm and Barbara: Love's farewell* about Malcolm Pointon, a composer and music lecturer with Alzheimer's disease. The film shows Pointon's continuing ability to improvise on the piano and on makeshift instruments despite his illness. He is still able to interact in rhythmic musical interplay, despite the fact that he is no longer able to read or write using musical notation (Watson, 1999/2007).

The activation of the body memory or strongly embodied skills is, of course, not confined to musical abilities. Thomas Fuchs cites the example of one of his own patients:

> A 78-year-old patient in an advanced stage of dementia was mostly incapable of recognizing his surroundings and his relatives any longer. He seemed lethargic, withdrawn, physically frail and was hardly in a position to move about independently any more. One day his two grandchildren visited him and were playing football in front of the house. As a youngster, the patient had played for a long while in a football club; now, he suddenly stood up and played with the boys. In contact with the ball, he appeared as if transformed and much younger; he showed them his skills at dribbling, demonstrated various ball tricks and gave expert explanations about these. For half an hour, almost nothing was discernible of the illness. (Fuchs, 2017, p. 301)

Such examples clearly demonstrate that the manifestation of embodied memory skills and habits in dementia are by no means stereotyped, preprogramed action schemas. When the grandfather starts to play football with his grandchildren or Dora begins to sing the lullaby, these are situation-specific embedded action patterns that depend on attention to and implicit understanding or know-how of the respective social context. One can therefore conclude that neither the second nature of these patients nor their selfhood has been destroyed; rather these persist in ways that still allow and sustain expressive and sense-making interactions. Embodied selfhood thus comprises two mutually co-constituting key facets: (1) the capacity of an individual embodied personal self and (2) a socially constituted self with intercorporeally acquired skills, who is able to (re) enact action patterns in embedded situations.

These key facets shed further light on the temporal continuity of selfhood in dementia. There is no reason to think that the basic temporal integration of phenomenal time-consciousness is interrupted in the examples given. Besides the ceaseless temporal experience of a phenomenally conscious selfhood, the skills and habits manifest in patients' interactions are inextricably linked to their individual biographies (former footballer or musician, etc.), despite the fact that the patients might not have voluntary access to declarative memories from their own past. Moreover, as indicated earlier, these temporal properties also have a foundation in the continuity of the body as an organism, as something that gains its identity over time by means of its dynamic life cycles and its continuing systemic form. This ceaseless energetic exchange implies not so much a material as a processual continuity. The dynamic processual continuity of *selfhood* is confirmed at the level of intercorporeal social activities that are manifested in the earlier examples too.

Does Embodied Selfhood Justify the Ascription of Embodied *Personal* Selfhood?

Do these considerations suffice to reject the cognitivist-inspired concept of personal identity? A cognitivist might respond to what I have argued as follows. Let us assume the validity of the embodied concept of selfhood in dementia you have set out. Does it actually support the conclusion that personal identity persists in dementia's late stages? What the strong embodied approach can only show, at best, is a continuity of selfhood in qualitative and numerical terms; it cannot prove a continuity of *personal* identity. This is so because the first-person perspective or expressive forms of interactions are necessary conditions for personal selfhood but not sufficient ones. Admittedly, the examples in the last section reveal that during the gradual loss of their personality people with dementia might retain more skills than are usually ascribed to them. Nevertheless, *declarative memories*, *narrative self-ascriptions*, and *reflexive moral evaluations* are essential ingredients of personhood. If the capacity to manifest these skills and properties is destroyed, then we are no longer justified in regarding these human beings as persons, despite the fact that they manifest *other forms* of embodied selfhood.

As it stands, this cognitivist response depends on the assumptions outlined in the first section, that the defining features of personhood consist of reflective capacities, declarative memories, and the narrative self-understanding of human beings. It is undeniable that these skills and properties disclose dimensions of personal existence that are central for human life, as Charles Taylor has explored and explained in detail (Taylor, 1989).

As I have shown, however, there are manifold sense-making dimensions that are still accessible for and enacted by people suffering from dementia even at late stages of their disease. These are based on acquired and entrenched cultural skills and habits in the process of enculturation. Such meaning dimensions are incorporated and facilitated by intercorporeal interactions and social "scaffolding," which is defined as integrating new information, cultural tools, and learning strategies with extant knowledge (Williams, Huang, & Bargh, 2009, p. 1257). The ability to acquire and *enact* such skills and habits in the cultural realm is a decisive feature of personhood. The manifestation of such skills in, for example, musical interactions, not only comforting others in distress but also in retaining narrative and gestural abilities (Hydén, 2018; McLean, 2006) depends on the *active engagement of the self* in creating *socially meaningful Gestalten* (holistic social action patterns).

Moreover, the manifestation of such skills and habits in the social context is based on body memories *and* the continuity of selfhood (perceiver self) in the stream of consciousness. This is so because the enacted meaningful Gestalten in dementia presupposes the first-person perspective of the patient, which is intertwined with the phenomenal continuity of the self. But are we actually entitled to ascribe a first-person perspective to Alzheimer's patients at the late stage of the disease? I conclude that we are, especially in the light of the expressive activities described earlier and the insights drawn from autopoetic research and an ecological-based affective neuroscience concerning the emergence of the self. Thus, the dementia patient is the same embodied self who in their past had the potential to develop those skills – including a declarative memory, language capacities, and a web of narrative structures – by means of scaffolded forms of enculturation. I therefore regard this embodied self with the potential to participate and engage in the different meaning dimensions of the cultural realm as the *essence of the personal self.*

Further Considerations and Conclusion

This approach discussed in this chapter has the advantage of integrating existential qualitative dimensions of personhood with the concept of personal identity over time. What does this mean? Accepting that "growth and decline" are decisive features of our personal life (Lesser, 2006) implies an acceptance that not only development but also the deterioration of one's own life and the approach of death are *integral* and not merely contingent parts of human personal existence. In precarious existential situations, subjects express a relation to fundamental meaning dimensions of human life: Loss and development are, on this view, defining traits of embodied personal selfhood. When people are confronted with illness, misfortune, or loss, personal selfhood is also disclosed in the way they try to cope with the boundary conditions of death and life over time by means of embodied interactions and their body memories too. As long as qualitative embodied personal selfhood is enacted in its existential manifold dimensions, numerical personal identity is preserved with it.

Admittedly, dementia has such a huge impact on the patient's entire individual and social life that it is understandable when a view prevails that with the loss of their narrative capacity and declarative memories, the dementia patient's embodied personal selfhood disappears too. Nevertheless, the sense-making activities discussed earlier show that this is not the case. When Dora, for instance, tries to comfort her coresident, she discloses compassion and implicit understanding of embedded social situations that one can construe as expressions of embodied personal selfhood.

Of course a cognitivist critic might still reply that though there are many *intermediate cases*, such as the one depicted earlier, where personal selfhood may or may not still exist, it is possible at least to imagine cases of dementia where *every* qualitative dimension of personhood has been lost. One cannot therefore rule out manifestations of dementia that result in the *entire deprivation* of qualitative and numerical personal selfhood.

My answer to this critic involves returning to the concept of strongly embodied selfhood set out earlier. If we accept that expressive forms of *personal* primordial intentionality comprise the stream of consciousness, as well as movements and interaffective and emotional forms of self-regulation (embodied affective neuroscience), then the loss of *every* qualitative property of embodied personal selfhood would indeed seem to imply the death of the living embodied person as such. Ascertaining whether this actually occurs, however, would require a discussion of further conceptual issues and empirical research – such as the criteria of "brain death" – a topic that exceeds the scope of this chapter. Drawing on the concept of "embodied selfhood" – introduced by Pia Kontos in her dementia research – proved a useful starting point for revising this one-sided picture. As has been shown, there are many neglected dimensions of embodied selfhood that are still present even in severe cases of late-stage dementia. One decisive task for embodied-oriented research on dementia is, however, to explore in greater detail how the manifold dimensions of embodied selfhood contribute to qualitative aspects of personhood and numerical personal identity over time. A goal of this chapter was to make headway on the question of how this can be accomplished with regard to the manifold aspects of embodied selfhood.

Acknowledgment

I am grateful for helpful comments on earlier versions of the chapter by Adrian Wilding, Daniel Vespermann, and Erik Norman Dzwiza-Ohlsen.

References

Bär, M. (2010). Sinn im Angesicht der Alzheimerdemenz. Ein phänomenologisch-existenzieller Zugang zum Verständnis demenzieller Erkrankung [Sense in the face of Alzheimers's disease. A phenomenological-existential approach to dementia]. In A. Kruse (Ed.), *Lebensqualität bei Demenz? Zum gesellschaftlichen und individuellen Umgang mit einer Grenzsituation im Alter* [Quality of living in dementia? How society and individuals cope with ultimate situations in old age] (pp. 249–259). Heidelberg, Germany: Akademische Verlagsgesellschaft.

Bourdieu, P. (1977). *Outline of a theory of practice.* Cambridge, UK: Cambridge University Press.

Brockmeier, J. (2014). Questions of meaning: Memory, dementia and the postautobiographical perspective. In L.-C. Hydén, H. Lindemann, & J. Brockmeier (Eds.), *Beyond loss: Dementia, memory, and identity* (pp. 69–90). Oxford, UK: Oxford University Press.

Butler, J. (1975). Of personal identity. In J. Perry (Ed.), *Personal identity* (pp. 99–106). Berkeley, CA: University of California Press. (Original work published 1736)

Casey, E. (2000). *Remembering: A phenomenological study.* Bloomington, IN: Indiana University Press. (Original work published 1984)

Connerton, P. (1989). *How societies remember*. Cambridge, UK: Cambridge University Press.

Csordas, T. J. (1990). Embodiment as a paradigm for anthropology. *Ethos*, 18(1), 5–47. doi:10.1525/eth.1990.18.1.02a00010

Dainton, B., & Bayne, T. (2005). Consciousness as a guide to personal persistence. *The Australasian Journal of Philosophy*, 83(4), 549–571. doi:10.1080/00048400500338856

Damasio, A. (1994). *Descartes's error: Emotion, reason and the human brain*. London, UK: Picador.

Deacon, T. (2016). On human (symbolic) nature: How the word became flesh. In G. Etzelmüller & C. Tewes (Eds.), *Embodiment in evolution and culture* (pp. 129–150). Tübingen, Germany: Mohr Siebeck.

Dennett, D. (1991). *Consciousness explained*. Boston, MA: Little, Brown.

Fuchs, T. (2012). The phenomenology of body memory. In S. C. Koch, T. Fuchs, M. Summa, & C. Müller (Eds.), *Body memory, metaphor and movement* (pp. 9–22). Amsterdam, Netherlands: John Benjamins.

Fuchs, T. (2017). Self across time: The diachronic unity of bodily existence. *Phenomenology and the Cognitive Sciences*, 16(2), 291–315. doi:10.1007/s11097-015-9449-4

Fuchs, T. (2018). *Ecology of the brain: The phenomenology and biology of the embodied mind*. Oxford, UK: Oxford University Press.

Hameed, S., Shah, J. M., Ting, S., Gabriel, C. J., Tay, S. Y., Chotphoksap, U., & Liong, A. (2018). Improving the quality of life in persons with dementia through a pilot study of a creative dance movement programme in an Asian setting. *International Journal of Neurorehabilitation*, 5(4), 1–4. doi:10.4172/2376-0281.1000334

Hughes, J., Louw, S., & Sabat, S. R. (2006). Seeing whole. In J. Hughes, S. Louw, & S. R. Sabat (Eds.), *Dementia: Mind, meaning, and the person* (pp. 2–39). Oxford, UK: Oxford University Press.

Husserl, E. (1991). *On the phenomenology of the consciousness of internal time* (J. B. Brough, Trans.). Dordrecht, Netherlands: Kluwer Academic. (Original work published 1966).

Hydén, L. C. (2018). Dementia, embodied memories, and the self. *Journal of Consciousness Studies*, 25(7–8), 225–241.

Jordan, S., & Mays, C. (2017). Wild meaning: The intercorporeal nature of bodies, objects, and words. In C. Meyer, J. Streeck, & S. Jordan (Eds.), *Intercorporeality: Emerging socialities in interaction* (pp. 361–378). Oxford, UK: Oxford University Press.

Kiverstein, J., & Miller, M. (2015). The embodied brain: Towards a radical embodied cognitive neuroscience. *Frontiers in Human Neuroscience*, 9, 1–11. doi:10.3389/fnhum.2015.00237

Kontos, P. C. (2004). Ethnographic reflections on selfhood, embodiment and Alzheimer's disease. *Ageing & Society*, 24(6), 829–849. doi:10.1017/S0144686X04002375

Kontos, P. C. (2005). Embodied selfhood in Alzheimer's disease: Rethinking person-centred care. *Dementia*, 4(4), 553–570. doi:10.1177%2F1471301205058311

Kontos, P. C. (2012). Alzheimer expressions or expressions despite Alzheimer's? Philosophical reflections on selfhood and embodiment. *Occasion: Interdisciplinary Studies in the Humanities*, 4, 1–12.

Kontos, P. C., & Martin, W. (2013). Embodiment and dementia: Exploring critical narratives of selfhood, surveillance, and dementia care. *Dementia*, 12(3), 288–302. doi:10.1017/S0144686X04002375

Lesser, A. H. (2006). Dementia and personal identity. In J. C. Hughes, S. J. Louw, & S. R. Sabat (Eds.), *Dementia: Mind, meaning, and the person* (pp. 55–62). Oxford, UK: Oxford University Press.

Lindemann, H. (2014). Second nature and the tragedy of Alzheimer's. In L.-C. Hydén, H. Lindemann, & J. Brockmeier (Eds.), *Beyond loss: Dementia, memory, and identity* (pp. 11–23). Oxford, UK: Oxford University Press.

Locke, J. (2017). *An essay concerning human understanding. Book II: Ideas*. Published electronically and edited by J. Bennett. Retrieved from www.earlymoderntexts.com/assets/pdfs/ (Original work published 1690)

McLean, A. H. (2006). Coherence without facticity in dementia: The case of Mrs. Fine. In A. Leibing & L. Cohen (Eds.), *Thinking about dementia: Culture, loss and the anthropology of senility* (pp. 157–179). New Brunswick, NJ: Rutgers University Press.

McMahan, J. (2002). *The ethics of killing. Problems at the margins of life*. Oxford, UK: Oxford University Press.

McMillan, J. (2006). Identity: Self and dementia. In J. Hughes, S. Louw, & S. R. Sabat (Eds.), *Dementia: Mind, meaning, and the person* (pp. 63–70). Oxford, UK: Oxford University Press.

Menary, R. (2015). Mathematical cognition – A case of enculturation. In T. Metzinger & J. M. Windt (Eds.), *Open MIND* (pp. 1–20). Frankfurt am Main, Germany: MIND Group.

Merleau-Ponty, M. (1968). *The visible and the invisible* (A. Lingis, Trans.). Evanston, IL: Northwestern University Press. (Original work published 1964)

Noonan, H. W. (2019). *Personal identity* (3rd ed.). London, UK: Routledge.

Parfit, D. (1971). Personal identity. *The Philosophical Review*, 80(1), 3–27.

Parfit, D. (1984). *Reasons and persons*. Oxford, UK: Oxford University Press.

Parfit, D. (2012). We are not human beings. *Philosophy*, 87(1), 5–28. doi:10.1017/S0031819111000520

Reid, T. (1975). Of Mr. Locke's account of personal identity. In J. Perry (Ed.), *Personal identity* (pp. 113–118). Berkeley, CA: University of California Press. (Original work published 1785)

Sabat, S. R., & Harré, R. (1994). The Alzheimer's disease sufferer as a semiotic subject. *Philosophy, Psychiatry, & Psychology*, 1(3), 145–160. doi:10.1353/ppp.0.0083

Schacter, D. (1987) Implicit memory: History and current status. *Journal of Experimental Psychology*, 13(3), 501–518. doi:10.1037/0278-7393.13.3.501

Schechtman, M. (1996). *The constitution of selves*. Ithaca, NY: Cornell University Press.

Schechtman, M. (2005). Personal identity and the past. *Philosophy, Psychiatry, & Psychology*, 12(1), 9–22. doi:10.1353/ppp.2005.0032

Stern, D. N. (1985). *The interpersonal world of the infant.* New York, NY: Basic Books.

Strawson, G. (2004). Against narrativity. *Ratio*, 17(4), 428–452.

Summa, M., & Fuchs, T. (2015). Self-experience in dementia. *Rivista internationale di filosofia e psicologia*, 6(2), 387–405. doi:10.4453/rifp.2015.0038

Sutton, J., McIlwain, D., Christensen, W., & Geeves, A. (2011). Applying intelligence to the reflexes: Embodied skills and habits between Dreyfus and Descartes. *Journal of the British Society for Phenomenology*, 42(1), 78–102. doi:10.1080/00071773.2011.11006732

Taylor, C. (1989). *Sources of the self. The making of modern identity.* Cambridge, UK: Cambridge University Press.

Taylor, R. (2007). *Alzheimer's from the inside out.* Baltimore, MD: Health Professions Press.

Tewes, C. (2018). The phenomenology of habits: Integrating first-person and neuropsychological studies of memory. *Frontiers in Psychology*, 9, 1–6. doi:10.3389/fpsyg.2018.01176

Tewes, C., & Fuchs, T. (2018). Editorial introduction: The formation of body memory. *Journal of Consciousness Studies*, 25(7–8), 8–19.

Thompson, E. (2007). *Mind in life. Biology, phenomenology, and the sciences of mind.* Cambridge, MA: Harvard University Press.

Tramoni, E., Felician, O., Barbeau, E. J., Guedj, E., Guye, M., Bartolomei, F., & Ceccaldi, M. (2011). Long-term consolidation of declarative memory: Insight from temporal lobe epilepsy. *Brain*, 134(3), 816–831. doi:10.1093/brain/awr002

Watson, P. (Director). (1999/2007). *Malcolm and Barbara: Love's farewell* [Film, Documentary]. Retrieved from www.youtube.com/watch?v=HYDxZQXYT5k

Williams, L. E., Huang, J. Y., & Bargh, J. A. (2009). The scaffolded mind: Higher mental processes are grounded in early experience of the physical world. *European Journal of Social Psychology*, 39(7), 1257–1267. doi:10.1002/ejsp.665

Zahavi, D. (2017). Thin, thinner, thinnest: Defining the minimal self. In C. Durt, T. Fuchs, & C. Tewes (Eds.), *Embodiment, enaction, and culture: Investigating the constitution of the shared world* (pp. 193–199). Cambridge, MA: Massachusetts Institute of Technology Press.

Zahavi, D., & Kriegel, U. (2016). For-me-ness: What it is and what it is not. In D. Dahlstrom, A. Elpidorou, & W. Hopp (Eds.), *Philosophy of mind and phenomenology: Conceptual and empirical approaches* (pp. 36–53). New York, NY: Routledge.

16.1

Commentary on "Embodied Selfhood and Personal Identity in Dementia" A Lifeworld Account of Personal Identity

Erik Norman Dzwiza-Ohlsen

The question of personal identity is of considerable societal importance. Its importance becomes particularly clear when discussing the experience of patients with terminal Alzheimer's dementia (P-TAD). Can such patients still be considered as persons even though they have forgotten essential facts about their lives? Is being a person compatible with the key symptoms of advanced Alzheimer's dementia (AD)? If this question is answered in the affirmative, it challenges the social function of the concept of the person, which is linked to juridical categories such as responsibility and accountability; if, on the other hand, this question is answered in the negative, depersonalization threatens to be accompanied by dehumanization, which devalues those affected and may exclude them from society.

Christian Tewes' contribution (2021) provides a comprehensive overview of the central research positions in the debate on personal identity. On the one hand, he distinguishes between cognitivistic and phenomenological approaches and, on the other, between narrow and broad versions of embodiment. In doing so, he makes it clear from the very beginning what he is interested in: to show that it makes sense to attribute personal identity to P-TAD. The reason why this contradicts many current research positions is that the latter overlook important aspects of the person. I would like to follow the argument of Tewes' text to a certain extent and work out in phenomenological terms what exactly the overlooked sources of personal identity are. I will then focus on the concept of the person to answer the crucial question: whether, in the final stage of AD, the status of *personhood* is retained or only the numerical and qualitative identity of a *self*.

Positions

Tewes' argument takes as its starting point the classic text for many cognitivist approaches to the debate on personal identity: Locke's *Essay concerning human understanding* from 1690. In the case of P-TAD, personal identity can no longer simply be assumed, since the patient no longer has the ability to explicitly reflect on past events as their own and thus create a diachronic identity. Locke's approach was criticized early on: Joseph Butler, for example, already pointed to a vicious circle involved in it, since every explicit reflection on identity is based on an implicit, "prereflective self-acquaintance or self-familiarity" (p. 373). It is precisely this prereflective familiarity with oneself that Dan Zahavi and colleagues have recently worked out in phenomenological ways, clarifying the experience from the first-person perspective.

According to Tewes, the representatives of *weak* embodied approaches fail to take advantage of this perspective in the debate on personal identity. Their (naturalistic and cerebrocentric) version of embodiment is simply too narrow to adequately deal with the problem of personal identity in the terminal stage of AD: Either it denies personal identity, without the psychological criterion for identity being clearly determinable (Parfit); or it assigns personal identity by means of a physical criterion, which has the virtue of clarity but which cannot make sense of the phenomenon of qualitative personal identity (McMahan, 2002). For Tewes, these limitations are to be overcome by phenomenologically oriented versions of *strong* embodied approaches. These have shown that both passive and active awareness can persist in the late stages of AD – such as perspectival ownership, self-awareness, habitual practice, expressive corporeality, emotional attunement, and a sense-making self (cf. pp. 383–386).

But do these findings justify the assumption not only of the identity of a self but also of a person? In order to answer this question, we must first define the difference between self and person; second, we must determine the features that justify why the latter goes beyond the former; and third, we must do so without reentering the waters of reductionist approaches.

Commentary

Does Tewes succeed in showing not only the numerical and qualitative identity of a self but also of a person? His argument succeeds insofar as we consider the embodied self as the "*essence of the personal self*" (p. 385, emphasis in original) and thus integrate the structures of the self still preserved in the final stage of AD into the more demanding experience of the person. Accordingly, Tewes first addresses the prereflective and habitualized practices associated with "embodied selfhood," in order to then outline the bodily foundations of the dynamic and meaningful interplay between organism and environment as elaborated by "enactivism." By illustrating their social and cultural function with the help of concepts of "expressivity, body memory, and intercorporeality," Tewes successfully integrates these findings with the sphere of the person, without getting into reductionist waters.

Even though the advantage of his approach is to highlight often-overlooked phenomenological evidence without losing contact with the main positions of this debate, I would like to propose a *reverse* research strategy and start directly *from the sphere of the person*. This has at least two advantages: *First*, the sphere of the person is the natural starting point of our lifeworld experience, which is also true in the case of conditions such as AD; *second*, a theory of the lifeworld captures the person as part of a social, cultural, historical, and expressive environment from the very beginning; that is, these elements do not have to be added afterward.

I would like to illustrate this approach by means of what I consider to be one of Husserl's most important texts, a text that was of considerable importance to phenomenologists such as Heidegger, Merleau-Ponty, and Ricoeur, but is largely unknown in the current debate about personal identity: the "Constitution of the Spiritual World" (CSW), that is, the third section of the *Ideas pertaining to a pure phenomenology and to a phenomenological philosophy, Book II* (Husserl, 1989, pp. 172–302).

Being a Person within the Lifeworld

In CSW, Husserl describes how it is to be a person in the spiritual world. To do so he distinguishes between the "naturalistic attitude," which is taken up by the natural sciences, and the "personalistic attitude," which is taken up by the person of the spiritual world. The latter is the attitude in which we are most of the time and on which the specialized attitudes of the sciences, be they natural or humanist, are founded (Husserl, 1989, p. 143). Because of this, we should not wonder that the "spiritual world" (*geistige Welt*) seems quite familiar to us. It is a cultural–historical world, in which we act as practical, valuing, judging, and expressive persons; as such, we are gifted with certain skills, which we develop, evaluate, and perform in concrete interactions within a complex society (which includes artifacts, institutions, etc.). This is why one can interpret this theory as Husserl's "first theory of the lifeworld" (Sommer, 1984, p. IX; cf. Dzwiza-Ohlsen, 2019).

Finally, I would like to apply this theory to the problem of personal identity in the final stage of AD by focusing on the relationship between personality and expressivity, and more precisely on the intertwining of *intrapersonal* and *interpersonal* identity within the framework of *situational orientation* and *habitualized expressivity*.

Situational Orientation

By drawing on Husserl, we can delineate how the lived body appears as the stable center of orientation in a lifeworldly situation, be it spatial, temporal, or personal (see Dzwiza-Ohlsen, 2019). If one considers that P-TAD still have the "capacity to adequately refer to … [themselves] as experiencing something" via indexical or gestural expression (Summa, 2014, p. 481), then one could argue that the rudimentary, three-dimensional orientation of the lifeworld is still functioning, which Bühler described as the "Origo": This is nothing other than the "here-now-I system of subjective orientation" structuring every kind of "situation" (Bühler, 1990, pp. 102, 149).

In order to foster this situational orientation, all forms of communication that are available in a face-to-face situation should be fully exploited, especially in the final stage of AD, whether they are mimic, gestural, vocal, or haptic; deictic, iconic, or habitual; or artistic, musical, or literary. That is because, with regard to Husserl, expression is the key for becoming and remaining a person within the lifeworld: First, because expression indicates a "unity of Body and spirit" (Husserl, 1989, p. 241) through which understandable sense appears for others; second, because what he calls "empathy into persons" (*Einfühlung in Personen*) is by this definition "nothing else than precisely that apprehension which understands the sense" (1989, p. 244); and third, this understanding through expression allows other persons to see me as I see them, so that I "fit myself into the family of men," as a "social man" (1989, p. 242). Thus, precisely through expressive communication, we become and remain a part of a spiritual world (see Husserl, 1989, pp. 196–197), of a "communal spirit" (1989, p. 243).

One could object that this approach to the social function of expressivity provides only the necessary and by no means the sufficient condition for being a person. But if the question is whether one can depart from what Husserl calls "the family of men" during one's lifetime due to the onset of AD, then we must be able to specify a criterion as to *when* this departure occurs. Since the classic criteria of personhood, such as symbolic-linguistic abilities or declarative memory, are no longer applicable, we must be able to specify a new criterion. This criterion of personhood must have an analogical function, that is, transcending the narrow limits of temporal presence as well as representing abstract sets of rules as we find them in our socioculturally shaped lifeworlds. As I would like to show, finally, a specific form of habitualization meets both these requirements, namely, *pluralistic* habitualization, which is the foundation of institutionalized practices.

Habitualized Expressivity

As Tewes and others have shown, habitualization is of special interest for the discussion of dementia in general and for personal identity in particular. I suggest that habitualized expressivity both transcends temporal presence and represents abstract sets of rules.

First of all, we can observe the "typical individuality" of the expressions of my fellow human beings. Like an amalgam, our affective, practical, and intellectual characteristics merge in the course of our lives, thereby relating self and others to an "individual habitus" (Husserl, 1989, p. 295). Though a self's spoken words, sayings, and jokes may seem predictable, their lifestyles, hairstyles, or cosmetic appearance ordinary, and the way they laugh or behave tiresome (see Husserl, 1989, pp. 270–271), nevertheless each of these forms of habitualized expression indicates the individuality of an identical human being over time. In this way, it is possible to understand why P-TAD recognize and interact with their loved ones, even if they are unable to retrieve seemingly essential information, such as names, professions, or ages – and this in turn offers their partners or family members a starting point for recognizing "the person they know from the past," at least in certain aspects.

The robust texture of this often-overlooked social bond becomes all the more tangible once we consider that habitualization is not only individual but always takes place in a pluralistic way, as in the case of friendship, partnership, or membership (see Husserl, 1989, p. 200). These structures shape our thinking, feeling, and acting, which is on the one hand of great importance for the interpersonal attribution of personal identity and the interpersonal constitution of a shared identity; on the other hand, it is of crucial importance for participation in abstract institutional practices. This does not only relate to juridical, scientific, or political institutions. Even the mastering of a complex, rule-based game, such as football, distinguishes humans from animals, or (in our case) persons from nonpersons. Since the idea of such abstract practices is also habitualized in objects of daily use, a football or badge or any other object can be enough to reactivate them (see Husserl, 1989, p. 182). My suggestion would be to use this concept of pluralistic habitualization for border questions of personal existence, as we find them in the debate on AD.

Conclusion

By uncovering these sources of our lifeworldly experience, phenomenology makes it possible to assess the question of numerical and qualitative personal identity in intrapersonal as well as interpersonal terms. Admittedly, there are disadvantages to starting with Husserl, for example, the lifeworldly and scientific understandings of nature can only be integrated with interpretative effort (see Dzwiza, 2018). At the same time, within the tradition of philosophical anthropology we find authors, such as Plessner (2019), who have provided just such a person-oriented philosophical biology. I see Christian Tewes' approach as an important contribution that succeeds in making phenomenological insights fruitful without losing touch with biologically and cognitively oriented approaches. As a result, the debate about personal identity benefits considerably.

References

Bühler, K. (1990). *The theory of language: The representational function of language* (D. F. Goodwin, Trans.). Amsterdam, Netherlands: John Benjamins.

Dzwiza, E. N. (2018). The situationality of the lifeworld. Reflections on key terms concerning human-animal relations. In T. Breyer & T. Widlok (Eds.), *The situationality of human-animal relations. Perspectives from anthropology and philosophy* (pp. 9–29). Bielefeld, Germany: Transcript.

Dzwiza-Ohlsen, E. N. (2019). *Die Horizonte der Lebenswelt. Sprachphilosophische Studien zu Husserls 'erster Phänomenologie der Lebenswelt'* [The horizons of the lifeworld. Linguistic-philosophical investigations in Husserl's 'first phenomenology of the lifeworld']. Paderborn, Germany: Wilhelm Fink.

Husserl, E. (1989). *Ideas pertaining to a pure phenomenology and to a phenomenological philosophy. Second book: Studies in the phenomenology of constitution* (R. Rojcewicz & A. Schuwer, Trans.). Dordrecht, Netherlands: Kluwer Academic Books.

McMahan, J. (2002). *The ethics of killing. Problems at the margins of life*. Oxford, UK: Oxford University Press.

Plessner, H. (2019). *Levels of organic life and the human. An introduction to philosophical anthropology* (M. Hyatt, Trans.). New York, NY: Fordham University Press.

Sommer, M. (1984). Husserls Göttinger Lebenswelt [Husserl's Göttingian lifeworld] [introduction]. In M. Sommer (Ed.), *E. Husserl, Die Konstitution der geistigen Welt* [The constitution of the spiritual world] (pp. IX–XLIV). Hamburg, Germany: Meiner.

Summa, M. (2014). The disoriented self: Layers and dynamics of self-experience in dementia and schizophrenia. *Phenomenology and the Cognitive Sciences*, 13(3), 477–496. doi:10.1007/s11097-013-9313-3

Tewes, C. (2021). Embodied selfhood and personal identity in dementia. In C. Tewes & G. Stanghellini (Eds.), *Time and body: Phenomenological and psychopathological approaches* (pp. 367–389). Cambridge, UK: Cambridge University Press.

Index

"The volume offers a rich cornucopia of articles that illuminate the experience of both time and the body: two domains of relative darkness, full of enigma and consequence, which are key topics in phenomenology and psychopathology. This superb book provides a bracing overview of many issues at the center of contemporary debate."

Louis Sass, Distinguished Professor of Clinical Psychology, Rutgers University, USA, and author of *Madness and Modernism* and *The Paradoxes of Delusion*

"*Time and Body* is a fascinating collection of essays that provides depth to the study of psychopathology. Every serious student of psychopathology, no matter what their theoretical preferences, will gain insights from the rich descriptions of psychosis, dementia, depression and bereavement, anorexia, and borderline personality offered herein."

Peter Zachar, Ida Belle Young Research Professor of Psychology. Auburn University Montgomery, USA

For EU product safety concerns, contact us at Calle de José Abascal, 56–1°,
28003 Madrid, Spain or eugpsr@cambridge.org.

www.ingramcontent.com/pod-product-compliance
Lightning Source LLC
LaVergne TN
LVHW011700200926
848484LV00004B/1008

* 9 7 8 1 1 0 8 4 8 9 3 5 5 *